P. Chanson   J. Epelbaum
S. Lamberts   Y. Christen (Eds.)

Endocrine Aspects of Successful Aging: Genes, Hormones and Lifestyles

With 40 Figures and 2 Tables

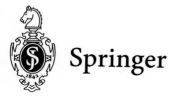 Springer

Philippe Chanson,
Service d'Endocrinologie
Hôpital Bicêtre
78, avenue de Géneral Leclerc
94275 Kremlin-Bicêtre
France
e-mail: pchanson@club-internet.fr

Steven Lamberts,
Deapartment of Internal Medicine
Erasmus MC
Dr Molewaterplein 40
3015 GD Rotterdam
The Netherlands
e-mail: lamberts@inw3.azr.nl

Jacques Epelbaum,
Institut National de la Santé
et de la Recherche Médicale U549
IFR Broca-Sainte Anne
2ter rue d'Alésia
75014 Paris
France
e-mail: epelbaum@broca.inserm.fr

Christen, Yves, Ph.D.
Fondation IPSEN
Pour la Recherche Thérapeutique
24, rue Erlanger
75781 Paris Cedex 16
France
e-mail: yves.christen@beaufour-ipsen.com

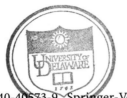

QP
187
.3
. A34
E 515
2004

ISBN 3-540-40573-9 Springer-Verlag Berlin Heidelberg New York

Cataloging-in-Publication Data applied for
Bibliographic information published by Die Deutsche Bibliothek
Die Deutsche Bibliothek lists this publication in the Deutsche Nationalbibliografie;
detailed bibliographic data is available in the Internet at <http://dnb.ddb.de>.

Springer-Verlag Berlin Heidelberg New York
a member of BertelsmannSpringer Science+Business Media GmbH

http://www.springer.de

© Springer-Verlag Berlin Heidelberg 2004
Printed in Germany

Production: PRO EDIT GmbH, D-69126 Heidelberg
Cover desing: Desing & Production, D-69126 Heidelberg
Typesetting: Satz & Druckservice, D-69181 Leimen
Printed on acid-free paper   27/3150Re   5 4 3 2 1 0

Preface

Endocrine Aspects of Successful Aging: of Genes, Hormones and Lifestyles

At the beginning of the 20th century, life expectancy at birth in North America and Western Europe was around 50 years of age. Nowadays, women have gained more than 30 years of age and men are trailing closer. Each year, new born babies still gain 3 months of life expectancy and sexagenarians are likely to live twenty more years. In 2025, the world population of people over sixty will reach 1.2 billion (14% of total) vs 0.2 billion in 1950 (8% of total). However, according to several sociologists, such as Louis Chauvel from "l'Institut des hautes études de Paris (IEP)", the notion of a "greying society" is not entirely adequate since aging people are physically and socially younger and more active for a longer time. Of course, the other side of the medal is to tackle the challenge of preventing age-associated chronic diseases (osteoarthritis, osteoporosis, neurodegenerative diseases, diabetes, obesity, etc ...).

This book is based on presentations made at the occasion of the second meeting of the series Research and Perspectives in Endocrine Interactions, organized in Paris by the Foundation IPSEN on December 3, 2002. The first goal of this meeting, and therefore of the book, was to review the extensive field of research on neuroendocrine aging which ranges on millions of years of Evolution. Indeed, many data gathered on simple organisms such as the nematode C. Elegans appears to be relevant in more complex mammalian models. One good example of such a conservation is the common involvement of the Insulin-like Growth Factor-I (IGF-I) / Insulin pathway in the control of energy expenditure and longevity from nematodes to mice and, possibly to Man (see contributions by Ruvkun et al; Bartke et al; Holzenberger et al; Janssen et al). Another good example is the clock gene arrays which contribute to the control of circadian rhythmicity across evolution (see contribution by Sassone-Corsi). The second goal was to provide a state of the Art report on human aging and the different tentative hormonal substitution strategies in order to postpone the effect of age in women (Estrogens, see contributions by Wise and Dubal and Sherwin), men (Testosterone, Basin et al), or in both genders (Growth Hormone, Shalet; Steroids, Schumacher; Finch et al. Finally, aging is one of the most complex biological processes determined by the interactions between genetic and environmental factors such as stress (see contribution by Pruessner et al). The evolutionary biological theory of aging implies that natural selection pressure is lower in low hazard ecological niches from which longer-lived species are more likely to emerge. In addition, gene alleles which are functionally active after the reproductive period will not be submitted to natural selection. Thus, genetic epidemiological analyses with a candidate endocrine gene approach appear as a good strategies to evaluate phenotypic endpoints of interest in a given population (see contributions by Uitterlinden et al; Jiang and Huhtaniemi; van den Beld et al).

In conclusion, we hope that this book testifies that the Neuroendocrinology of Aging has gone a long way since 1888 when Charles Edouard Brown-Sequard, at the age of 72, injected himself with testicular extracts in order to regain his youth. As indicated by Jonathan Swift when he turned sixty: "Every man desires to live long but no man wishes to be old".

September 2003

Philippe Chanson
Jacques Epelbaum
Steven Lamberts
Yves Christen

Contents

List of Contributors

Bartke, A.
Southern Illinois University School of Medicine, P.O. Box 19636,
Springfield, IL 62794-9636, USA

Bhasin, S.
Division of Endocrinology, Metabolism, and Molecular Medicine,
Charles R. Drew University of Medicine and Science,
Los Angeles, CA 90059, USA

Dominici, F.
Instituto de Química y Fisioquímica Biológicas (UBA-CONICET),
Facultad de Farmacia y Bioquímica, Junín 956, 1113 Buenos Aires, Argentina

Dubal, D.B.
Division of Biological Sciences, University of California Davis,
One Shields Avenue, Davis, CA 95616-8536, USA

Finch, C.E.
Department of Biological Sciences, Andrus Gerontology Center USC,
Los Angeles, CA 90089-191, USA

Franklin, R.
University of Cambridge, Cambridge CB3 OES, UK
and
Division of Biological Sciences, University of California Davis,
One Shields Avenue, Davis, CA 95616-8536, USA

Garcia-Segura, L.M.
Instituto Cajal, Avenida del Doctor Arce 37, 28002 Madrid, Spain

Holzenberger, M.
INSERM U515, Hôpital Saint-Antoine, 75571 Paris 12, France

Huhtaniemi, I.
Department of Physiology, University of Turku, Kiinamyllynkaatu 10,
20520 Turku, Finland
and
Institute of Reproductive and Developmental Biology (IRDB),
Faculty of Medicine, Imperial College London, Du Cane Road,
London W12 ONN, UK

Ibanez, C.
INSERM U488, 80 rue du Général Leclerc, 94276 Kremlin-Bicêtre, France

Janssen, J.A.M.J.L.
Department Internal Medicine, Erasmus University, Dr Molewaterplein 40,
3015 GD Rotterdam, The Netherlands

Jiang, M.
Department of Physiology, University of Turku, Kiinamyllynkaatu 10,
20520 Turku, Finland

Kopchick, J.
Edison Biotechnology Institute and Department of Clinical Research,
Ohio University, Athens, OH 45701, USA

Lamberts, S.W.J.
Department Internal Medicine, Erasmus University, Dr Molewaterplein 40,
3015 GD Rotterdam, The Netherlands

Lord, C.
Douglas Hospital Research Centre, Brain Imaging Division, McGill University,
6875 Boulevard LaSalle, Verdun QC H4H 1R3
and
McConnell Brain Imaging Center, Montreal Neurological Institute,
McGill University, 845 Sherbrooke St., W. Montreal, Quebec, Canada H3A 2T5

Lupien, S.
Douglas Hospital Research Centre, Brain Imaging Division, McGill University,
6875 Boulevard LaSalle, Verdun QC H4H 1R3, Canada

Meaney, M.
Douglas Hospital Research Centre, Brain Imaging Division, McGill University,
6875 Boulevard LaSalle, Verdun QC H4H 1R3, Canada

Melcangi, R.
Department of Endocrinology, Center of Excellence on Neurodegenerative
Diseases, University of Milan, Via Balzaretti 9, 20133, Milan, Italy.

Morgan, T.E.
Department of Biological Sciences, Andrus Gerontology Center USC,
Los Angeles, CA 90089-191, USA

Pols, H. A. P.
Genetic Laboratory Internal Medicine, Department of Internal Medicine,
Erasmus Medical Center, P.O. Box 1738, 3000 DR Rotterdam, The Netherlands

Pruessner, J.C.
Douglas Hospital Research Centre, Brain Imaging Division, McGill University,
6875 Boulevard LaSalle, Verdun QC H4H 1R3
and
McConnell Brain Imaging Center, Montreal Neurological Institute,
McGill University, 845 Sherbrooke St. W. Montreal, Quebec, Canada H3A 2T5

Renwick, R.
McConnell Brain Imaging Center, Montreal Neurological Institute,
McGill University, Montreal, Canada

Robert, F.
INSERM U488, 80 rue du Général Leclerc, 94276 Kremlin-Bicêtre, France

Rozovsky, I.
Department of Biological Sciences, Andrus Gerontology Center USC,
Los Angeles, CA 90089-191, USA

Ruvkun, G.
Department of Genetics, Massachusetts General Hospital,
Harvard Medical School,
50 Blossom Street, Wellman 901, Boston, MA 02114, USA

Sassone-Corsi, P.
Institut de Génétique et de Biologie Moléculaire et Cellulaire, 1 rue Laurent Fries,
67404 Illkirch, Strasbourg, France

Schumacher, M.
INSERM U488, 80 rue du Général Leclerc, 94276 Kremlin-Bicêtre, France

Shakoor, S.K.A.
Department of Endocrinology, Christie Hospital,
Wilmslow Road, Manchester M20 4BX, UK

Shalet, S.M.
Department of Endocrinology, Christie Hospital NHS Trust,
Wilmslow Road, Manchester M20 4BX, UK.

Sherwin, B.B.
McGill University, Department of Psychology,
1205 Dr. Penfield Ave., Montreal, Quebec, Canada H3X 1B1

Toogood, A.A.
Division of Medical Sciences, University of Birmingham, Edgbaston,
Birmingham B15 2TH, UK

Turyn, D.
Instituto de Química y Fisioquímica Biológicas (UBA-CONICET),
Facultad de Farmacia y Bioquímica, Junín 956, 1113 Buenos Aires, Argentina

Uitterlinden, A.G.
Genetic Laboratory Internal Medicine, Department of Internal Medicine,
Erasmus Medical Center, P.O. Box 1738, 3000 DR Rotterdam, The Netherlands

Van den Beld, A.
Department of Internal Medicine, Erasmus Univ. MC, Room D-433,
Dr Molewaterplein 40, 3015 GD Rotterdam, The Netherlands

Wei, M.
Department of Biological Sciences, Andrus Gerontology Center
USC, Los Angeles, CA 90089-191, USA

Wise, P.M.
Division of Biological Sciences, University of California Davis,
One Shields Avenue, Davis, CA 95616-8536, USA

Regulation of C. elegans Life Span
by Insulin-Like Signaling

Gary Ruvkun

Insulin control of metabolism, development, and longevity

An insulin signaling pathway couples feeding and nutritional status in mammals to the tempo and mode of metabolism in most tissues of the animal (Kahn 1994; Kahn and Weir 1994). Insulin secretion by the pancreas is regulated by nutritional and autonomic neural inputs, and this endocrine signal of metabolic status is detected by target tissues to regulate the activities of metabolic enzymes that synthesize or break down glucose, amino acids, fat, etc. We have shown that an insulin-like signaling pathway regulates longevity and metabolism in *C. elegans* (Kimura et al. 1997). This regulation may be mechanistically related to the longevity increase caused by caloric restriction in mammals. Our genetic analysis has also revealed outputs of *C. elegans* insulin -like signaling. We identified human homologs of many of these components in genome databases; many of these homologs have now been shown to transduce insulin and insulin-like signaling in humans.

The *C. elegans* insulin-like signaling pathway genes control metabolism as part of a global endocrine system that controls whether the animals grow reproductively or arrest at the dauer larval stage. Dauer arrest is normally regulated by a combination of a high dauer pheromone (an unidentified fatty acid), high temperature, and low bacterial food (Golden and Riddle 1984). Genes that regulate the function of this neuroendocrine pathway were identified by two general classes of mutants: dauer-defective and dauer-constitutive mutants (Georgi et al. 1990: Golden and Riddle 1984; Gottlieb and Ruvkun 1994; Larsen

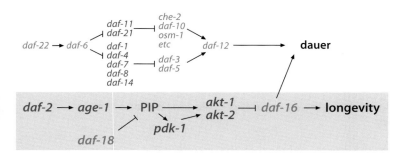

daf-c = dauer constitutive   *daf-d* = dauer defective

Fig. 1. Genetic pathway for dauer arrest

Chanson et al.
Endocrine Aspects of Successful Aging
© Springer-Verlag Berlin Heidelberg 2004

1993; Ren et al. 1996; Patterson et al. 1997; Schackwitz et al. 1996; Thomas et al. 1993; Dorman et al. 1995; Estevez et al. 1993; Kenyon et al. 1993; Klass 1983; Larsen et al. 1995; Morris et al. 1996; Ogg et al. 1997). For example, *daf-2* dauer-constitutive mutant animals form dauers in the absence of high pheromone levels. Conversely, *daf-16* dauer-defective mutants do not form dauers under normal dauer pheromone induction conditions and suppress the dauer-constitutive phenotype induced by *daf-2* mutations. Based on genetic epistasis and synergistic interactions, most of the dauer-defective and dauer-constitutive genes have been ordered into a genetic pathway. The most important conclusion from this genetic analysis is that the *daf* genes constitute multiple parallel signaling pathways that converge to regulate *C. elegans* diapause. The *daf-2/age-1/pdk-1/daf-18/akt-1/akt-2/daf-16* subpathway corresponds to an insulin-like signaling pathway, and the *daf-7/daf-1/daf-4/daf-8/daf-14/daf-3* subpathway corresponds to a TGF-beta-like neuroendocrine signaling pathway. We have also discovered a large number of worm insulin genes that couple to this pathway, as well as a variety of sensory pathways that also couple to the pathway. These genes are likely to couple environmental and nutritional status to the activity of the pathway.

Mammalian orthologs of the *C. elegans* insulin-signaling pathway may be key components of a mammalian longevity-determining pathway. The *C. elegans* insulin signaling genes may also reveal components of insulin signaling in mammals that are important for the understanding and eventual treatment of diabetes. Diabetes is a common disease that affects the production or response to insulin, causing devastating metabolic dysregulations. The molecular basis of the defective insulin response in the more common adult onset or type II diabetes is unknown (Kahn 1994; Kahn and Weir 1994). It is clear that it is at least in part a genetic disease, but it is likely to be multifactorial, based on pedigree analysis. In addition, it is clear that both genetically and environmentally induced obesity are major modulators of diabetes symptoms. The usual route of pedigree analysis and positional cloning to reveal the mechanism of the lack of insulin response in type II diabetics has proven cumbersome for a multifactorial disease like diabetes. However, saturation genetic analysis of the homologous *C. elegans* metabolic control pathway has revealed genes that act downstream of the insulin-like receptor, as well as other neuroendocrine signals that converge with insulin. The *C. elegans* genetics strongly argues that activation of the particular kinases AKT or PDK or inhibition of DAF-16 or DAF-18 activity by drugs may bypass the need for upstream insulin signaling. These signal transduction components identified by *C. elegans* genetic analysis are, therefore, targets for pharmaceutical development of diabetes therapies.

An insulin signaling pathway regulates C. elegans metabolism and longevity

daf-2 encodes the worm ortholog of the insulin/IGF-I receptor gene and is necessary for reproductive development and metabolism. *daf-2* mutant animals arrest development at the dauer larval stage and shift metabolism to fat storage

(Kimura et al. 1997). Many DAF-2 tyrosines bear flanking sequence motifs, suggesting that they are autophosphorylated and likely to mediate interaction with the AGE-1 PI 3-kinase as well as other signaling pathways. We have recently found that null mutations in *daf-2* (nonsense alleles in the ligand-binding domain or upstream of the kinase domain) also cause dauer arrest, showing that the only *daf-2* function is in this pathway. DAF-2 is the only member of the insulin receptor family in the essentially complete *C. elegans* genome sequence.

The AGE1 PI-3 kinase acts downstream of the DAF-2 insulin receptor

age-1 acts at the same point in the genetic epistasis pathway as *daf-2*. Based on sequence comparisons (but not interspecies gene activity), AGE-1 is the worm ortholog mammalian phosphatidylinositol 3-kinase (PI 3-kinase) p110 catalytic subunit (Morris et al. 1996). PI 3-kinases generate a membrane-localized signaling molecule, phosphatidylinositol P_3 (PIP$_3$), that is thought to transduce signals from upstream receptors to effector molecules such as AKT/PKB (Alessi et al. 1996).

Longevity regulation by *daf-2* weak *daf-2* and *age-1* mutants that do not arrest at the dauer stage nevertheless live much longer than wild type (Dorman et al. 1995; Kenyon et al. 1993; Larsen et al. 1995). And this longevity increase is dependent on *daf-16* gene activity (Dorman et al. 1995; Larsen et al. 1995). The connection between longevity and diapause control may not be parochial to *C. elegans*. Diapause arrest is an essential feature of many vertebrate and invertebrate life cycles, especially in regions with seasonal temperature and humidity extremes (Tauber et al. 1986). Animals in diapause arrest slow their metabolism and their rates of aging and can survive for periods much longer than their reproductive life span.

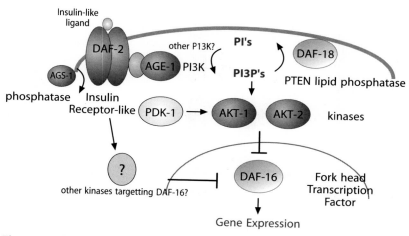

Fig. 2. An insulin-like receptor to PI-3 kinase, PTEN, PDK-1, AKT-1, AKT-2, to DAF-16 signaling cascade controls C. elegans aging and metabolism.

Reproductive senescence is delayed in weak *daf-2* mutants and is also dependent on *daf-16* gene activity (Sze et al. 2002). The coregulation of reproductive senescence and longevity of the entire animal is reminiscent of their co-regulation in humans: female centenarians tend to continue to bear children much later (after 45 years of age) than non-centenarian females (Alessi et al. 1997). The late reproduction phenotype is very handy for genetic screens, since we can select for fertility much later than normal animals and we can test secondarily for long life span.

IRS and p55 PI3K adaptor proteins in worm insulin signaling. We have detected a very weak worm homolog of mammalian IRS (Kahn and Weir 1994) but an excellent homolog of the PI3K adaptor subunit (Alessi et al. 1996). Consistent with our failure to detect these genes by simple genetic screens for dauer arrest or lack of arrest, RNA inhibition of these gene products in wild type does not cause dauer arrest, as would be predicted from their action in the mammalian insulin signaling pathway. However, RNA inhibition of these genes in a weak *age-1(hx546)* mutant is strongly synergistic, causing about 10 to 20x more dauer arrest than the parent *age-1* mutant strain. These results are important for demonstrating further congruence between worm and mammalian insulin signaling and important for the precedent of showing that we should be able to detect mutations in such adaptor proteins by using an *age-1(hx546)* mutant as a sensitized screen.

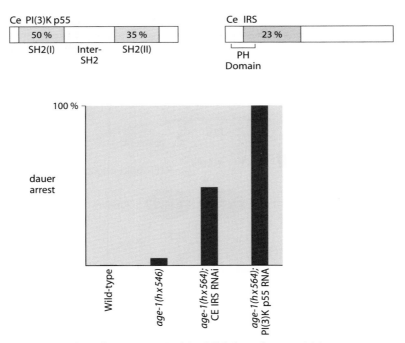

Fig. 3. PI(K) p55 and IRS are required for full daf-2 pathway activitiy

pdk-1 transduces PIP₃ signals to AKT/PKB

Activated PI3K generates 3-phosphoinositides such as phosphatidylinositol-3,4-bisphosphate (PtdIns-3,4-P2) and phosphatidylinositol-3,4,5-trisphosphate (PtdIns-3,4,5-P3), which bind to the pleckstrin homology domain of Akt/PKB and are required for its activation (Alessi et al. 1996). One of the kinases that phosphorylates Akt/PKB and is required for its activation is 3-phosphoinositide-dependent kinase-1 (PDK1; Alessi et al. 1997).

Loss of function mutations in *C. elegans pdk-1* emerged from genetic screens for mutants that arrest at the dauer stage constitutively, and two gain of function alleles emerged from a screen for suppression of the dauer-constitutive phenotype of an *age-1(mg44)* null mutant. We found a *pdk-1* Gly295Arg substitution in the loss-of-function mutant and Ala303Val substitution in the gain-of-function mutant, both conserved residues in the kinase domain. Another *pdk-1*-activating mutation maps to the unconserved linker region between the PH and kinase domains, as in the case of *akt-1* (see below). The genetic evidence that *pdk-1(mg142)* mutation activates PDK1 kinase activity towards Akt/PKB was biochemically verified using mammalian PDK1. The Alal303Val substitution in hPDK1 has a significantly higher protein kinase activity (2.9-fold) toward the AKT substrate than wild type hPDK1 (Paradis et al. 1999). Genetic epistasis experiments showed that *pdk-1(mg142)* activates *akt-1* and *akt-2* signaling in the absence of upstream AGE-1 PI3K inputs.

A loss-of-function mutation in *pdk-1* increases *C. elegans* life span almost two-fold, similar to a mutation in *age-1*. *daf-16* suppresses the longevity phenotype of *pdk-1(sa680)*. These results show that longevity regulation signals from the DAF-2 and AGE-1 signaling pathway are propagated by PDK-1, via AKT-1 and AKT-2, to the DAF-16 transcriptional outputs.

akt-1 and akt-2 transduce to the DAF-16 transcription factor

The *akt-1(mg144)*-activating mutation was identified in a genetic screen for mutations that suppress the dauer arrest phenotype of the *age-1(mg44)* null mutant. *akt-1(mg144)* alone does not activate the PI3K signaling pathway to the point that normal dauer arrest is affected but does activate the pathway sufficiently to alleviate the requirement for AGE-1 PI3K outputs (Kulik et al. 1997). *akt-1 (mg144)* is a Ala183Thr substitution in an unconserved region of the protein that links the N-terminal pleckstrin homology domain to the C-terminal kinase domain. An analogous gain-of-function mutation that we have detected in *pdk-1* points to the generality of such regulatory regions in unconserved linkers.

There are two Akt/PKB orthologs in *C. elegans*. Simultaneous inhibition of both *akt-1* and *akt-2* activities causes nearly 100% arrest at the dauer stage, whereas RNAi of either does not. This dauer arrest is fully suppressed by *daf-16* but not by *daf-3*. DAF-16 contains four consensus sites for phosphorylation by Akt/PKB, and three of these sites are conserved in the human DAF-16 homologs AFX, FKHR, and FKHRL1. Mutation of those Akt sites causes nuclear localization in the presence of insulin or IGF-I signaling (Durham et al. 1999; Guo et al. 1999; Rena et al, 19999' Tang et al, 1999; Nakae et al. 1999). We have shown that human AKT will phosphorylate *C. elegans* DAF-16 in vitro and that this phosphorylation is dependent on these conserved sites. DAF-16 with these sites changed to alanine causes some dauer arrest but also embryonic lethality. The daf-2 null phenotype has some embryonic lethality, so this finding is reasonable.

The PTEN homolog DAF-18 acts
in the insulin receptor-like signaling pathway

The dauer arrest, fat accumulation, and longevity phenotypes of age-1 null mutants are suppressed by *daf-18(e1375)* and by the *daf-18(mg198)* null allele. Both mutations map to the *C. elegans* ortholog of mammalian PTEN lipid phosphatase gene: *daf-18(e1375)* is a stop codon downstream of the phosphatase domain in the C terminal half of the protein. Several oncogenic human PTEN mutations have been identified in the carboxyl-terminal half of the protein (analogous to *daf-18(e1375)*); these regions, though unconserved, may be critical for phosphatase localization or function (Ogg and Ruvkun 1998). The *daf-18(mg198)* allele is a stop codon upstream of the kinase domain and thus defines the null phenotype. We have recently shown that human PTEN can rescue a worm *daf-18* mutant, proving the orthology (unpublished).

As determined by genetic epistasis experiments, *daf-18* acts downstream of the AGE-1 PI3K but upstream of AKT-1 and AKT-2 in this signaling cascade. The DAF-18 lipid phosphatase may normally decrease the level of PIP3 signals, perhaps insulating signals emanating from the DAF-2/AGE-1 signaling complex from other PIP$_3$ signals in the cell or resolving insulin-like signaling episodes. It is not clear from the genetic analysis whether DAF-18/PTEN activity is regulated during insulin-like or other signaling.

A mutation in the lipid phosphatase would not be expected to suppress a null mutation in the PI3K if it was the only source of PIP$_3$; there must be a source of PIP3 that is normally too low in abundance (because an *age-1* mutation has a mutant phenotype) but whose abundance (AMOUNT, increases in the absence of DAF-18 PTEN. Other PI kinases revealed by the genome sequence may be an alternative source of 3-phosphorylated PIP$_3$.

The DAF-16 forkhead protein transduces DAF-2 signals

Mutations in *daf-16* completely suppress the dauer arrest and metabolic shift of animals bearing *daf-2, age-1, pdk-1* mutations, or RNAi inhibited *akt-1* and akt-2 activity. Thus DAF-16 is activated in the absence of these upstream inputs. We showed that *daf-16* encodes two proteins with forkhead DNA binding domains. The mammalian orthologs to DAF-16 are human FKHR, FKHRL1, and AFX (Ogg et al. 1997). FKHR, FKHRL1 and AFX activities are regulated by AKT phosphorylation; these transcription factors are nuclearly localized only when insulin-like signaling (AKT activity) is low (Granner et al. 1983; Schmoll et al. 2000; Hall et al. 2000; Tomizawa et al. 2000; Durham et al. 1999; Guo et al. 1999; Rena et al. 1999; Tang et al. 1999; Nakae et al. 1999). The nuclear localization of a DAF-16/GFP fusion protein that is functional is controlled by upstream pathway activity. This reporter gene is very useful for discerning where a new mutation acts in the pathway: thus, if DAF-16 GFP is nuclearly localized in a dauer or long-lived mutant, the gene revealed by that mutation acts upstream; if DAF-16/GFP localization is unaffected, the new gene acts in parallel or downstream. Similarly, the tissue specificity of an upstream mutant can be ascertained by where DAF-16 nuclear localization is affected, for example, in neurons or gonad.

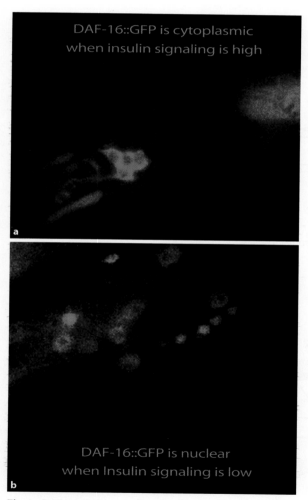

Fig. 4.a DAF-16: GFP is cytoplasmic when insulin signaling is high
Fig. 4.b DAF-16: GFP is nuclear when insulin signaling is low

Our molecular genetic analysis suggests that DAF-2, AGE-1, DAF-18, AKT-1, AKT-2, and DAF-16 act in the same cells to regulate *C. elegans* metabolism and longevity, though we have not yet proven this. Under reproductive growth conditions, high DAF-2 receptor signaling activates AGE-1 and PDK-1 to in turn

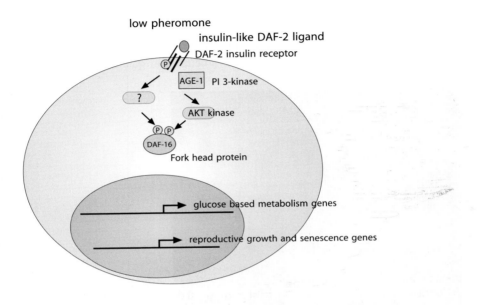

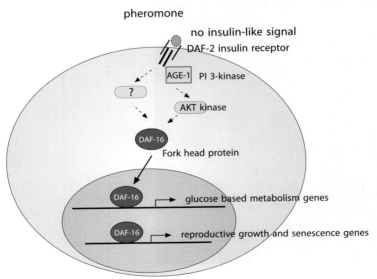

Fig. 5. Model : DAF-2 receptor signaling regulates DAF-16 transcriptional activity

activate the AKT-1 and AKT-2 kinases, as well as molecules from the parallel pathway, which negatively regulate DAF-16 activity. Phosphorylated DAF-16 is excluded from the nucleus and therefore does not activate the genes necessary for dauer arrest and energy storage or repress the genes that inhibit reproductive growth and metabolism. Under dauer-inducing conditions, these kinase cascades are inactive, and DAF-16 is active and nuclear. Active DAF-16 either represses genes required for reproductive growth and metabolism and/or activates genes necessary for dauer arrest and energy storage.

The mammalian DAF-16 orthologs have also been shown to regulate the expression of target genes such as the metabolic genes PEPCK and glucose 6 phosphatase (Granner et al. 1983; Schmoll et al. 2000; Hall et al. 2000; Tomizawa et al. 2000; Durham et al. 1999; Guo et al. 1999; Rena et al. 1999; Tang et al. 1999; Nakae et al. 1999). DAF-16 binds to this same insulin response sequence in vitro (Nasrin et al. 2000.) C. elegans DAF-16 may regulate the C. elegans homologs of these and other metabolic genes.

The *ctl-1* catalase and *sod-3* superoxide dismutase genes are expressed at higher levels in a *daf-2* mutant than in a *daf-2; daf-16* double mutant (Honda and Honda 1999; Taub et al. 1999). We detect probable DAF-16 binding sites upstream of *sod-3*. In support of that model, mutations in *ctl-1* are epistatic to the longevity enhancement of *daf-2* mutants (Taub et al. 1999).

The unusually large and diverse C. elegans insulin gene family

Insulin and its related proteins define a superfamily of secreted proteins that share a structural motif stabilized by a set of stereotypical disulfide bonds (Blundell and Humbel 1980). Seven members of the insulin superfamily have been identified in humans. Insulin superfamily genes that regulate metabolism have also been identified in invertebrates, implicating insulin-like proteins in metabolic control across animal phylogeny.

We analyzed the C. elegans genome sequence for insulins. This procedure revealed 37 genes with structural features and intron exon organization typical of the gene superfamily. Many members of the C. elegans ins gene family are organized into clusters. The tandem arrangement of the worm insulin superfamily genes suggests that these clusters arose relatively recently by gene duplication. Clusters of linked insulin superfamily genes are also found in humans. We constructed GFP fusions to the regulatory regions for 14 of the *ins* genes and found that they are expressed primarily in subsets of sensory neurons.

Since all of the INS proteins are predicted to adopt a similar tertiary structure, they may all bind to DAF-2, the only member of this receptor superfamily in the worm genome. Some INS proteins may be DAF-2 agonists whereas others may be antagonists.

Two of the 37 C. elegans insulin superfamily members, INS-1 and INS-18, are predicted to have a cleaved C peptide. The INS-1 protein is the most closely related to human insulin. High gene dosages of *ins-1* and *ins-18* act antagonistically to DAF-2. We expressed human insulin in the same cells that express *ins-1*, using

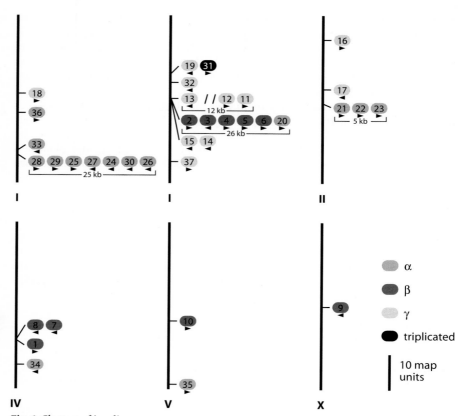

Fig. 6. Clusters of insulin genes

the 5' flanking region of *ins-1* to drive a human insulin cDNA. Human insulin expressed in this way also causes dauer arrest. In contrast, increased gene dosage of the *ins* genes tested without predicted C peptide cleavage sites does not antagonize *daf-2*. A deletion of *ins-1* does not enhance or suppress *daf-2*. Thus *ins-1* may be redundant with one or more of the other 36 *C. elegans* insulin superfamily members.

Cleavage of the C peptide is associated with loading of insulin into vesicles for regulated secretion, in contrast, for example, to IGF-I secretion, which is not vesicular (Kahn and Weir 1994). *ins-1* and *ins-18* are expressed in many neuronal cells that may have features in common with beta cells, including the ability to process out the C peptide, load processed INS-1 into vesicles, and regulate the secretion of this hormone based on dauer pheromone and other sensory inputs (Rigler et al.1999).

A TGF-beta neuroendocrine signal from the ASI dauer regulatory neuron

In addition to the *daf-2* insulin-like signaling pathway, dauer arrest is also regulated by the *daf-7/daf-1/daf-4/daf-8/daf-14/daf-3* TGF-beta signaling pathway. The signals in these two pathways are not redundant and not sequential: animals missing either of these two signals shift their metabolism and arrest at the dauer stage. *daf-7* encodes a TGF-beta neuroendocrine signal that is produced by the ASI neuron. *daf-7* expression in this neuron is inhibited by dauer-inducing pheromone (Ren et al. 1996; Schackwitz et al. 1996). *daf-1* encodes a type I TGF beta class ser/thr receptor kinase, *daf-4* encodes a type II TGF-beta class ser/thr receptor kinase , and *daf-8* and *daf-14* encode Smad proteins (Georgi et al. 1990; Estevez et al. 1993; Inoue and Thomas 2000), which couple TGF-beta signals from receptor kinases to the control of transcription.

daf-3 is a unique TGF-beta signaling pathway gene in that it is antagonized, rather than activated by the *daf-7* pathway. A *daf-3* null allele completely suppresses the dauer constitutive phenotype of mutations in *daf-1, daf-4, daf-7, daf-8,* and *daf-14.* Thus mutations in *daf-3* bypass the need for any of the DAF-7 signal transduction pathway genes, suggesting that the major function of this signaling pathway is to antagonize DAF-3 gene activity. The DAF-3 Smad protein is most closely related to vertebrate DPC4, which is a cofactor for Smad1, Smad2 and Smad3 (Patterson et al. 1997).

The DAF-16 Forkhead and the DAF-3 Smad proteins are active in the absence of upstream signaling to induce arrest at the dauer stage and a shift to energy storage metabolism. DAF-16 may interact with DAF-3 on the promoters of genes that regulate metabolism and reproductive vs dauer development. The genes regulated by the Forkhead/Smad transcriptional regulatory complex may

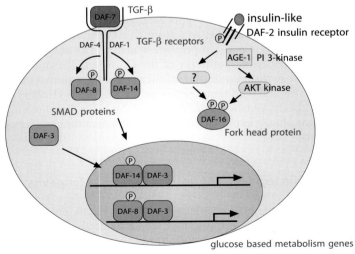

Fig. 7. The model: Convergent TGF-ß and insulin signaling activates glucose metabolism genes

correspond to the *C. elegans* homologs of mammalian genes, such as those that encode PEPCK, GAPDH, and the Glut4 glucose transporter, that are known to be transcriptionally regulated by insulin (Granner et al. 1983; Schmoll et al. 2000; Hall et al. 2000; Tomizawa et al. 2000; Durham et al. 1999; Guo et al. 1999; Rena et al. 1999; Tang et al. 1999; Nakae et al. 1999). *C. elegans* homologs of these genes are found in the genome sequence and studies are underway to explore their regulation in various daf mutants.

Only mutations in the insulin-like pathway genes cause dramatic increases in longevity. The increase in longevity induced by decreased insulin-like signaling activity is suppressed by mutations in *daf-16* but not by mutations in *daf-3*. This finding suggests that the transcriptional program for longevity does not depend on TGF-beta transcriptional cofactors in the same manner that the metabolic switch to fat storage depends on both pathways.

Thermosensory input to endocrine control of metabolism

Temperature is a potent regulator of dauer arrest (Golden and Riddle 1984). All mutations in the DAF-7 TGF-beta pathway, including *daf-7* null mutations, are temperature sensitive, whereas null mutations in the insulin pathway cause dauer arrest at all temperatures; they are not temperature sensitive (Hobert et al. 1997). We have shown that there is explicit temperature sensory input to this endocrine pathway. This pathway includes the AFD thermosensory neurons which connect to the interneurons AIY and AIZ, that may connect to secretory as well as motor control neurons. *ttx-3* encodes a LIM homeodomain protein that is expressed specifically in the AIY interneuron. In *ttx-3* mutant animals, the AIY interneuron is generated but exhibits patterns of abnormal axonal outgrowth. Similarly, the *lin-11* LIM transcription factor specifies AIZ interneuron identity. The temperature sensitivity of dauer arrest is due to an AIY-mediated enhancement of dauer arrest at high temperature and suppression of dauer arrest at low temperature. The *ttx-3* mutation decouples AIY from this thermoregulation of dauer arrest, rendering dauer arrest non-temperature sensitive. The antagonistic high and low temperature-processing pathways of the *C. elegans* thermotactic response pathway are similar to the organization of the vertebrate hypothalamus, which contains distinct warm and cold temperature-processing units (Hobert et al. 1997). The coupling of thermosensory input to the *daf-2* insulin-like signaling pathway may be homologous to the hypothalamic modulation of autonomic input to the pancreatic beta cells.

Serotinergic input to insulin regulation of worm reproductive longevity

Serotonin is synthesized by an enzymatic pathway from tryptophan. Tryptophan hydroxlyase (TPH) catalyzes the rate-limiting first step (Sze et al. 2000). There is one probable tryptophan hydroxylase in the *C. elegans* genome, *tph-1*. A GFP fusion to *tph-1* is expressed in the *C. elegans* serotonergic neurons. We generated a

1.3 kb deletion in *tph-1* that removes conserved amino acids in both the regulatory and catalytic domains. Mutant animals accumulate no detectable serotonin and display several behavioral defects that are associated with starvation: on abundant food the mutant feeds more slowly, retains more eggs, and accumulates larger stores of fat, and 10-15% arrest at the dauer stage. The metabolic phenotypes are due to serotonin inputs to both the TGF-beta and insulin-like pathways. The expression of a *daf-7:GFP* fusion gene is decreased in the *tph-1(mg280)* mutant, and dauer arrest of *daf-7(e1372)* at low temperature is enhanced. In addition, high gene dosage of tph-1 suppresses dauer arrest of *daf-7(e1372)* at high temperature. This finding suggests that temperature may modulate serotonin levels to influence dauer arrest. For example, the AIY interneuron may connect to serotinergic neurons. There is also serotonergic input to the parallel insulin-like signaling pathway. A *daf-16(mgDf50)* null mutation suppresses the dauer arrest and fat accumulation phenotypes of *tph-1(mg280)*. Moreover, like *daf-2* insulin-receptor mutants (but unlike *daf-7* pathway mutations), *tph-1(mg280)* hermaphrodites have an extended reproductive life span that is dependent on *daf-16* gene activity. Consistent with the effect on reproductive life span, we have recently found that *tph-1* animals have 25% longer life spans, which is suppressed by *daf-16*.

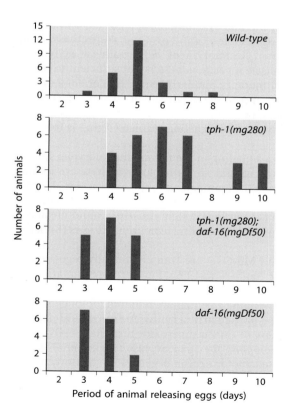

Fig. 8. Increase in reproductive longevity in the tph-1 mutant

Bacterial food and low temperature may normally up-regulate serotonin signaling to in turn up-regulate DAF-7 and insulin-like neuroendocrine signals. In the *tph*-1 mutant, these hormones may be decoupled from such food signaling. Serotonin signaling has also been implicated in the control of mammalian feeding and metabolism.

C. elegans life span is regulated by insulin-like signaling in the nervous system

Insulin-like signaling may regulate metabolism and free radical production directly in aging skin and muscle, or in signaling centers that then in coordination control the senescence of the entire organism. *age-1, daf-18, akt-1* and *daf-16* are all expressed in neurons and throughout much of the animal, consistent with their function either in signaling cells or target tissues. Studies of *daf-2* genetic mosaic animals showed that *daf-2* can act non-autonomously to regulate lifespan, but did not assign *daf-2* longevity control to particular cell types (Apfeld and Kenyon 1998).

We restored *daf-2* pathway function only to restricted cell types by using distinct promoters to express *daf-2* or *age-1* cDNAs in either neurons, intestine or muscle cells of a *daf-2* or *age-1* mutant. The long life span of *daf-2* and *age-1* mutants is rescued by neuronal expression of *daf-2* or *age-1*, respectively, using the pan-neuronal *unc-14* promoter. Restoration of *daf-2* pathway activity to muscles from the promoter for muscle myosin, *unc-54*, is not sufficient to rescue the long life span of *daf-2* or *age-1* mutants. Similarly, expression of *daf-2* or *age-1* in the intestine from the *ges-1* promoter, the major site of fat storage, does not rescue life span as efficiently as neural expression of these genes. These data argue that the key tissue where *daf-2* insulin-like signaling regulates aging is from the nervous system.

There are precedents for insulin signaling in the mammalian nervous system. While the target tissue responses to insulin are better known, there are feeding and metabolic responses to insulin in the mammalian brain (Schwartz et al. 2000). In addition, insulin receptor signaling defects in the neurosecretory beta cells of the mouse pancreas or only in the nervous system cause profound metabolic defects, also suggestive of a role for insulin signaling in neuronal tissues (Kulkarni et al. 1999; Bruning et al. 2000).

The expressions of catalase and Mn-SOD are transcriptionally regulated by DAF-16 (Honda and Honda 1999; Taub et al. 1999). Furthermore, mutations in *ctl-1* cytosolic catalase reduce the life span of *daf-2* mutants, showing that *ctl-1* and possibly other free radical-scavenging enzymes are required for long life span (Taub et al. 1999). Neurons may be particularly sensitive to free radical damage during aging. In fact, overexpression of Cu/Zn superoxide dismutase (SOD) only in motor neurons can extend *Drosophila* life span by 48% (Parkes et al. 1998), And perhaps mechanistically related, motor neuron degeneration in amyotrophic lateral sclerosis is caused by mutations in Cu/Zn SOD (Esteban et al. 1994). It is striking that aging in two different organisms can be controlled from neurons and is correlated with increased free radical protection in those neurons. By this model, neuronal *daf-2* signaling might regulate an organism's life span by controlling the integrity of specific neurons that secrete neuroendocrine signals, some of which may regulate the life span of target tissues in the organism. Our results, together with those from *Drosophila*, suggest that oxidative damage to neurons may be a primary determinant of life span.

References

Alessi DR, Andjelkovic M, Caudwell B, Cron P, Morrice N, Cohen P, Hemmings BA (1996) Mechanism of activation of protein kinase B by insulin and IGF-1. EMBO J 15:6541–6551

Alessi DR, James SR, Downes CP, Holmes AB, Gaffney PRJ, Reese CB, Cohen P (1997) Characterization of a 3-phosphoinositide-dependent protein kinase which phosphorylates and activates protein kinase B. Current Biol 7:261–269

Apfeld J, Kenyon C (1998) Cell nonautonomy of C. elegans daf-2 function in the regulation of diapause and life span. Cell 95:199–210

Blundell TL, Humbel RE (1980) Hormone families: pancreatic hormones and homologous growth factors. Nature 287:781–787

Bruning JC, Gautam D, Burks DJ, Gillette J, Schubert M, Orban PC, Klein R, Krone W, Muller-Wieland D, Kahn CR (2000) Role of brain insulin receptor in control of body weight and reproduction. Science 289:2122–2125

Dorman JB, Albinder B, Shroyer T, Kenyon C (1995) The *age-1* and *daf-2* genes function in a common pathway to control the lifespan of *Caenorhabditis elegans*. Genetics 14: 1399–1406

Dudek H, Datta SR, Franke TF, Birnbaum MJ, Yao R, Cooper GM, Segal RA, Kaplan DR, Greenberg ME (1997) Regulation of neuronal survival by the serine-threonine protein kinase Akt. Science 275:661–665

Durham SK, Suwanichkul A, Scheimann AO, Yee D, Jackson JG, Barr FG Powell DR (1999) FKHR binds the insulin response element in the insulin-like growth factor binding protein-1 promoter. Endocrinology 140:3140–3146

Esteban J, Rosen DR, Bowling AC, Sapp P, McKenna-Yasek D, O'Regan JP, Beal MF, Horvitz HR, Brown RH Jr (1994) Identification of two novel mutations and a new polymorphism in the gene for Cu/Zn superoxide dismutase in patients with amyotrophic lateral sclerosis. Human Mol Genet 3:997–998

Estevez, M, Attisano L, Wrana JL, Albert PS, Massague J, Riddle DL (1993) The *daf-4* gene encodes a bone morphogenetic protein receptor controlling C. elegans dauer larva development. Nature 365:644–649

Georgi LL, Albert PS, Riddle DL (1990) daf-1, a C. elegans gene controlling dauer larva development, encodes a novel receptor protein kinase. Cell 61:635–645

Golden JW, Riddle DL (1984) A pheromone-induced developmental switch in *Caenorhabditis elegans*: Temperature-sensitive mutants reveal a wild-type temperature-dependent process. Proc. Natl. Acad. Sci. USA 81:819–823

Gottlieb S, Ruvkun G (1994) *daf-2*, *daf-16*, and *daf-23*: genetically interacting genes controlling dauer formation in *Caenorhabditis elegans*. Genetics 137:107–120

Granner D, Andreone T, Sasaki K, Beale E (1983) Inhibition of transcription of the phosphoenolpyruvate carboxykinase gene by insulin. Nature 305:549–551

Guo S, Rena G, Cichy S, He X, Cohen P, Uterman T (1999) Phosphorylation of serine 256 by proteiun kinase B disrupts transactivation by FKHR and mediates effects of insulin on insulin-like growth factor-binding protein-1 promoter activity through a conserved insulin response sequence. J Biol Chem174:17184–17192

Hall RK, Yamasaki T, Kucera T, Waltner-Law,M, Obrien R,Granner DK (2000) Regulation of phosphoenolpyruvate carboxykinase and insulin-like growth factor-binding protein-1 gene expression by insulin. The role of winged helix/forkhead proteins. J Biol Chem 275: 30169–30175

Hobert O, Mori I, Yamashita Y, Honda H, Ohshima Y, Liu Y, Ruvkun G (1997) Regulation of interneuron function in the C. elegans thermoregulatory pathway by the ttx-3 LIM homeobox gene. Neuron 19: 345–357

Honda Y, Honda S (1999) The daf-2 gene network for longevity regulates oxidative stress resistance and Mn-superoxide dismutase gene expression in Caenorhabditis elegans. FASEB J13(:1385–1393)

Inoue T, Thomas JH (2000) Targets of TGF-beta signaling in Caenorhabditis elegans dauer formation. Dev Biol 217:192–204

Kahn CR (1994) Insulin action, diabetogenes, and the cause of Type II Diabetes. Diabetes 43: 1066–1084

Kahn CR, Weir GC (eds) (1994) Joslin's Diabetes Mellitus. 13th Edition. Lea & Febiger

Kenyon C, Chang J, Gensch E, Rudner A, Tabtlang R (1993) A C. elegans mutant that lives twice as long as wild type. Nature 366:461–464

Kimura K, Tissenbaum HA, Liu Y, Ruvkun G (1997) daf-2, an insulin receptor-like gene that regulates longevity and diapause in Caenorhabditis elegans. Science 277:942–946

Klass M (1983) A method for the isolation of longevity mutants in the nematode C. elegans and initial results. Mech Ageing Dev 22:279–286

Kulik G, Klippel A, Weber MJ (1997) Antiapoptotic signalling by the insulin-like growth factor I receptor, phophatidylinositol 3-kinase, and Akt. Mol Cell Biol 17:1595–1606

Kulkarni RN, Brüning JC, Winnay JN, Postic C, Magnuson MA, Kahn CR (1999) Tissue-specific knockout of the insulin receptor in pancreatic beta cells creates an insulin secretory defect similar to that in type 2 diabetes.Cell 96: 329

Larsen P (1993) Aging and resistance to oxidative damage in Caenorhabditis elegans. Proc Natl Acad Sci USA 90:8905–8909

Larsen PL, Albert PS, Riddle DL (1995) Genes that regulate both development and longevity in Caenorhabditis elegans. Genetics 139:1567–1583

Morris JZ, Tissenbaum HA, Ruvkun G (1996) A phsophatidylinositol-3-OH kinase family member regulating longevity and diapause in Caenorhavditis elegans. Nature 382:536–539

Nakae J, Park BC Accili D (1999) Insulin stimulates phosphorylation of the forkhead transcription factor FKHR on serine 253 through a Wortmannin-sensitive pathway. J Biol Chem 274:15982–15985

Nasrin N, Ogg S, Cahill C, Biggs W, Nui S, Dore J, Calvo D, ShiY, Ruvkun G, Alexander-Bridges M (2000) DAF-16 recruits the CBP co- activator to the IGFBP-1 promoter in HepG2 cells. Proc Natl Acad Sci USA97:10412–10417

Ogg S,Ruvkun G (1998) The C. elegans PTEN homolog daf-18 acts in the insulin receptor-like metabolic signaling pathway. Mol Cell 2: 887–893

Ogg S, Paradis S, Gottlieb S, Patterson GI, Lee L, Tissenbaum HA, RuvkunG (1997) The Fork head Transcription factor DAF-16 transduces insulin-like metabolic and longevity singals in C. elegans. Nature 389: 994–999

Paradis S, Ailion M, Toker A, Thomas JH, Ruvkun G (1999) A PDK1 homolog is Necessary and Sufficient to Transduce AGE-1 PI3 Kinase Signals that Regulate Diapause in C. elegans Genes Devel 13: 1438–1452

Parkes TL, Elia AJ, Dickinson D, Hilliker AJ, Phillips JP, Boulianne GL Extension of Drosophila lifespan by overexpression of human SOD1 in motorneurons. Nat Genet 19: 171

Patterson G, Koweek A, Wong A, Liu Y, Ruvkun G (1997) The DAF-3 Smad protein antagonizes TGF-beta-related receptor signaling in the Caenorhabditis elegans dauer pathway. Genes Dev 11:2679–2690

Perls TT, Alpert L, Fretts RC (1997) Middle-aged mothers live longer. Nature 389:133

Rena G, Guo S, Cichy SC, Unterman TG, Cohen P (1999) Phosphorylation of the transcription factor forkhead family member FKHR by protein kinase B. J Biol Chem 274:17179–17183

Ren P, Lim CS, Johnsen R, Albert PS, Pilgrim D, Riddle DL (1996) Control of C. elegans larval development by neuronal expression of a TGF-beta homolog. Science 274:1389–1392

Rubin GM, Yandell MD, Wortman JR, Gabor Miklos GL, Nelson CR, Hariharan IK, Fortini ME, Li PW, Apweiler R, Fleischmann W, Cherry JM, Henikoff S, Skupski MP, Misra S, Ashburner M, Birney E, Boguski MS, Brody T, Brokstein P, Celniker SE, Chervitz SA, Coates D, Cravchik A, Gabrielian A, Galle RF, Gelbart WM, George RA, Goldstein LS, Gong F, Guan P, Harris NL, Hay BA, Hoskins RA, Li J, Li Z, Hynes RO, Jones SJ, Kuehl PM, Lemaitre B, Littleton JT, Morrison DK, Mungall C, O'Farrell PH, Pickeral OK, Shue C, Vosshall LB, Zhang J, Zhao Q, Zheng XH, Lewis S (2000). Comparative genomics of the eukaryotes. Science 287: 2204–2215

Schackwitz WS, Inoue T, Thomas JH (1996) Chemosensory neurons function in parallel to mediate a pheromone response in C. elegans. Neuron 17:719–728

Schmoll D, Walker KS, Alessi DR, Grempler R, Burchell A, Guo S, Walther R, Unterman TG (2000) Regulation of glucose-6-phosphatase gene expression by protein kinase Balpha and the forkhead transcription factor FKHR: Evidence for insulin response unit (IRU)-dependent and independent effects of insulin on promoter activity. J Biol Chem 275: 36324–36333

Schwartz MW, Woods SC, Porte D Jr, Seeley RJ, Baskin DG (2000) Central nervous system control of food intake Nature 404: 661

Tauber MJ, Tauber CA, Masaki S (1986) Seasonal adaptation of insects. Oxford University Press, New York

Taub J, Lau JF, Ma C, Hahn JH, Hoque R, Rothblatt J, Chalfie M (1999) A cytosolic catalase is needed to extend adult lifespan in C. elegans dauer constitutive and clk-1 mutants. Nature 399:162–166

Thomas JH, Birnby DA, Vowels JJ (1993) Evidence for parallel processing of sensory information controlling dauer formation in Caenorhabditis elegans. Genetics 134:1005–1117

Tang ED, Nunez G, Barr FG, Guan KL (1999) Negative regulation of the forkhead transcription factor FKHR by Akt. J Biol Chem 274(24):16741–16746

Thacker C, Peters K, Srayko M, Rose AM (1995) The bli-4 locus of Caenorhabditis elegans encodes structurally distinct kex2/subtilisin-like endoproteases essential for early development and adult morphology. Genes Devel 9: 956–971

Tomizawa M, Kumar A, Perrot V, Nakae J, Accili D, Rechler MM, Kumaro A (2000) Insulin inhibits the activation of transcription by a C-terminal fragment of the forkhead transcription factor FKHR. A mechanism for insulin inhibition of insulin-like growth factor-binding protein-1 transcription. J Biol Chem 275: 7289–7295

IGF-1 and Insulin Signaling in the Control of Longevity

A. Bartke[1], J. Kopchick[2], F. Dominici[3] and D. Turyn[3]

Summary

In the laboratory mouse, there are three spontaneous mutations and one gene knockout that induce primary deficits in endocrine signaling and prolong life. Increased life expectancy appears to be due to delayed aging in at least three of these four mutants. Ames dwarf (Prop1^{df}) and Snell dwarf (Pit1^{dw}) mice have primary deficiency of growth hormone (GH), prolactin and thyrotropin, little (GHRHR^{lit}) mice have GH releasing hormone resistance, and GHR-KO mice are GH resistant. Reduced GH secretion or action leads, in each case, to the expected precipitous decline in peripheral levels of insulin-like growth factor-1 (IGF-1), the key mediator of GH actions. The role of reduced IGF-1 signaling in mediating the effects of these four "longevity genes" in the mouse is consistent with the findings in *Caenorhabditis elegans* and *Drosophila melanogaster*. However, the formal proof of a cause-effect relationship between reduced IGF-1 levels and delayed aging remains to be obtained, and the mechanisms of IGF-1 action on aging remain to be identified.

As expected from the anti-insulin actions of GH and from its effects on the pancreatic islets, insulin regulation of peripheral glucose levels is significantly altered in dwarf and GHR-KO mice. These alterations include reductions in basal and glucose-stimulated insulin levels, enhanced sensitivity of the liver to insulin, and reduced plasma glucose levels. Surprisingly, indices of enhanced sensitivity to insulin coexist with reduced ability to dispose of a glucose load. As in the case of IGF-1 signaling, a role of reduced insulin signaling in extending longevity is strongly supported by data from invertebrates. In Ames dwarf mice, there is evidence for increased activity of antioxidant enzymes and reduced oxidative damage of mitochondrial DNA and other cell components.

Data derived from animals subjected to caloric restriction (CR) suggest that there is considerable overlap of phenotypic characteristics of long-lived dwarf and GHR-KO mice with those of normal (wild type) animals subjected

[1] Southern Illinois University School of Medicine, PO Box 19636, Springfield, IL 62794-9636;
[2] Edison Biotechnology Institute and Department of Clinical Research, Ohio University Athens, OH 45701;
[3] Instituto de Química y Fisicoquímica Biológicas (UBA-CONICET), Facultad de Farmacia y Bioquímica, Junín 956, (1113) Buenos Aires, Argentina

Chanson et al.
Endocrine Aspects of Successful Aging
© Springer-Verlag Berlin Heidelberg 2004

to CR. These include reductions in plasma insulin and glucose levels, core body temperature, growth, adult body size, and fertility. However, there are also considerable differences, including discordant changes in body composition and in spontaneous locomotor activity and differences in the profiles of hepatic gene expression. Ongoing studies of the interactions of CR and longevity genes suggest additive effects on longevity in at least one of these mutants, the Ames dwarf. Effects of CR on plasma insulin and glucose levels in GHR-KO mice resemble its actions in wild type animals, while CR effects on corticosterone levels are distinctly different.

In summary, results available to date suggest that reduced function of the somatotropic axis and reduced IGF-1 and insulin signaling mediate the action of several mutations on aging and life span of laboratory mice. The mechanisms linking these neuroendocrine changes to delayed aging remain to be identified, but it is reasonable to suspect that reduced generation of reactive oxygen species and reduced oxidative damage to DNA and other macromolecules are involved and ultimately responsible for prolonged longevity.

Introduction

Although the process of aging affects most, if not all, living organisms, identifying the mechanisms that are responsible has been difficult. Results obtained during the last decade in experimental animals ranging from microscopic worms to mice indicate that the rate of aging and the life span may be controlled by genetic differences in insulin-like growth factor (IGF) and insulin signaling. Studies in nematodes, insects, and rodents provided numerous examples of increased longevity of animals that either produce reduced amounts of IGF-I, insulin, or analogous signaling molecules or are resistant to their actions. These findings attracted considerable attention because they imply the existence of an evolutionarily conserved mechanism that links food intake, metabolism, growth, and reproduction to regulation of aging and life expectancy. However, the suggestion that reduced IGF/insulin signaling promotes longevity is not easy to accept. Both IGF-I and insulin are necessary for normal development and intimately involved in the control of reproduction. In mammals, insulin action is necessary for life. In the human, deficiency of insulin or IGF-I as well as insulin resistance represent serious endocrine diseases. Moreover, insulin resistance is a major risk factor for cardiovascular disease. In this chapter, we will briefly review the data that link IGF/insulin-like signaling to the control of longevity in invertebrates, list key endocrine characteristics of long-lived mutant and gene knock-out mice, and discuss evidence that findings concerning control of aging in experimental animals may apply to the human. Finally, we will attempt to reconcile concepts presented in this article with the current interest in diagnosing and treating somatopause in elderly subjects and in using growth hormone as an anti-aging agent.

Longevity genes in invertebrates

The microscopic soil-dwelling roundworm, *Caenorhabditis elegans* (*C. elegans*), has been studied extensively by developmental biologists and geneticists. The complete sequence of its genome, as well as the derivation of each of approximately 1000 somatic cells in its body, is known, and effects of many mutations have been studied extensively. In this organism, food intake stimulates secretion of insulin-like ligands that act on a receptor encoded by daf-2, a gene homologous to IGF-I and insulin receptor genes in mammals (Kimura et al. 1997). Other genes in the daf-2 signaling pathway also exhibit homology to genes involved in insulin/IGF signaling in higher organisms (Paradis and Ruvkun 1998). Several mutations of daf-2, daf-16, and other genes that control this pathway cause striking extension to life span. Some of the *C. elegans* mutants live more than three times longer than the wild type (normal) worms (Guarente and Kenyon 2000). Although unique characteristics of *C. elegans* biology and its life cycle complicate comparisons with other animals, results obtained in this interesting and well-studied organism clearly indicate that reduced IGF/insulin-like signaling can prolong life. This novel and important conclusion received strong support from results obtained in insects.

In a fruit fly, *Drosophila melanogaster*, another extensively studied invertebrate, there are many insulin-like hormones, and several steps of insulin signaling, as well as their genetic control, exhibit clear homology to mammals. Mutations of insulin receptor-like gene and mutations of insulin receptor substrate were recently reported to cause significant extension of the life span of *Drosophila* (Tatar et al. 2001; Clancy et al. 2001). These exciting findings provided strong support of the concept that reduced insulin/IGF signaling can prolong life and suggested an unexpected conclusion that insulin resistance can delay aging. We will return to this issue in the discussion of findings obtained in mice.

Long-lived mutant mice

The importance of IGF-I and insulin signaling in the control of aging in mammals was deduced from results obtained in long-lived mutant mice. In laboratory stocks of house mice (*Mus musculus*), two spontaneous mutations, Ames dwarf (Prop-1[df]) and Snell dwarf (Pit-1[dw]), cause congenital deficiency of growth hormone (GH), prolactin (PRL), and thyrotropin (TSH; Bartke 1979; Li et al. 1990; Sornson et al. 1996) along with a major, approximately 40-60% increase in life span (Brown-Borg et al. 1996; Flurkey et al. 2001). As expected from GH deficiency, plasma IGF-I levels in Ames and Snell dwarf mice are very low, near or below the levels of detectability of radioimmunoassay systems (van Buul-Offers et al. 1986; Chandrashekar and Bartke 1993). Plasma insulin levels in Ames and Snell dwarf mice are significantly reduced (Borg et al. 1995; Hsieh et al. 2002), presumably as a secondary consequence of GH, IGF-I and PRL deficiency. We strongly suspect that the prolonged longevity of Ames and Snell dwarf mice is due to GH deficiency and reduced IGF-I levels rather than to deficiency of PRL and/or TSH, because a comparable extension of life span was described in GH receptor/GH binding protein knock-out (GHR-KO) mice (Coschigano et al. 2000; Bartke et al. 2002) in which GH action is eliminated but release of PRL and thyroid function are not suppressed (Zhou et al. 1997; Chandrashekar et al. 1999; Hauck et al. 2001). GHR-KO mice are GH resistant and consequently have severely suppressed peripheral IGF-I levels (Zhou et al. 1997; Chandrashekar et al. 1999). Moreover, longevity is significantly increased in mutant "little" (GHRHR[lit]) mice with isolated GH deficiency, providing they are fed a low-fat diet (Flurkey et al. 2001).

Ames dwarf, Snell dwarf, and GHR-KO mice share many phenotypic and physiological characteristics, some of which may represent mechanisms of prolonged longevity. These characteristics include reduced postnatal growth, greatly reduced adult body size, reduced total food intake (while food intake per unit of body weight is increased), reduced body core temperature, reduced plasma insulin and plasma glucose levels, delayed puberty, and reduced fertility (Bartke 1979; Flurkey et al. 2001; Borg et al. 1995; Zhou et al. 1997; Hauck et al. 2001; Hunter et al. 1999). These phenotypic characteristics are not equally pronounced in these mutants. For example, insulin levels are much lower in GHR-KO than in dwarf mice, while puberty is delayed by several days in GHR-KO (Danilovich et al. 1999; Keene et al. 2002) and by several weeks or indefinitely (depending on the genetic background) in dwarf mice (Bartke, unpublished data). Female GHR-KO mice have various indices of reduced fertility but can produce live young and raise them to weaning (Zhou et al. 1997; Danilovich et al. 1999; Zaczek et al. 2002). In contrast, female Ames and Snell dwarf mice are infertile due to PRL deficiency and the resulting luteal failure (Bartke 1966).

Importantly, increased longevity of Ames dwarf, Snell dwarf, and GHR-KO mice is associated with, and perhaps due to, delayed aging. This finding is suggested by significant increases in both the average and the maximal life span, by delayed aging of immune system and collagen (Flurkey et al. 2001), by delay in age-related decline in cognitive function (Kinney et al. 2001a, b), and by the apparent delay in development of neoplastic and non-neoplastic lesions (Ikeno et al., 2003). Interestingly, many of the phenotypic characteristics of the long-lived mutant and GHR-KO mice resemble those of genetically normal ("wild type") mice subjected to caloric restriction (CR), a procedure that is well known to delay aging and prolong life in laboratory rodents (Weindruch and Sohal 1997; Masoro 2001). These characteristics include reduced body size and body core temperature, as well as reduced circulatory levels of IGF-I, insulin and glucose. However, major differences also exist, suggesting that genetic dwarf and GHR-KO mice are not merely CR mimetics (Mattison et al. 2000; Bartke et al. 2001). For example, spontaneous locomotor activity is increased in CR and reduced in dwarf mice (Mattison et al. 2000), and CR animals are lean, whereas body fat content in GHR-KO and in young (but not middle-aged or old) Ames dwarfs is increased (Heiman et al., 2003). Hereditary dwarfism, GH resistance, and CR have markedly different effects on the profile of gene expression in the liver (Dozmorov et al. 2001; Miller et al. 2002a). Moreover, subjecting Ames dwarf mice to CR causes a further extension of their remarkably long life span (Bartke et al. 2001a).

Comparison of the effects of mutations at the Prop1, Pit1, and GHRHR loci, targeted disruption of the GHR/GHBP gene and CR in genetically normal animals identifies the reduction of peripheral IGF-I levels as a likely common denominator. In other words, chronic reduction in GH/IGF-I signaling emerges as a primary alteration in endocrine function that delays aging and prolongs life. Final proof of the cause-effect relationship between reduced IGF-I signaling and delayed aging would require hormone replacement or "genetic rescue" studies in which a wild type (i.e., shorter living) phenotype could be produced in dwarf, GHR-KO, or wild-type CR animals by experimentally restoring normal IGF-I levels. Such studies are yet to be performed. However, the proposed causal association between reduced IGF signaling and prolonged longevity in mutant, GHR-KO and normal CR mice is entirely consistent with results obtained in C. elegans and Drosophila and with the association of small body size with prolonged longevity in mice (Eklund and Bradford 1977; Miller et al. 2002b) and other species (Eigenmann et al. 1988; Patronek et al. 1997; Rollo 2002).

The suspected role of reduced insulin signaling in extending the life span of Ames dwarf, Snell dwarf, and GHR-KO mice is more difficult to relate to results obtained in lower organisms. In Drosophila, mutations interfering with insulin action, i.e., conditions of insulin resistance, are associated with prolonged longevity (Tatar et al, 2001; Clancy et al. 2001). In Ames dwarf, Snell dwarf, and GHR-KO mice, plasma levels of both insulin and glucose are reduced (Borg et al. 1995; Hauck et al. 2001; Hsieh et al. 2002), indicating that sensitivity to insulin is enhanced rather than reduced. In support of this conclusion, administration of identical doses of insulin (in terms of mIU/g bwt) causes greater suppression of plasma glucose levels in Ames dwarf and in GHR-KO mice than in the normal animals from the same strain (Coschigano et al. 1999; Dominici et al. 2002). Thus, it would appear that, while the role of insulin signaling in the control of longevity is evolutionarily conserved, the relationship of insulin sensitivity to life expectancy may be opposite in insects and mammals. However, an alternative and, we believe, more plausible interpretation of these findings is that insulin signaling is reduced in both long-lived invertebrates and long-lived mice, but this reduction is achieved by different mechanisms. In long-lived insulin receptor and insulin receptor substrate (Chico) mutants in Drosophila, insulin action is reduced by disruption of early steps in its signaling pathway. In dwarf and GHR-KO mice, insulin signaling is attenuated due to reduced release of insulin under both basal and stimulated conditions. In support of this interpretation, plasma insulin levels are reduced in both fasted and fed dwarf and GHR-KO mice (Borg et al. 1995; Dominici et al. 2000; Hauck et al. 2001), and insulin response to an acute glucose challenge is dramatically reduced in Ames dwarf as compared to normal mice (Grier and Bartke, unpublished). In further support of this concept, Hsieh et al. (2002) recently reported numerous indications of reduced insulin signaling in Snell dwarf mice. Reduced secretion of insulin in dwarf and GHR-KO mice is consistent with stimulatory actions of GH, IGF-I and PRL on the insulin-producing cells in the pancreas (Garcia-Ocana et al. 2001; Freemark et al. 2002; Nielsen et al. 1999) and with morphological studies of the islets of Langerhans in Ames dwarf, as compared to normal mice (Parsons et al. 1995).

The relationship between insulin signaling and longevity in mammals appears to be further complicated by differential alterations in insulin sensitivity in different insulin target tissues. We have shown that insulin sensitivity is enhanced in the liver of Ames dwarf mice in association with increased levels of the insulin receptor and its substrates, IRS-1 and IRS-2 (Dominici et al. 2002). Unexpectedly, our recent findings indicate that sensitivity of the skeletal muscles of these animals to the action of insulin is reduced rather than enhanced (Dominici et al., unpublished). The physiological importance of insulin resistance in skeletal muscle of Ames dwarf mice is suggested by the observation that these animals have limited capacity to dispose of an injected glucose load (Dominici et al. 2002). Insulin resistance of skeletal muscle was previously reported in animals with liver-specific knockout of the IGF gene (Yakar et al. 2001). Apparently, chronic GH/IGF-I deficiency produces changes in the rate of insulin biosynthesis and release and induces organ-specific alterations in responsiveness to insulin action. Further research will be required to determine which of these alterations link mutations of "longevity genes" to increased life expectancy.

The mechanisms that are ultimately responsible for delayed aging and prolonged longevity of dwarf and GHR-KO mice remain to be positively identified, but several possibilities are supported by the available data. Thus, reduced body core temperature and reduced levels of anabolic hormones and glucose suggest reduction in metabolic rate. Life-long maintenance of low glucose levels predicts reduced damage from non-enzymatic glycation (Baynes and Monnier 1989). Reduced levels of insulin may also have a direct role in reducing the rate of aging (Parr 1997). Finally, and perhaps most importantly, oxidative damage of mitochondrial DNA (Sanz et al., 2002) and other macromolecules (Brown-Borg et al. 2001) is reduced in several tissues of Ames dwarf mice. This probably reflects reduced generation of free oxygen radicals (consistent with reduced levels of glucose and anabolic hormones) as well as improved anti-oxidant defenses, including increased activity of catalase and superoxide dismutase (Brown-Borg et al. 1999, 2001; Hauck and Bartke 2000).

Insulin, somatotropic axis and human aging

Most of the evidence linking GH, IGF-I and insulin actions to the control of aging and longevity in the human is indirect and some of it is controversial. However, there is increasing evidence that in men, similarly to mice, enhanced sensitivity to insulin predicts long life. Moreover, there are numerous indications that reduced activity of the somatotropic axis may be associated with extended longevity in the human.

Detailed studies of a large cohort of centenarians in Italy revealed that increased sensitivity to insulin is among the most consistent physiological characteristics of this remarkable group of individuals (Paolisso et al. 1996). In these studies, people over 100 years of age were much more sensitive to insulin that elderly (70-90 year old) subjects from the same population, and, in fact, the average insulin responsiveness of centenarians resembled values measured in individuals half their age. Apparently, people predisposed (presumably genetically) to be very insulin sensitive are most likely to survive to a very advanced age. Moreover, insulin resistance is a recognized, important risk factor for various age-related diseases, including cardiovascular problems and cancer (Facchini et al. 2001).

Elevated levels of IGF-I in acromegalic patients with pathologic hypersecretion of GH are associated with reduced life expectancy (Orme et al. 1998). However, acromegalics have an increased incidence of diabetes, cardiovascular disease, and probably also cancer, and thus their reduced life expectancy may not be due to acceleration of aging per se. In transgenic mice overexpressing GH, lifelong elevation of GH and IGF-I levels is associated with indices of premature aging as well as an increased incidence of pathological lesions that can be linked directly to GH excess (Wanke et al. 1992; Pendergrass et al. 1993; Miller et al. 1995; Bartke et al. 2001b). In one prospective study of endocrinologically normal men, high GH levels were identified as a risk factor for early mortality (Maison et al. 1998). Additional support for the concept that reduced activity of the somatotropic axis may promote longer survival is derived from negative correlation of body size and longevity. The existence of such a negative relationship is supported by results of many, although not all, studies in humans (Samaras and Elrick 2002) and is very well documented for other species, in particular domestic dogs (Patronek et al. 1997) and laboratory mice (Rollo, 2002; Miller et al. 2002a). In the human, height has been identified as a cancer risk (Tretli 1989). The correlation of IGF-I levels and previous GH therapy with incidence of several types of tumors (Werner and LeRoith 1996; Swerdlow et al. 2002) offers a plausible causal explanation for this finding. However, it is interesting and difficult to explain that, when comparisons are made between, rather than within, species, it is the larger animals that usually live longer than the small animals.

We are not aware of any systematic studies of longevity in humans afflicted with GH deficiency, GH resistance, or other syndromes that produce dwarfism. Many of these patients exhibit insulin resistance, presumably as a consequence of increased adiposity and particularly central (abdominal) fat accumulation (Rosen and Bengtsson 1990), and this would predict reduced life expectancy. However, no evidence for early deaths or premature aging was noticed in GH-resistant patients with Laron dwarfism (Kopchick and Laron 1999), and several individuals with hypopituitarism due to mutations at the Prop 1 locus (the same locus that is mutated in long-lived Ames dwarf mice) were reported to reach a very advanced age (Krzisnik et al. 1999).

Additional support for the importance of GH, IGF-I, and insulin signaling in the control of longevity in mammals, including humans, is provided by studies of the effects of caloric restriction on endocrine function and longevity. In rats and mice, reducing caloric intake suppresses plasma insulin, IGF-I and glucose levels, delays onset of age-related disease and reliably prolongs life (Weindruch and Sohal 1997; Masoro 2001). Comparable results were recently obtained in dogs (Kealy et al. 2002), and ongoing studies in rhesus monkeys indicate that the response to caloric restriction in primates is similar (Roth et al. 2001). Epidemiologic studies suggest that reduced caloric intake may prolong longevity also in humans (reviewed in Roth et al. 1999), and several characteristics of calorically restricted animals, including reduced insulin levels, were found to be associated with prolonged longevity in humans (Roth et al. 2002).

Thus it would appear that the association of delayed aging and increased life expectancy with reduced activity of the somatotropic axis, reduced insulin levels, and enhanced responsiveness to insulin which was demonstrated in mutant, knock-out and calorically restricted rodents is related to fundamental mechanisms of aging and likely to apply to other species, including humans.

Conceptually, the association of enhanced sensitivity to insulin with delayed aging is not surprising in view of the age-related decline in responsiveness to insulin and the role of insulin resistance in the development of type 2 diabetes. However, the association of reduced GH levels or action with prolonged longevity is difficult to reconcile with some findings concerning secretion and effects of GH and with the recent interest in GH as an "anti-aging" agent. This controversial area will be discussed below.

Age-related suppression of GH release and "anti-aging" effects of GH replacement therapy.

Secretion of GH and circulating GH levels begin to decline in early adulthood and this decrease continues during aging (Corpas et al. 1993). Consequently, plasma IGF-1 levels also decline with age (Ghigo et al. 2000). These well-documented effects of aging on the somatotropic axis and the similarity of some of the symptoms of aging to the symptoms of GH deficiency provided impetus for evaluating the effects of GH therapy in the elderly. The landmark study of Rudman and his colleagues (1990) reported that treatment of men over 60 years of age with recombinant human GH led to reduction in adiposity and increases in lean body mass and bone mineral density. These effects are consistent with the well-established lipolytic and anabolic effects of GH and produced a more "youthful" body composition. These findings attracted considerable attention and continue to be used in promoting GH as well as various GH-releasing or "GH-related" products. Results of subsequent studies indicated that GH treatment in unselected elderly patients does not consistently produce the desired effects, that an increase in muscle mass in GH-treated subjects is not accompanied by an increase in strength, and that prolonged GH administration can lead to many side effects. Currently, the prevailing opinion of endocrinologists is that administration of GH to normal (i.e., not GH-deficient) middle aged or elderly individuals is an experimental treatment with few if any proven benefits (Papadakis et al. 1996; von Werder 1999). However, some physicians feel that the age-related decline in GH levels, the so-called somatopause, is an endocrine deficiency that, similar to the menopause and the andropause, constitutes an indication for replacement therapy. The risks and benefits of long-term GH therapy remain to be evaluated, and the results of ongoing studies in this area may either alleviate or substantiate the concerns that GH treatment may induce insulin resistance (even though it often initially improves insulin sensitivity by reducing adiposity) or that it will increase the risk of cancer (Swerdlow et al. 2002).

In the context of our discussion of the role of the somatotropic axis in the control of aging, it is important to distinguish between the effects of GH on age-related changes in body composition and its promised or implied effects on aging. Aging is notoriously difficult to define and the rate of aging is difficult to measure. Analysis of survival curves and alterations in maximal life span in particular are considered most reliable, but sufficient data are hard to obtain in clinical trials. It is a consensus of gerontologists that there is currently no treatment that has been shown to slow the rate of aging in humans, and thus any claims of anti-aging effects of GH (or any other) therapy are false and misleading (Olshansky et al. 2002). Admittedly, the concept of biological aging as a process that can be distinguished from age-related disease is somewhat difficult to grasp and, to those not working in this field, may seem largely semantic. Currently there is no information on the effects (positive or negative) of GH therapy on life expectancy in humans. Data on longevity of experimental animals chronically treated with GH are very limited and results are not consistent (Khansari and Gustad 1991; Kalu et al, 1998). By selecting different sets of data from what has been published in this field, one could make seemingly well-supported predictions of both life-extending and life-shortening effects of prolonged treatment with GH. Research in experimental animals continues to provide new evidence supporting each of these opposing points of view by documenting the benefits of both GH/IGF-I therapy and congenital absence of the GH signal. A series of studies in aged normal rats and in GH-deficient dwarf rats provided very convincing evidence for neurotropic and neuroprotective effects of IGF-I and for the ability of GH treatment to improve vascular supply of the brain and cognitive function of old animals (Sonntag et al. 1999, 2000; Markowska et al. 1998). However, studies in GH-resistant GHR-KO mice and in hypopituitary dwarf mice revealed normal performance of these animals in a battery of behavioral tests used to assess cognitive function, as well as a marked delay and/or attenuation of cognitive aging and reduced oxidative damage to brain mitochondrial DNA (Kinney et al. 2001a,b; Sanz et al., 2002).

In the concluding section of this chapter, we will try to reconcile conflicting findings in this area and put them in the broader context of hormonal control of life histories, including growth, maturation, reproduction and aging.

Role of IGF-I/insulin signaling in the control of aging vs. utility of GH therapy in the elderly

Cumulative evidence from studies of gene mutations and knock-outs that extend life in organisms ranging from yeast to mice, and from the studies of caloric restriction, suggests that reduced IGF /insulin signaling leads to delayed aging and increased longevity. The evidence obtained from the latter studies is particularly convincing because caloric restriction is the only intervention repeatedly proven to delay aging in mammals (Weindruch and Sohal 1997; Masoro 2001), and because it appears to be effective in primates and has excellent potential for extending human life also (Roth et al. 1999). Evidence that suppression of signaling by GH, a hormone that exerts anabolic effects and promotes growth, development, sexual maturation and reproductive function, could be beneficial and prolong life seems counterintuitive and difficult to accept. However, it is entirely consistent with the well-documented trade-offs between reproduction and longevity (Kirkwood 1987; Partridge and Barton 1993) and with the current understanding of the ability of different organisms to adjust their life strategies to optimize chances for successful reproduction. The evolutionarily conserved IGF-1/insulin signaling pathway figures prominently among potential mechanisms that link available food supply and energy intake to regulation of growth and reproductive effort. Thus the animals can react to reduced nutritional intake by altering partitioning of available energy resources toward maintenance and repair and away from growth and reproduction. Release of IGF-1 and insulin increases in direct response to dietary intake, and both hormones stimulate somatic growth and sexual maturation and synergize with gonadotropins to enhance gonadal function. Thus, it is not surprising that alterations in the somatotropic axis and in insulin release, as well as changes in tissue responsiveness to insulin, play a prominent role in executing these adjustments in developmental program and/or life history. The result of reduced IGF-1/insulin signaling would thus be prolonged survival and improved chances for reproducing when environmental conditions improve. This interpretation of the available data explains why extension of life by caloric restriction or by mutation of different "longevity genes" generally involves some "costs" in terms of reproductive development and/or competence.

Viewed in this light, the beneficial effects of GH treatment of elderly individuals - on body composition, fat distribution, muscle mass, and brain vascularity - may not be related to the physiological role of GH in the control of aging but rather to the well-documented anabolic and lipolytic action of this hormone and to the normal decline of its release during aging. There are interesting analogies of these findings to the age-related decline in the levels of gonadal steroids and the ability of these hormones to improve the appearance and quality of life of elderly individuals.

We realize that this explanation of the relationship of endogenous GH and GH therapy to aging is oversimplified in that it ignores many complexities in which environmental, genetic and hormonal factors interact to control aging and life span. For example, GH influences insulin action and release, GH and IGF-1 have generally opposite effects on insulin sensitivity, and the usefulness of extrapolating physiological information from mice and rats to humans is limited by physiological differences between these species as well as differences in the environment in which they are studied.

Evidence that lifelong reduction in GH signaling can prolong life does not preclude the possibility that judicious treatment with low doses of GH may find its place among therapies designed to improve functionality and quality of life of the elderly. Additional research in this area will undoubtedly allow clearer definition of the role of GH, IGF-1, and insulin in mediating   the effect of genes and environment in aging, as well as detailed evaluation of the risks and benefits of various hormonal therapies, including treatment with GH or GH-releasing agents.

Acknowledgments

Our studies were supported by NIH (AG 19899) and by Illinois CFAR. We thank Ms. Nancy Cowan for her help in formatting and typing this manuscript. We also wish to apologize to those whose work, pertinent to this topic, was not mentioned due to inadvertent omissions or limitations of space.

Note added in proof

After preparation of this manuscript, Holzenberger et. al. (2003) reported prolonged longevity of mice heterozygous for knock-out of the IGF-1 receptor and Bluher et. al. (2003) reported increase in the life span of mice with selective deletion of insulin receptor in the adipose tissue. These exciting findings provide strong support of the proposed role of IGF-1 and insulin in the control of mammalian aging.

References

Bartke A (1966) Reproduction of female dwarf mice treated with prolactin. J Reprod Fertili 11: 203–206

Bartke A (1979) Genetic models in the study of anterior pituitary hormones. In: Shire JGM (ed) Genet Variation in Hormonal System Boca Raton, CRC Press, pp. 113–126

Bartke A, Coschigano K, Kopchick J, Chandrashekar V, Mattison J, Kinney B,

Bartke A, Turyn D (2001a) Mechanisms of prolonged longevity: mutants, knock-outs, and caloric restriction. J Anti-Aging Med 4: 197–203

Bartke A, Wright JC, Mattison JA, Ingram DK, Miller RA, Roth GS (2001b) Extending the lifespan of long-lived mice. Nature 414: 412

Bartke A, Chandrashekar V, Bailey B, Zaczek D, Turyn D (2002) Consequences of growth hormone (GH) overexpression and GH resistance. Neuropeptides 36: 201–208

Baynes JW, Monnier VM (1989) The maillard reaction in aging, diabetes and nutrition. New York, Alan R. Liss.

Bluher M, Kahn B, Kahn CR: Extended Longevity in Mice Lacking the Insulin Receptor in Adipose Tissue. Science 299: 572, 2003.

Borg KE, Brown-Borg HM, Bartke A (1995) Assessment of the primary adrenal cortical and pancreatic hormone basal levels in relation to plasma glucose and age in the unstressed Ames dwarf mouse. Proc Soc Exp Biol Med 210: 126–133

Brown-Borg HM, Borg KE, Meliska CJ, Bartke A (1996) Dwarf mice and the ageing process. Nature 384: 33

Brown-Borg HM, Bode AM, Bartke A (1999) Antioxidative mechanisms and plasma growth hormone levels. Endocrine 11: 41–48

Brown-Borg H, Johnson W, Rakoczky S, Romanick M (2001) Mitochondrial oxidant generation and oxidative damage in Ames dwarf and GH transgenic mice. Am Aging Assoc 24: 85–96

Chandrashekar V, Bartke A (1993) Induction of endogenous insulin-like growth factor-I secretion alters the hypothalamic-pituitary-testicular function in growth hormone-deficient adult dwarf mice. Biol Reprod 48: 544–551

Chandrashekar V, Bartke A, Coschigano KT, Kopchick JJ (1999) Pituitary and testicular function in growth hormone receptor gene knockout mice. Endocrinology 140: 1082–1088

Clancy D J, Gems D, Harshman LG, Oldham S, Stocker H, Hafen E, Leevers SJ, Partridge L (2001) Extension of life-span by loss of CHICO, a Drosophila insulin receptor substrate protein. Science 292: 104–106

Corpas E, Harman SM, Blackman MR (1993) Human growth hormone and human aging. Endocrine Rev 14: 20–39

Coschigano KT, Riders ME, Bellush LL, Kopchick JJ (1999) Glucose metabolism in growth hormone receptor/binding protein gene disrupted mice. Annual Meeting, The Endocrine Society, San Diego, CA, USA, Abstract P3-537, p. 553

Coschigano KT, Clemmons D, Bellush LL, Kopchick JJ (2000) Assessment of growth parameters and life span of GHR/BP gene-disrupted mice. Endocrinology 141: 2608–2613

Danilovich N, Wernsing D, Coschigano KT, Kopchick JJ, Bartke A (1999) Deficits in female reproductive function in GH-R-KO mice; role of IGF-I. Endocrinology 140(6): 2637–2640

Dominici FP, Arostegui Diaz G, Bartke A, Kopchick JJ, Turyn D (2000) Compensatory alterations of insulin signal transduction in liver of growth hormone receptor knockout mice. J Endocrinol 166: 579–590

Dominici FP, Hauck S, Argentino DP, Bartke A, Turyn D (2002) Increased insulin sensitivity and upregulation of insulin receptor, insulin receptor substrate (IRS)-I and IRS-2 in liver of Ames dwarf mice. J Endocrinol 173: 81–94

Dozmorov I, Bartke A, Miller RA (2001) Array-based expression analysis of mouse liver genes: Effect of age and of the longevity mutant Prop 1df. J Gerontol: Biol Sci 56A: B72–B80

Eigenmann JE, Amador A, Patterson DF (1988) Insulin-like growth factor I levels in proportionate dogs, chondrodystrophic dogs and in giant dogs. Acta Endocrinol 118: 105–108

Eklund J, Bradford CE (1977) Longevity and lifetime body weight in mice selected for rapid growth. Nature 265: 48–49

Facchini FS, Hua N, Abbasi F, Reaven GM (2001) Insulin resistance as a predictor of age-related diseases. J Clin Endocrinol Metab 86: 3574–3578

Flurkey K, Papaconstantinou J, Miller RA, Harrison DE (2001) Lifespan extension and delayed immune and collagen aging in mutant mice with defects in growth hormone production. Proc Natl Acad Sci USA 98: 6736–6741

Freemark M, Avril I, Fleenor D, Driscoll P, Petro A, Opara E, Kendall W, Oden J, Bridges S, Binart N, Breant B, Kelly PA (2002) Targeted deletion of the PRL receptor: effects on islet development, insulin production, and glucose tolerance. Endocrinology 143(4): 1378–1385

Garcia-Ocana A, Vasavada R, Takane KK, Cebrian A, Lopez-Talavera JC, Stewart AF (2001) Using B cell growth factors to enhance human pancreatic islet transplantation. J Clin Endocrinol Metab 86: 984–988

Ghigo E, Arvat E, Gianotti L, Lanfranco F, Broglio F, Aimaretti G, Maccario M, Camami F (2000) Hypothalamic growth hormone-insulin-like growth factor-I axis across the human life span. J Pediatr Endocrinol Metab 13: 1493–1502

Guarente L, Kenyon C (2000) Genetic pathways that regulate ageing in model organisms. Nature 408: 255–262

Hauck S (2001) Genes that prolong life: Relationships of growth hormone and growth to aging and life span. J Gerontol: Biol Sci 56A: B340–B349

Hauck S, Bartke A (2000) Effects of growth hormone on hypothalamic Catalase and Cu/Zn superoxide dismutase. Free Rad Biol Med 28: 970–978

Hauck SJ, Hunter WS, Danilovich N, Kopchick J, Bartke A (2001) Reduced levels of thyroid hormones, insulin, and glucose, and lower body core temperature in the growth hormone receptor/binding protein knockout mouse. Exp Biol Med 226: 552–558

Heiman M, Tinsley F, Mattison J, Hauck S, Bartke A (2003) Body composition of prolactin-, growth hormone-, and thyrotropin-deficient Ames dwarf mice. Endocrine 20: 149–154

Holzenberger M, Dupont J, Ducos B, Leneuve P, Geloen A, Evens P, Cervera P, LeBouc Y: IGF-1 receptor regulates lifespan and resistance to oxidative stress in mice. Nature 421: 182–187, 2003..

Hsieh CC, DeFord JH, Flurkey K, Harrison DE, Papaconstantinou J (2002) Effects of the Pit 1 mutation on the insulin signaling pathway: implications on the longevity of the long-lived Snell dwarf mouse. Mech Ageing Devel 123: 1244–1255

Hunter WS, Croson WB, Bartke A, Gentry MV, Meliska CJ (1999) Low body temperature in long-lived Ames dwarf mice at rest and during stress. Physiol Behav 67: 433–437

Ikeno Y, Bronson RT, Hubbard GB, Lee S, Bartke A (2003) Delayed occurrence of fatal neoplastic diseases in Ames dwarf mice: correlation to extended longevity. J Gerontol A Biol Sci Med Sci 58A: 291–296

Kalu DN, Orhii PB, Chen C, Lee DY, Hubbard GB, Lee S, Olatunjibello Y (1998) Aged-rodent models of long-term growth hormone therapy - lack of deleterious effect on longevity. J Gerontol: Biol Sci Med Sci 53: B452-B463

Kealy RD, Lawler DF, Ballam JM (2002) Effects of diet restriction on life span and age-related changes in dogs. J Am Vet Med Assoc 220: 1315–1320

Keene DF, Suescun M, Bostwick M, Chandrashekar V, Bartke A, Kopchick J (2002) Puberty in male growh hormone receptor gene disrupted mice. JAndrology 23: 661–668

Khansari DN, Gustad T (1991) Effects of long-term, low-dose growth hormone therapy on immune function and life expectancy of mice. Mech Ageing Devel 57: 87–100

Kimura K D, Tissenbaum HA, Liu Y, Ruvkun G (1997) daf-2, an insulin receptor-like gene that regulates longevity and diapause in Caenorhabditis elegans. Science 277: 942–946

Kinney BA, Meliska CJ, Steger RW, Bartke A (2001a) Evidence that Ames dwarf mice age differently from their normal siblings in behavioral and learning and memory parameters. Horm Behav 39: 277–284

Kinney BA, Coschigano KT, Kopchick JJ, Bartke A (2001b) Evidence that age-induced decline in memory retention is delayed in growth hormone resistant GH-R-KO (Laron) mice. Physiol Behav 72: 653–660

Kirkwood T (1987) Immortality of the germ-line versus disposability of the soma.In: Woodhead AD,Thompson KH (eds), London, England. Evolution of longevity in animals; a comparative approach, pp.209–213

Kopchick JJ, Laron Z (1999) Is the Laron mouse an accurate model of Laron Syndrome? (Minireview). Mol Genet Metab 68: 232–236

Krzisnik C, Kolacio Z, Battelino T, Brown M, Parks JS, Laron Z (1999) The "Little People" of the island of Krk – revisited. Etiology of hypopituitarism revealed. J Endocrine Genet 1: 9–19

Li S, Crenshaw III BE, Rawson EJ, Simmons DM, Swanson LW, Rosenfeld MG (1990) Dwarf locus mutants lacking three pituitary cell types result from mutations in the POU-domain gene pit-1. Nature 347: 528–533

Maison P, Balkau B, Simon D, Chanson P, Rosselin G, Eschwège E (1998) Growth hormone as a risk for premature mortality in healthy subjects: data from the Paris prospective study. BritMed J 316: 1132–1133

Markowska AL, Mooney M, Sonntag WE (1998) Insulin-like growth factor-I (IGF-I) ameliorates age-related behavioral deficits. Neuroscience 87: 559–569

Masoro EJ (2001) Dietary restriction: an experimental approach to the study of the biology of aging. In: Masoro EJ, Austad SN (eds) Handbook of the biology of aging. Fifth Ed.. San Diego, Academic Press, pp. 396–420

Mattison JA, Wright JC, Bronson RT, Roth GS, Ingram DK, Bartke A (2000) Studies of aging in Ames dwarf mice: Effects of caloric restriction. J Am Aging Assoc 23: 9–16

Miller DB, Bartke A, O'Callaghan JP (1995) Increased glial fibrillary acidic protein (GFAP) levels in the brains of transgenic mice expressing the bovine growth hormone (bGH) gene. Experimental Gerontology 30: 383–400

Miller R A, Harper JM, Galecki A, Burke DT (2002a) Big mice die young: early life body weight predicts longevity in genetically heterogeneous mice. Aging Cell 1: 22–29

Miller R, Chang Y, Galecki A, Al-Regaiey K, Kopchick J, Bartke A (2002b) Gene Expression Patterns in Calorically Restricted Mice: Partial Overlap with Long-Lived Mutant Mice. Molecular Endocrinology 16

Nielsen J, Svensson C, Galsgaard ED, Moldrup A, Billestrup N (1999) B Cell proliferation and growth factors. J Mol Med 77: 62–66

Olshansky SJ, Hayflick L, Carnes BA (2002) Position Statement on Human Aging. Journal of Gerontology 57A(No. 8): B292–B297

Orme SM, McNally RJQ, Cartwright RA, Belchetz PE (1998) Mortality and cancer incidence in acromegaly: a retrospective cohort study. Journal of Clinical Endocrinology and Metabolism 83: 2730–2734

Paolisso G, Gambardella A, Ammendola S, D'Amore A, Balbi V, Varricchio M, D'Onofrio F (1996) Glucose tolerance and insulin action in healthy centenarians. American Journal of Physiology 270: E890–E894

Papadakis MA, Grady D, Black D, Tierney MJ, Gooding GA, Schambelan M, Grunfeld C (1996) Growth hormone replacement in healthy older men improves body composition but not functional ability. Annual of Internal Medicine 124: 708–716

Paradis S, Ruvkun G (1998) Caenorhabditis elegans Akt/PKB transduces insulin receptor-like signals from AGE-1 PI3 kinase to the DAF-16 transcription factor. Genes & Development 12: 2488–98

Parr T (1997) Insulin exposure and aging theory. Gerontology 43: 182–200.

Parsons J A, Bartke A, Sorenson RL (1995) Number and size of islets of langerhans in pregnant, human growth hormone-expressing transgenic, and pituitary dwarf mice: Effect of lactogenic hormones. Endocrinology 136: 2013–2021

Partridge L, Barton N (1993) Optimality, mutation and the evolution of ageing. Nature 362: 305–311

Patronek GJ, Waters DJ, Glickman LT (1997) Comparative longevity of pet dogs and humans: implications for gerontology research. Journal of Gerontology 52A: B171–B178

Pendergrass WR, Li Y, Jiang D, Wolf NS (1993) Decrease in cellular replicative potential in "giant" mice transfected with the bovine growth hormone gene correlates to shortened life span. Journal of Cellular Physiology 156: 96–103

Rollo CD (2002) Growth negatively impacts the life span of mammals. Evol. Dev. 4: 55–61

Rosen T, Bengtsson BA (1990) Premature mortality due to cardiovascular disease in hypopituitarism. Lancet 336: 285–288

Roth GS, Ingram DK, Lane, M.A (1999) Calorie restriction in primates: Will it work and how will we know? Journal of American Geriatric Society 47: 896–903

Roth GS, Lane M, Ingram DK, Mattison J, Elahi D, Tobin JD, Muller D, Metter EJ (2002) Biomarkers of Caloric Restriction May Predict Longevity in Humans. Science 297: 811

Roth GS, Lesnikov V, Lesnikov M, Ingram DK, Lane M (2001) Dietary caloric restriction prevents age related decline in plasma melatonin levels of rhesus monkeys. J Clin Endo Metab 86: 392–3295

Rudman D, Feller AG Nagraj HS, Gergans GA, Lalitha PY, Goldberg AF, Schlenker RA, Cohn L, Rudman IW, Mattson DE (1990) Effects of human growth hormone in men over 60 years old. New England Journal of Medicine 323: 1–6

Samaras TT, Elrick H (2002) Less is better. Journal of the National Medical Association 94: 88–99

Sanz A, Bartke A, Barja G (2002) Long-lived Ames dwarf mice: oxidative damage to mitochondrial DNA in heart and brain. Journal of the American Aging Association 25: 119–122

Sonntag WE, Cefalu WT, Ingram RL, Bennett SA, Lynch CD, Cooney PT, Thornton PL, Khan AS (1999) Pleiotropic effects of growth hormone and insulin-like growth factor (IGF) on biological aging: Inferences from moderate caloric restricted animals. Journal of Gerontology 54A: B521–B538

Sonntag WE, Lynch C, Thornton P, Khan A, Bennett S, Ingram R (2000) The effects of growth hormone and IGF-I deficiency on cerebrovascular and brain ageing. Journal of Anatomy 4: 575–585

Sornson MW, Wu W, Dasen JS, Flynn SE, Norman DJ, O'Connell SM, Gukovsky I, Carriére C, Ryan AK, Miller AP, Zuo L, Gleiberman AS, Anderson B, Beamer WG, Rosenfeld MG (1996)

Pituitary lineage determination by the prophet of pit-1 homeodomain factor defective in Ames dwarfism. Nature 384: 327–333

Swerdlow AJ, Higgins CD, Adlard P, Preece MA (2002) Risk of cancer in patients treated with human pituitary growth hormone in the UK, 1959–85: a cohort study. Lancet 360: 273–77

Tatar M, Kopelman A, Epstein D, Tu MP, Yin CM, Garofalo RS (2001) A mutant Drosophila insulin receptor homolog that extends life-span and impairs neuroendocrine function. Science 292: 107–110

Tretli S (1989) Height and weight in relation to breast cancer morbidity and mortality. A prospective study of 570,000 women in Norway. Int J Cancer 44: 23–30

van Buul-Offers S, Veda I, van den Brande JL (1986) Biosynthetic somatomedin C (SM-C/IGF-I) increases the length and weight of Snell dwarf mice. Pediatric Research 20: 825–827

von Werder K (1999) The somatopause is no indication for growth hormone therapy. J Endocrinol Invest 22(suppl 5): 137–141

Wanke R, Wolf E, Hermanns W, Folger S, Buchmuller T, Brem G (1992) The GH-transgenic mouse as an experimental model for growth research: clinical and pathological studies. Hormone Research 37: 74–87

Weindruch R, Sohal SS (1997) Caloric intake and aging. New England Journal of Medicine 337: 986–994

Werner H, LeRoith D (1996) The role of the insulin-like growth factor system in human cancer. Advances in Cancer Research 68: 183–223

Yakar S, Liu JL, Fernandez AM, Wu Y, Schally AV, Frystyk J, Chernausek SD, Mejia W, LeRoith D (2001) Liver-specific igf-I gene deletion leads to muscle insulin insensitivity. Diabetes 50: 1110–1118

Zaczek D J, Hammond JM, Suen L, Wandji S, Service D, Bartke A, Chandrashekar V, Coschigano K, Kopchick J (2002) Impact of growth hormone resistance on female reproductive function: New insight from growth hormone receptor knockout mice. Biology of Reproduction 67: 1115–1124

Zhou Y, Xu BC, Maheshwari HG, He L, Reed M, Lozykowski M, Okada S, Wagner TE, Cataldo LA, Coschigano K, Baumann G, Kopchick JJ (1997) A mammalian model for Laron syndrome produced by targeted disruption of the mouse growth hormone receptor/binding protein gene (The Laron mouse). Proc Nat Acad Sci USA 94: 13215–13220

IGF-1 Receptors in Mammalian Longevity: Less is More

Martin Holzenberger

Summary

Recent advances in research into ageing mechanisms have revealed that the cellular receptors InR and DAF-2 control the life span of fruit flies and roundworms, respectively. Comparative studies have identified these structurally and evolutionarily related tyrosine kinase receptors as orthologues of the mammalian insulin receptor (IR) and insulin-like growth factor receptor type 1 (IGF-1R). We investigated whether IGF-1R also regulates life span in mammals, by targeting the gene encoding this receptor in the mouse. Mice with a homozygous null mutation of this gene (IGF-1R$^{-/-}$) were not viable because of severe growth retardation and developmental immaturity at birth. Heterozygous knockout mice (IGF-1R$^{+/-}$) were, however, fully viable, and we studied life span and a number of age-related physiological parameters in this model (Holzenberger et al. 2003). Heterozygous knockout mice presented a 50% decrease in the number of IGF-1 receptors in all tissues but were healthy despite this defect. Life span analysis, comparing IGF-1R$^{+/-}$ mice with their wild-type littermates, showed that this mutation significantly increased longevity, by 26%, when both sexes were analysed together. Evaluated separately, IGF-1R$^{+/-}$ females lived 33% longer than wild-type females, whereas male mutants lived 16% longer than wild-type males. Growth and development were normal in long-lived IGF-1R$^{+/-}$ mice. They displayed no dwarfism, had normal energy metabolism and nutrient uptake, and physical activity identical to that of their wild-type control littermates. Moreover, no change was observed in male and female fertility and reproduction. IGF-1R$^{+/-}$ mutants displayed a high level of resistance in vivo to oxidative stress, a widely accepted key determinant of the ageing process. This finding was reproduced in vitro in experiments with mutant embryonic fibroblasts with hydrogen peroxide treatment used to generate oxidative stress. We tried to unravel the molecular mechanisms involved in life span control via IGF signalling by examining the major intracellular pathways involved. We found that levels of Akt and Erk1/2 MAP kinase activation were clearly diminished in cells derived from long-lived mutants. Moreover, the signal transduction molecule p66 Shc (one of the isoforms of Shc, and also a major substrate of IGF-1R), previously shown to control both the cellular response to oxidative stress and life span in mice, also showed a clear lack of activation in IGF-1R$^{+/-}$ cells. This finding provides the first mechanistic evidence for a link between IGF-1R activation and the regulation of stress resistance. Overall, our results strongly suggest a possible role for the IGF-1 receptor as a major regulator of mammalian longevity. There is also circumstantial evidence of a relationship

Chanson et al.
Endocrine Aspects of Successful Aging
© Springer-Verlag Berlin Heidelberg 2004

between growth and longevity in humans, but further studies are required to formally identify the human genes determining life span. Recent studies in *C. elegans* have shown that life span is regulated in a non cell-autonomous fashion, and that the nervous system may play a central role in these processes. Together, these exciting findings open up new avenues of research, including the possibility of extending life span pharmacologically.

Introduction

In non-vertebrate species, systematic screening has recently identified a number of genes involved in life span regulation. Interestingly, several of these genes encode proteins of the CLK family of proteins or proteins involved in insulin/insulin-like signalling (IIS) pathways (Guarente and Kenyon 2000; Kenyon 2001; Gems and Partridge 2001). The genes encoding IIS pathway proteins include those for DAF-2 from *C. elegans* and its homologue in *Drosophila*, InR. Numerous mutants of these genes have been produced and tested, revealing that the partial inactivation of these genes efficiently increased longevity in the worm (Kenyon et al. 1993; Kimura et al. 1997; Tissenbaum and Ruvkun 1998) and fruit fly (Tatar et al. 2001; Bartke 2001), respectively (Fig. 1). Other molecules from the IIS pathway may also be involved in life span regulation: knocking out the *Drosophila* insulin-receptor substrate CHICO, for example, also prolongs life span (Clancy et al. 2001). Unlike some of the long-lived *daf-2* and *Inr* mutants, which were hypofertile dwarfs, some of the *Inr* mutants showed normal growth and fertility. Thus, under certain circumstances, longevity may be controlled independently of growth regulation and reproduction. Analyses comparing the structures of DAF-2 and InR have shown that these two molecules are closely related to a group of tyrosine kinase receptors in vertebrate species that includes the insulin receptor (IR) and the insulin-like growth factor type 1 receptor (IGF-1R). Both receptors have been extensively studied, revealing that IR is a key regulator of energy metabolism (Kulkarni et al. 1999) and IGF-1R is an important receptor for the stimulation of somatic growth (Lupu et al. 2001). The principal ligand of IGF-1R is IGF-I, a peptide that is produced in the liver and other tissues in response to pituitary growth hormone (GH) secretion. IR and IGF-1R seem to have developed from a common ancestral receptor, but it is unknown whether one of these receptors has taken over the function of life span regulation in vertebrate species (Gems and Partridge 2001 ; Clancy et al. 2001). However, a study of the phenotypes of long-lived spontaneous mouse mutants provided indirect evidence suggesting that growth and longevity are partly co-regulated in this species. These spontaneously long-lived mouse strains, including the Prop1[df/df] mutant mouse (or Ames dwarf) and the Pit1[dw/dw] mutant (Snell dwarf; Flurkey et al. 2001; Brown-Borg et al. 1996), develop functional insufficiency of the anterior pituitary gland resulting in a lack of GH, but they also lack other pituitary hormones. Growth and fertility are strongly impaired in these mutants. The recently described targeted null mutation of the GH receptor gene, which severely reduces serum IGF-I levels and strongly affects somatic growth, also increases life span (Coschigano et al. 2000), further implicating IIS pathways in the control of mammalian life span. Similarly, caloric restriction, the only efficient treatment known today to increase life span in mammals, invariably reduces circulating IGF-I levels and, if begun in juveniles, also engenders dwarfism. These findings suggest that mammalian life span may be regulated by IGF-1R (Carter et al. 2002).

Further investigation of this issue in mammalian systems will necessarily involve the consideration of additional aspects and will certainly raise many new questions. This is partly because the mammalian family of IGF genes is more complex than its insect and worm counterparts. In addition to IGF-1R, mammals possess a second receptor, the IGF type 2 receptor, which, although not directly involved in transmembrane signalling, potently regulates ligand bioactivity. There are also six additional high-affinity IGF binding proteins, ubiquitous in the extracellular space and bloodstream, that add a new level of complexity to IGF regulation. Intracellular signalling cascades also appear to be more complex in

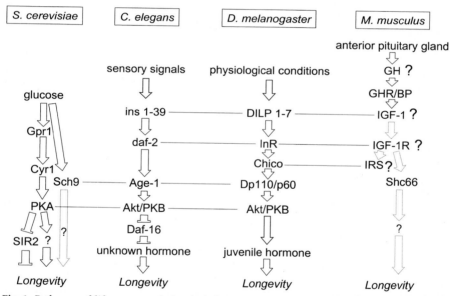

Fig. 1. Pathways of life span regulation in eukaryotes. An evolutionarily conserved signalling pathway, termed IIS for insulin/insulin-like signalling, regulates life span in yeast, worms and flies. There is some evidence that this pathway also regulates ageing in mammalian species. In simpler organisms, this mechanism seems to sense and to integrate environmental conditions essential for energy metabolism and to enable individuals to switch homeostasis between reproductive activity and the capacity to endure harsh environmental conditions. IGF-1R, which has now been shown to regulate lif espan in the mouse, is the mammalian orthologue of Daf-2 and InR. Whereas in *C. elegans* and *D. melanogaster* many genes have been found that potentially encode extracellular ligands of IIS receptors, there seem to be only two ligands, IGF-I and embryonic IGF-II, in mammals. Question marks and dashed arrows indicate molecules and pathways for which involvement in life span control has not yet been firmly established.

higher vertebrates, given the multiplication of signalling molecules (e.g., IRS-1 to -4 in mammals). The relationship between this complexity and longevity is currently unclear.

Constitutive reduction of IGF-1 receptor levels prolongs life span

We investigated the role of the IGF-1R in life span regulation by targeting the essential exon 3 of the gene by homologous recombination, using the Cre-lox system (Holzenberger et al. 2000b, 2001). Nullizygous (IGF-1R$^{-/-}$) newborns, which completely lack the IGF-1 receptor, invariably died at birth, as previously described by Efstratiadis and co-workers (Liu et al. 1993) in a study involving classical insertional mutagenesis. In the search for an appropriate model of receptor inactivation, we first tested an IGF-1R knockdown mutation (Holzenberger et al. 2000a) that decreases the number of receptors to 80% or to 60% of that in the wild type, but we concluded that this model was not optimal for the projected ageing study. We then tried compound heterozygous receptor inactivation, which left cells with only about 30% of wild-type receptor levels, but we found that the development of fat tissue, in particular, was negatively affected in animals with such small numbers of receptors (Holzenberger et al. 2000a). We therefore decided to use the heterozygous null mutant IGF-1R$^{+/-}$, which should give 50% receptor inactivation, for a life span study (Holzenberger et al. 2003). As transcripts from the IGF-1R^{-} allele do not encode a functional protein, the IGF-1 receptor levels in IGF-1R$^{+/-}$ mice were indeed found to be only 50% those in the wild-type, IGF-1R$^{+/+}$ mice. The number of receptors was halved in all tissues, as shown by ligand binding assay and IGF-1 receptor autoradiography. Body weight increased normally during the first three weeks of life, until the time of natural weaning. Thereafter, IGF-1R$^{+/-}$ males developed a slight growth deficit, showing 8% less growth than their IGF-1R$^{+/+}$ littermates. A similar growth deficit, of 6%, was observed in IGF-1R$^{+/-}$ females. These modest decreases in body weight affected all tissues to similar degrees, persisted in the adult, and resembled the growth pattern described previously in a similar model of partial IGF-1R knockout (Holzenberger et al. 2001).

Mice had free access to a regular rodent diet and were maintained under standard conditions until their death from natural causes. At the end of the experiment, IGF-1R$^{+/-}$ mice had lived significantly longer (+26%) than their wild-type littermates. Interestingly, mutant females lived 33% longer than wild-type females, whereas the gain in mutant males was only 16%. This finding suggests that, in IGF-1R$^{+/-}$ mutants, the increase in life span depended on sex, as has been described for *Drosophila* mutants with impaired IIS-signalling (Tatar et al. 2001; Clancy et al. 2001). Tumours were rare in our ageing mice [5%, a typical tumour incidence for mice from a 129 background (Stevens and Little 1954)] and unrelated to genotype. Necropsy revealed a number of different diseases at death, consistent with the results of previous studies showing that mice with this background do not develop specific age-related diseases (Smith et al. 1973).

Routine blood biochemistry tests were normal. However, as expected, the concentration of circulating IGF-I was one third higher in adult IGF-1R$^{+/-}$ mice than in wild-type mice, probably due to weaker feedback control of IGF-I production. As the IGF receptor has a tissue-specific role in the regulation of glucose homeostasis (Kulkarni et al. 1999), we performed intraperitoneal glucose tolerance tests in fasted animals. We found that IGF-1R$^{+/-}$ males specifically lacked tight blood glucose control, whereas females did not. This finding again represents a clear sex-dimorphic response to the decrease in IGF-1R levels and requires further clarification. The ß-cell mass in IGF-1R$^{+/-}$ mice is known to be reduced (Withers et al. 1999) but it is unclear whether this is directly related to the hyperglycaemic effect in males.

Energy metabolism may have a major influence on the ageing process. We therefore studied several aspects of energy expenditure in mutant IGF-1R$^{+/-}$ mice. Body surface and core temperature, which have been reported to be low in long-lived Ames dwarfs (Hunter et al. 1999), appeared to be normal in IGF-1R$^{+/-}$ mice. Circadian profiles of physical activity were also identical for IGF-1R$^{+/-}$ and IGF-1R$^{+/+}$ mice. Furthermore, as decreasing food intake efficiently increases mammalian life span, we explored the possibility that our mutant mice had restricted their own nutrient consumption, but we found very similar mean food and water intakes in males and females from both genotypes. We then measured metabolic rates (MR) to exclude the possibility that mutant mice displayed a different efficiency of food use. Mean 24-hour MR in the fed state, resting MR and basal MR, measured in fasted animals, did not differ between IGF-1R$^{+/-}$ mice and their controls. Thus, differences in metabolism could not account for the observed longevity.

Many ageing studies carried out in recent decades have provided evidence for the existence of a trade-off between longevity and reproduction in a number of species. Long-lived *daf-2* mutant worms and long-lived dwarf mice, in particular, display reduced fertility. This finding led us to explore fertility and the reproductive phenotype of IGF-1R mutant mice. The onset of male and female fertility was unaffected in these mutants, providing evidence that the lower levels of IGF-1R did not postpone sexual maturation, as has been observed in GH receptor-knockout mice (Coschigano et al. 2000). The number of pups per litter was also identical in young IGF-1R$^{+/-}$ and control females. We also explored the decline of fertility in females from 5 to 13 months of age, comparing IGF-1R$^{+/-}$ with control females. The frequency of pregnancies after three-week mating periods was similar in mutant and wild-type females and declined as a function of age. The number of live newborns per litter also strongly decreased with age in both groups, but with no obvious difference between genotypes. Mating behaviour, which was assessed based on the frequency of copulation plugs following mating with fertile male partners, was also highly similar in IGF-1R$^{+/-}$ and control females. Oestrus cycle length, as determined from vaginal smear cytology, increased significantly with age, indicating normal age-related changes in the hormonal regulation of ovarian function, with no difference between genotypes. Finally, the interval from one copulation plug to the next, following mating with a sterile male, indicative of the capacity of the ovaries to maintain pseudogestation, decreased significantly with age in both groups. In summary, female fertility, as expected, decreased drastically with age, but IGF-1R$^{+/-}$ females and their controls were indistinguishable for all characteristics tested.

Mutations in genes encoding proteins functioning downstream from IGF-1R (see Fig. 1) increase longevity. The proteins concerned include the *Drosophila* IRS homologue CHICO (Clancy et al. 2001), the mouse isoform p66 of Shc (Migliaccio et al. 1999 and the *C. elegans* PI(3)K (known as AGE-1; Guarente and Kenyon 2000), together with the Forkhead transcription factor daf-16. We therefore investigated the way in which diminished IGF-1R levels in this model affected subsequent intracellular signalling events (Fig. 2). We analysed IGF-dependent signalling in embryonic fibroblasts from WT, IGF-1R$^{+/-}$ and IGF-1R$^{-/-}$ mice (Holzenberger et al. 2000a, 2001) by Western blotting. As expected, cells with the IGF-1R$^{+/-}$ genotype had 50% fewer receptors than did wild-type cells. Combined immunoprecipitation and Western blotting also revealed much lower levels of IGF-I-induced phosphorylation of the receptor and of its substrate, IRS-1. The level of phosphorylation of the Shc isoforms p52 and p66, both of which are major substrates of IGF-1R, was also halved. The lack of p66 Shc activation in IGF-1R$^{+/-}$ cells may be one mechanism by which IGF-I regulates oxidative stress resistance. For signalling through the IIS pathway, it is essential for the Grb2 molecule to associate with Shc and IRS-1 in response to phosphorylation. This association may induce a mitogenic response in cells, via activation of the MAP kinase pathway. We found that the amount of Grb2 co-immunoprecipitated with Shc or with IRS-1 in IGF-1R$^{+/-}$ cells was indeed about 50% that in the wild type. Moreover, the level of IGF-I-induced phosphorylation of the downstream kinases ERK1/2 and Akt was decreased by 50 to 60% in mutant cells. In summary, these findings suggested that mutations causing IGF-1R heteroinsufficiency halved the signalling capacities of the major pathways normally activated by IGF-I.

Lack of IGF-1R increases resistance to oxidative stress in vivo and in vitro

Cellular ageing involves an accumulation of oxidative damage. In numerous ageing models, it has been shown that reactive oxygen species (ROS) degrade proteins and DNA, and it is generally accepted that ageing is at least in part caused by the consequences of oxidative stress (Finkel and Holbrook 2000). Consequently, transgenic mice and flies with increased resistance to oxidative stress may have extended life spans (Migliaccio et al. 1999; Sun and Tower 1999). To test whether long-lived IGF-1R$^{+/-}$ mice also displayed enhanced resistance to acute oxidative stress, adult mutant mice and their controls received a single intraperitoneal injection of methyl viologen (paraquat), a chemical that induces the intracellular production of ROS in large quantities. Survival time after the paraquat bolus was measured, and subsequent Kaplan-Meier analysis revealed that IGF-1R$^{+/-}$ mutants resisted this intense oxidative stress significantly longer than did the controls. When the sexes were evaluated separately, the female IGF-1R$^{+/-}$ mice displayed

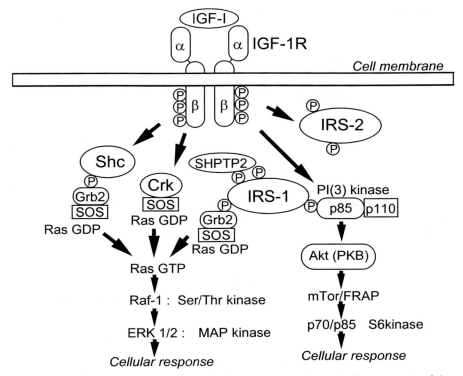

Fig. 2. Intracellular signalling from the IGF-1R follows two principal pathways, one involving the MAP kinases ERK 1 and ERK 2, and the other involving Akt (for review see Butler et al. 1998). Western blot analysis showed that decreasing IGF-1R levels on the cell membrane by 50% decreases the inducibility of both pathways to about 50% of normal values. This decrease concerned receptor phosphorylation, Shc and IRS-1 and IRS-2 phosphorylation, the association of Shc and IRS with Grb2, and the activation of ERK 1/2 and Akt. The intracellular levels of these signalling molecules were, however, found to be unaffected (Holzenberger et al. 2003). We observed higher levels of resistance to oxidative stress in heterozygous (IGF-1R[+/-]) and homozygous (IGF-1R[-/-]) cells in vitro, probably due to changes in the phosphorylation of Shc (Migliaccio et al. 1999). Interestingly, IGF-1R[-/-] cells proliferated at a much lower rate in culture than did heterozygous and wild-type cells.

much greater increases in stress resistance than did males. This situation resembled the sex-dimorphism of the Kaplan-Meier curves previously observed in survival analysis (Holzenberger et al. 2003). We determined whether this effect was cell autonomous by experiments with mouse embryo fibroblasts (MEF) from female embryos. These cultured cells were subjected to oxidative stress by adding 100 µM hydrogen peroxide to the culture medium. As expected, the percentage of cells surviving after 24 and 72 hours of this treatment was considerably higher in IGF-1R[+/-] MEF than in wild-type MEF.

Discussion

The findings presented here show that the ubiquitous down-regulation of IGF-1 receptor expression can increase mean life span in the mouse. Thus, the connection between IIS signalling and life span, which was first reported in studies using non-vertebrate models (Kenyon et al. 1993; Kimura et al. 1997; Tissenbaum and Ruvkun 1998; Tatar et al. 2001) is also likely to exist in vertebrates (Fig. 3). Surprisingly, IGF-1R[+/-] mutants did not develop dwarfism or hypofertility,and are thus phenotypically very different from long-lived mouse mutants with hypopituitarism (Flurkey et al. 2001; Brown-Borg et al. 1996; Bartke et al. 2001) or mutants totally lacking GHR/BP (Coschigano et al. 2000). IGF-1R[+/-] mutant mice also displayed normal nutrient consumption, and had normal motor activity and energy expenditure, traits that together excluded metabolic changes as an explanation for their increased life span. Calorie restriction, on the other hand, may exert its life-prolonging effects partly via large decreases in serum IGF-I levels, imitating features produced in this study by directly targeting the receptor gene.

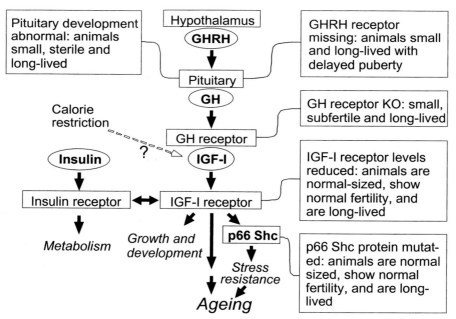

Fig. 3. Mammalian longevity may be regulated via a hormonal axis similar to the hypothalamic-pituitary pathways that control somatic growth, as shown here. Phenotypes of mutant mice are summarised in large boxes. Calorie restriction may modify signalling through this axis by lowering circulating IGF-I levels. A horizontal arrow indicates cross-talk between insulin and IGF receptors in mammals and its importance for life span control. (Modified from Lithgow and Gill, 2003 and Holzenberger et al. 2003)

The recently reported knockout mutation of the Shc isoform p66 (p66 Shc[-/-]) increases life span without marked secondary effects (Migliaccio et al. 1999). Shc is, together with the IRS signalling molecules, one of the principal intracellular signal transducers downstream from the IGF-1R. The p66 isoform of Shc has a special task in this pathway: to initiate the cellular responses that act as specific reactions to acute oxidative stress. The observation of an increase in stress resistance in mutants is therefore of considerable interest. The demonstration that p66 Shc showed a lack of phosphorylation under conditions of IGF-1R deficiency, revealed a potential mechanism connecting the IGF pathway to oxidative stress regulation. Studies with *Drosophila* CHICO[1] mutants (Clancy et al. 2001) have indicated that these mechanisms function independently to produce longevity. Nevertheless, the interactions between calorie restriction, IGF and oxidative stress involved in the extension of life span are not yet well understood (Bartke et al. 2001; Clancy et al. 2002; Honda and Honda 2002), and more detailed studies in vertebrate models are required.

The results presented here also inevitably raise the question as to whether the observed effects are specific to mice or whether they also apply to other mammals, humans in particular. There is currently at least circumstantial evidence for a similar relationship between the physiology of growth and longevity in humans. This evidence comes from retrospective studies directly investigating human lifespan and growth (Holzenberger et al. 1991; Samaras and Storms 1992). In one of these studies, the authors found an inverse relationship between body height and life span among men from the general population. However, the authors also included a set of data obtained from previous studies for a large group of American baseball players. Analysis of the data from these selected individuals clearly showed a very similar negative relationship between mean body height and life span, resulting in a highly significant correlation. Moreover, we reported several years ago a very similar, negative regression between the height of the Spanish male population and their life span (Holzenberger et al. 1991; Fig. 4). One merit of such studies is that they help provide the basis of a hypothesis. The principal problem with such studies is that any potential inverse relationship between body size and longevity is likely to be masked by superimposed changes in the opposite direction prevailing in modern society: the steady increase in life expectancy due to better hygiene and disease prevention, and the steady increase in the mean height of the general population, referred to as a *secular growth trend*, in developed countries. This secular growth trend is thought to be a direct consequence of socio-economic advances and improvements in the quality and quantity of food. Another very interesting study reports human genetic syndromes affecting the anterior pituitary gland in a group of people living on the Adriatic island of Krk (Krzisnik et al. 1999). These men and women suffer from a pituitary defect similar to that observed in long-lived Prop1[df/df] and Pit1[dw/dw] mutant mice (Flurkey et al. 2001; Brown-Borg et al. 1996). Despite the lack of hormones other than GH, the life span of this group of men and women was surprisingly high with respect to their reference population.

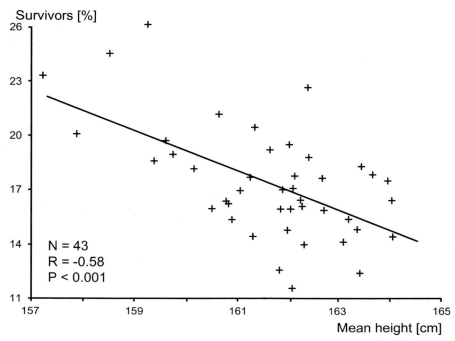

Fig. 4. Studies in humans have provided circumstantial evidence for a relationship between human growth and life span. The data shown here are extracted from our study of the Spanish male population (Holzenberger et al. 1991). Analysis of these data revealed linear regression between male body height and longevity index. Body height was taken from military statistics for young conscripts from the years 1858-1861 (birth cohorts 1840-1843) and corresponding survival data from general population censuses 50 years later. Data points indicate the means obtained for each of the evaluated 43 Spanish provinces. Their distribution shows a significant negative correlation between mean body height and the proportion of long-lived male individuals in the study cohorts

The identification of IGF-1R as a potential regulator of human life span makes this molecule a potentially interesting therapeutic target for slowing the ageing process. Given the nature of the relationship between IGF-1R and life span, it would be interesting to inhibit the receptor or IGF signalling specifically, in a dose-dependent fashion. With the recent crystallisation of the ligand-binding domain of the receptor and molecular dissection of the interaction of this domain with its ligand (De Meyts and Whittaker 2002), it is only a question of time before designed drugs become available for anti-ageing testing in laboratory animals. However, the question of how to administer this treatment, remains unresolved. It already seems clear that systemic treatment with substances inhibiting IGF function may not be necessary and that a topical application could be sufficient. This is because life span may be regulated in a tissue-specific manner. It was recently shown that the control of longevity through insulin-like signals in non-vertebrates may occur in a non-cell autonomous fashion and that this function may be associated with a particular organ or cellular compartment (Apfeld and Kenyon 1998; Wolkow et al. 2000). Results from worms and flies are consistent with the existence of such a central control of life span and with this control having a neuroendocrine basis (Wolkow 2002). It has been suggested that neurons in the CNS may sense the concentration of ligands in the bloodstream and regulate the rate of ageing in other tissues accordingly, by means of unknown endocrine mechanisms. As growth in mammals also has a strong central component (see Fig. 5), this neuroendocrine control of ageing may apply to mammalian life span regulation, too. Yet, things may be more complicated than that, since other tissues do control longevity as well. Endocrine signals with life span-promoting capacity may come from the gonads (Hsin and Kenyon 1999). Moreover, very recent work, performed in genetically modified mice, suggests that the inactivation of the insulin receptor, specifically in adipose tissue, also provides with additional longevity (Blüher et al. 2003).

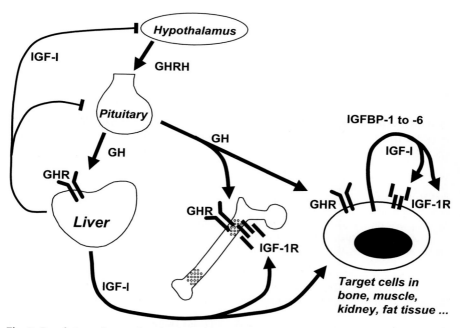

Fig. 5. Regulation of somatic growth by growth hormone (GH). Classical understanding of endocrine growth control centres on the hypothalamic-pituitary axis responsible for GH secretion. Circulating GH stimulates IGF-I production in the liver and in many other tissues. Circulating IGF-I, in turn, promotes the growth of target tissues and exerts negative feedback control on hypothalamic releasing hormones and pituitary GH secretion. Autocrine and paracrine effects on cell proliferation contribute substantially to tissue growth, as deduced from tissue-specific inactivation of the IGF-I gene (Liu et al. 1998; Yakar et al. 1999). The complexity of IGF bioactivity control is increased by the presence of IGF-binding proteins (IGFBP-1 to -6) in almost all tissues. The principle action of these proteins is the inhibition of IGF signalling via its receptor, IGF-1R. The potential involvement of IGFBPs in the regulation of ageing has yet to be explored.

Finally, the IGF system in mammals is quite complex, comprising multiple levels that control IGF bioactivity. The tissue-specific regulation of IGF function involves interplay between receptor availability, IGF binding protein activity — which may up- or down-regulate IGF signalling — and, particularly in the brain, active transport of IGF to target regions distant from the producing cells. Thus, mammalian longevity is probably controlled by IGF signals that exert their effects via complex neuroendocrine pathways, which may be organised in a hierarchical fashion, similar to that in other integrated endocrine systems. Although transposition of the findings reported here from lower organisms to mammals settled some issues, it immediately raises many new and exciting questions that will require a considerable research effort before the potential application of these results to humans can be addressed.

Materials and Methods

For materials, methods and mutant strains used, please refer to the following publications: Holzenberger et al. 1991, 2000a, 2000b, 2001, 2003; Dupont et al. 2000; Kulkarni et al. 2002; Leneuve et al. 2001.

Acknowledgements

I would like to thank J. Dupont, B. Ducos, P. Leneuve, P. Cervera, P.C. Even and Y. Le Bouc for their contributions, J. Sappa for language revision, and MENRT and ATC ageing 2002 for financial support.

References

Apfeld J, Kenyon C (1998) Cell nonautonomy of *C. elegans* daf-2 function in the regulation of diapause and lifespan. Cell 95: 199–210

Bartke A (2001) Mutations prolong life in flies; implications for aging in mammals. Trends Endocrinol Metab 12: 233–234

Bartke A, Wright JC, Mattison JA, Ingram DK, Miller RA, Roth GS (2001) Extending the lifespan of long-lived mice. Nature 414: 412

Blüher M, Kahn B, Kahn CR (2003) Extended longevity in mice lacking the insulin receptor in adipose tissue. Science 299: 572–574

Brown-Borg HM, Borg KE, Meliska CJ, Bartke A (1996) Dwarf mice and the ageing process. Nature 384: 33

Butler AA, Yakar S, Gewolb IH, Karas M, Okubo Y, LeRoith D (1998) Insulin-like growth factor-I receptor signal transduction: at the interface between physiology and cell biology. Comp Biochem Physiol B Biochem Mol Biol 121: 19–26

Carter CS, Ramsey MM, Sonntag WE (2002) A critical analysis of the role of growth hormone and IGF-1 in aging and lifespan. TIGS 18: 295–301

Clancy DJ, Gems D, Harshman LG, Oldham S, Stocker H, Hafen E, Leevers SJ, Partridge L (2001) Extension of life-span by loss of CHICO, a *Drosophila* insulin receptor substrate protein. Science 292: 104–106

Clancy DJ, Gems D, Hafen E, Leevers SJ, Partridge L (2002) Dietary restriction in long-lived dwarf flies. Science 296: 319

Coschigano KT, Clemmons D, Bellushi LL, Kopchick JJ (2000) Assessment of growth parameters and life span of GHR/BP gene-disrupted mice. Endocrinology 141: 2608–2613

De Meyts, Whittaker J (2002) Structural biology of insulin and IGF1 receptors: implications for drug design. Nat Rev Drug Discov 1: 769–783

Dupont J, Karas M, LeRoith D (2000) The potentiation of estrogen on insulin-like growth factor I action in MCF-7 human breast cancer cells includes cell cycle components. J Biol Chem 275: 35893–35901

Finkel T, Holbrook NJ (2000) Oxidants, oxidative stress and the biology of ageing. Nature 408: 239–247

Flurkey K, Papaconstantinou J, Miller RA, Harrison DE (2001) Lifespan extension and delayed immune and collagen aging in mutant mice with defects in growth hormone production. Proc Natl Acad Sci USA 98: 6736–6741

Gems D, Partridge L (2001) Insulin/IGF signalling and ageing: seeing the bigger picture. Curr Opin Genet Dev 11: 287–292

Guarente L, Kenyon C (2000) Genetic pathways that regulate ageing in model organisms. Nature 408: 255–262

Holzenberger M, Martín-Crespo RM, Vicent D, Ruiz-Torres A (1991) Decelerated growth and longevity in men. Arch Gerontol Geriat 13: 89–101

Holzenberger M, Leneuve P, Hamard G, Ducos B, Périn L, Binoux M, Le Bouc Y (2000a) A targeted partial invalidation of the insulin-like growth factor I receptor gene in mice causes a postnatal growth deficit. Endocrinology 141: 2557–2566

Holzenberger M, Lenzner C, Leneuve P, Zaoui R, Hamard G, Vaulont S, Le Bouc Y (2000b) Cre-mediated germ-line mosaicism: a method allowing rapid generation of several alleles of a target gene. Nucleic Acids Res 28: e92

Holzenberger M, Hamard G, Zaoui R, Leneuve P, Ducos B, Beccavin C, Périn L, Le Bouc Y (2001) Experimental IGF-I receptor deficiency generates a sexually dimorphic pattern of organ-specific growth deficits in mice, affecting fat tissue in particular. Endocrinology 142: 4469–4478

Holzenberger M, Dupont J, Ducos B, Leneuve P, Géloën A, Even PC, Cervera P, Le Bouc Y (2003) IGF-1 receptor regulates lifespan and resistance to oxidative stress in mice. Nature 421: 182–187

Honda Y, Honda S (2002) Oxidative stress and life span determination in the nematode *Caenorhabditis elegans*. Ann NY Acad Sci 959: 466–474

Hsin H, Kenyon C (1999) Signals from the reproductive system regulate the lifespan of *C. elegans*. Nature 399: 362–366

Hunter WS, Croson WB, Bartke A, Gentry MV, Meliska CJ (1999) Low body temperature in long-lived Ames dwarf mice at rest and during stress. Physiol Behav 67: 433–437

Kenyon C (2001) A conserved regulatory system for aging. Cell 105: 165–168

Kenyon C, Chang J, Gensch E, Rudner A, Tabtiang R (1993) A *C. elegans* mutant that lives twice as long as wild type. Nature 366: 461–464

Kimura KD, Tissenbaum HA, Liu Y, Ruvkun G (1997) Daf-2, an insulin receptor-like gene that regulates longevity and diapause in *Caenorhabditis elegans*. Science 277: 942–946

Krzisnik C, Kolacio Z, Battelino T, Brown M, Parks JS and Laron Z (1999) The "Little People" of the island of Krk – revisited. Etiology of hypopituitarism revealed. J Endocrine Genet 1: 9–19,

Kulkarni RN, Brüning JC, Winnay JN, Postic C, Magnuson MA, Kahn CR (1999) Tissue-specific knockout of the insulin receptor in pancreatic beta cells creates an insulin secretory defect similar to that in type 2 diabetes. Cell 96: 329–339

Kulkarni RN, Holzenberger M, Shih DQ, Ozcan U, Stoffel M, Magnuson MA, Kahn CR (2002) β-cell specific deletion of the IGF-1 receptor leads to hyperinsulinemia and glucose intolerance but does not alter β-cell mass. Nat Genet 31: 111–115

Leneuve P, Zaoui R, Monget P, Le Bouc Y, Holzenberger M (2001) Genotyping of *Cre-lox* mice and detection of tissue-specific recombination by multiplex PCR. Biotechniques 31: 1156–1162

Liu JL, Grinberg A, Westphal H, Sauer B, Accili D, Karas M, LeRoith D (1998) Insulin-like growth factor-I affects perinatal lethality and postnatal development in a gene dosage-dependent manner: manipulation using the Cre/loxP system in transgenic mice. Mol Endocrinol 12: 1452–1462

Liu JP, Baker J, Perkins AS, Robertson EJ, Efstratiadis A (1993) Mice carrying null mutations of the genes encoding insulin-like growth factor I (Igf-1) and type 1 IGF receptor (Igf1r). Cell 75: 59–72

Lupu L, Terwilliger JD, Lee K, Segre GV, Efstratiadis A (2001) Roles of growth hormone and insulin-like growth factor 1 in mouse postnatal growth. Dev Biol 229: 141–162

Migliaccio E, Giorgio M, Mele S, Pelicci G, Reboldi P, Pandolfi PP, Lanfrancone L, Pelicci PG (1999) The p66[shc] adaptor protein controls oxidative stress response and life span in mammals. Nature 402: 309–313

Samaras TT, Storms LH (1992) Impact of height and weight on life span. Bull World Health Org 70: 259–267

Smith GS, Walford RL, Mickey MR (1973) Lifespan and incidence of cancer and other diseases in selected long-lived inbred mice and their F1 hybrids. J Natl Cancer Inst 50: 1195–1213

Stevens LC, Little CC (1954) Spontaneous testicular teratomas in an inbred strain of mice. Proc Natl Acad Sci USA 40: 1080–1087

Sun J, Tower J (1999) FLP recombinase-mediated induction of Cu/Zn-superoxide dismutase transgene expression can extend the life span of adult *Drosophila melanogaster* flies. Mol Cell Biol 19: 216–228

Tatar M, Kopelman A, Epstein D, Tu MP, Yin CM, Garofalo RS (2001) A mutant *Drosophila* insulin receptor homolog that extends life-span and impairs neuroendocrine function. Science 292: 107–110

Tissenbaum HA, Ruvkun G (1998) An insulin-like signaling pathway affects both longevity and reproduction in *Caenorhabditis elegans*. Genetics 148: 703–717

Withers DJ, Burks DJ, Towery HH, Altamuro SL, Flint CL, White MF (1999) Irs-2 coordinates IGF-1 receptor-mediated ß-cell development and peripheral insulin signalling. Nat Genet 23: 32–39

Wolkow CA (2002) Life span: getting the signal from the nervous system. Trends Neurosci 25: 212–216

Wolkow CA, Kimura KD, Lee MS, Ruvkun G (2000) Regulation of *C. elegans* life-span by insulin-like signaling in the nervous system. Science 290: 147–150

Yakar S, Liu JL, Stannard B, Butler A, Accili D, Sauer B, LeRoith D (1999) Normal growth and development in the absence of hepatic insulin-like growth factor I. Proc Natl Acad Sci USA 96: 7327–7329

IGF-1 Gene Polymorphisms and Disease in the Elderly

J.A.M.J.L. Janssen and *S.W.J. Lamberts*

Summary

Age is a major determinant of circulating total IGF-I levels. After a peak in puberty, mean circulating IGF-I levels decrease 2.5-fold by the third decade, while a further two-fold decrease occurs between the third and eighth decades. Besides growth hormone (GH), age, nutrition and a number of other factors, individual circulating IGF-I concentrations are also influenced by a number of genetic factors. Twin studies have shown that at least 38% of the interindividual variability in circulating IGF-I levels is genetically determined. The IGF-I gene contains a microsatellite polymorphism approximately 1 kb upstream from the IGF-I gene transcription site. This IGF-I gene polymorphism may directly influence the IGF-I production.

This IGF-I gene polymorphism has the potential to influence the expression of IGF-I and could therefore serve as a better indicator for chronic IGF-I exposure in the body, both locally and systemically, than the actual circulating IGF-I concentrations. This IGF-I gene polymorphism makes it possible to characterize, on a genetic basis, subjects who are chronically (i.e.,life-long) exposed to low IGF-I levels throughout the body.

In the Rotterdam Study, a population-based study in a Caucasian population aged 55 years and over, 10 different alleles of a genetic polymorphism were observed in the regulatory region of the IGF-I gene. Genotype and allele frequencies were in Hardy-Weinberg equilibrium. When considering genotypes, 88% of the studied subjects from this population-based sample were homozygous or heterozygous for a 192-bp allele, suggesting that this is the wild-type allele from which all other alleles originated. The frequency of the other alleles was low and therefore it was decided to pool these other alleles in the further analyses. This pooling resulted in three possible genotypes: 1) carriers homozygous for the 192-bp allele (46.7%), 2) carriers heterozygous for the 192-bp allele (41.7%), and 3) non-carriers for the 192-bp allele (11.6 %).

Mean circulating total IGF-I levels increased with the number of 192-bp alleles carried. In non-carriers of the 192-bp allele, the mean circulating total IGF-I level was 18% lower (16.7 nmol/L) than in those homozygous for the allele (20.5 nmol/L, P=0.003). In addition, body height significantly increased with the number of 192-bp alleles present.

In those homozygous and heterozygous for the 192-bp allele, fewer subjects with type 2 diabetes or myocardial infarction were observed than in non-carriers. Although the IGF-I genotype was not associated with known cardiovascular

Chanson et al.
Endocrine Aspects of Successful Aging
© Springer-Verlag Berlin Heidelberg 2004

risk factors, such as age, male gender, smoking, body mass index, WHR, total cholesterol, HDL-cholesterol and hypertension, both the risk of type 2 diabetes and myocardial infarction were significantly increased in non-carriers of the 192-bp allele when compared with carriers of this polymorphism. This finding suggests that the genetically determined exposure to relatively low IGF-I plays a role in the pathogenesis of both type 2 diabetes and myocardial infarction.

An age-related decline in circulating total IGF-I levels was only observed in those homozygous for the 192-bp allele, but such decline was not found in heterozygotes and non-carriers of the 192-bp allele. We hypothesize that this IGF-I gene polymorphism directly or indirectly influences GH-mediated regulation of IGF-I secretion with aging.

In conclusion, circulating IGF-I levels are determined to a considerable extent by genetic factors. Genetically determined chronic exposure to low IGF-I levels is associated with an increased risk for type 2 diabetes mellitus and myocardial infarction.

Introduction

Insulin-like growth factor-I (IGF-I) has both anabolic and mitogenic effects in vivo and vitro that often overlap with the biological effects of insulin (Jones and Clemmons 1995; Froesch et al., 1985). In vitro, glucose uptake and amino acid uptake are increased by IGF-I (Kiess et al. 1993). IGF-I infusions in healthy volunteers increase glucose uptake, reduce free fatty acid and triglyceride levels, and decrease protein breakdown (Kiess et al., 1993). In calorically restricted patients, administration of IGF-I improves nitrogen balance (Clemmons et al. 1992). IGF-I stimulates cell differentiation and is a mitogen for most cells, stimulating [3H] thymidinine incorporation into DNA and [3H] uridine incorporation into RNA (Kiess et al. 1993). IGF-I thus influences many cell functions and is considered to be a growth factor with important anabolic and metabolic regulatory functions. Another action of IGF-I that is complementary to its stimulatory effect on cell proliferation is its capacity to inhibit programmed cell death in certain cells, known as apoptosis (Hadsell and Abdel-Fattah 2001).

The circulating plasma IGF-I concentration (nmol/L) is about a factor 50-100 higher than circulating free insulin (Froesch and Zapf 1985). However, in contrast to insulin, only 0.5-1.0% of circulating IGF-I is present in the free form in the healthy state, whereas the majority of plasma circulating IGF-I (99%) is bound by the insulin-like growth factor-binding proteins (the so-called IGFBPs). Six IGFBPs have been described to date (Jones and Clemmons 1995). IGFBPs have been proposed to have four major functions that are essential to coordinate and regulate the bioactivity of IGF-I: 1) to act as transport proteins in the plasma and to control the efflux of IGF-I from the circulation to the extravascular space, 2) to prolong the half-life of IGF-I and thereby regulate its metabolic clearance, 3) to provide a means of tissue- and cell-specific delivery of IGF-I, and 4) to directly modulate (stimulating or inhibiting) interaction between IGF-I and the IGF-I receptor, thereby indirectly controlling its biological actions (Jones and Clemmons 1995).

IGF-1, glucose tolerance, type 2 diabetes and aging.

Aging is associated with a decline in function in many, if not all, human systems. Age is a major determinant of plasma IGF-I concentrations (Clemmons 1992). After puberty, a 2.5- fold decline occurs in the mean IGF-I values by the third decade, and a further two-fold decrease occurs between the third and eighth decade (Clemmons 1992). In the Baltimore Longitudinal Study on Aging, a marked inter-individual variation in circulating IGF-I levels was observed at every age (Hochberg et al. 1994). The circulating levels for IGF-I in some elderly (over 70 years of age) men or women are comparable or even higher than in some young (up to 40 years of age) men and women (Ruiz-Torres et al. 2002). There is substantial evidence that increasing age is also associated with a decreased glucose tolerance (DeFronzo 1981; Reaven et al. 1989). In the above-mentioned Baltimore Longitudinal Study on aging, oral glucose tolerance tests performed in healthy, non-diabetic individuals across the age range showed a progressive decline in glucose tolerance from the third decade to the ninth decade (Elahi andMuller, 2000). Paolisso et al. (1999) suggested that the decline in glucose tolerance with increasing age is related to the changes in circulating IGF-I levels. They observed that low plasma IGF-1 concentrations predicted a decline in whole blood glucose disposal (WBGD) in an elderly population during the 12 months follow-up, independent of body fat, free fatty acids, waist/hip ratio, and basal adjusted respiratory quotient (Paolisso et al. 1999). They concluded, therefore, that plasma IGF-I concentration may have a modulatory role on insulin action in older people (Paolisso et al. 1999).The Ely study, a 4.5-year follow-up study among 615 participants aged 45-65 years, showed that higher circulating total IGF-I levels were associated with a reduced risk of development of impaired glucose tolerance and type 2 diabetes in individuals with normal glucose tolerance at baseline (Sandhu et al. 2002).

IGF-I levels in diabetes type 2 patients are significantly lower in every age range than those in age-matched normal subjects (Tan and Baxter 1986). This extra reduction occurs independently of age-related changes in IGF-I (Tan and Baxter 1986). In addition, type 2 diabetes circulating levels of IGF-I decrease with diabetes duration and with increased blood glucose (Clauson et al. 1998). Treatment of type II diabetic patients with recombinant human IGF-I increases insulin sensitivity and improves glycemic control (Moses et al. 1996). Although insulin might control glucose concentrations overall, it has been also suggested that IGF-I might fine-tune insulin sensitivity (Holt 2002).

All these data show that circulating IGF-I could be important in glucose homeostasis and provide further evidence for a protective role of IGF-I against the development of glucose tolerance and type 2 diabetes mellitus.

Are reduced insulin and IGF-1 levels also involved in human longevity?

Several recent studies have demonstrated evidence for the involvement of insulin and IGF-I signaling in the control of aging and longevity in worms, mice and calorically restricted rodents (Bartke 2001). It has been suggested that deficiency of GH and the resulting suppression of circulating IGF-I levels play a key role in delayed aging and prolonged longevity because life extension has been reported in animals with GH resistance and/or IGF-I deficiency (Coschigano et al. 2000). Aging might be controlled by similar mechanisms in organisms ranging from unicellular yeast to mammals and even humans (Bartke 2001).

Common phenotypic characteristics of long-lived mutant mice, GHR-knockout mice and calorically restricted rodents are reduced levels of IGF-I, insulin and glucose. But how does this explain why diabetes mellitus in humans, which is characterized by increased glucose and reduced insulin signaling and IGF-I levels. tends to shorten life expectancy ? As Mobbs et al. and others have pointed out, there are extensive data that suggest that the cumulative exposure to glucose may drive key aspects of the aging process (Mobbs et al. 2001; Cerami 1985; Cerami et al. 1985; Masoro et al. 1989). In addition, the above-discussed studies in worms, mice and calorically restricted rodents have not resolved the critical question regarding whether it is the neuroendocrine response to caloric restriction that leads to increased life span or whether caloric restriction acts by protecting nutrition-sensitive neuroendocrine cells from metabolism-induced damage. Mobbs et al. (2001) suggested that glucose economy is fundamentally regulated by, and in turn regulates, neuroendocrine function. The above-discussed decline in glucose tolerance with aging suggests that, in humans, cumulative nutritional stimulation (especially by glucose) drives age-related impairments of essential neuroendocrine functions (such as GH, insulin and IGF-I) over the life span.

Low IGF-1 and cardiovascular disease

Because IGF-I is important for tissue repair and cell proliferation, it has been suggested that IGF-I may be involved in the pathogenesis of atherosclerosis (Ferns et al. 1991). Adults with hypopituitarism have a reduced life expectancy and a two-fold increased mortality from cardiovascular disease (CVD) compared to healthy controls (Rosen and Bengtsson 1990). This report by Rosen and Bengtsson was the first to suggest that GH deficiency (which is often accompanied by lowered circulating IGF-I levels) could be the factor responsible for the observed increased mortality from CVD in adults with hypopituitarism. In a cross-sectional study in relatively young, non-obese and non-diabetic men, Spallarossa et al. (1996) observed an association between circulating IGF-I concentrations and the presence of angiographically demonstrated coronary artery disease. In this study by Spallorossa et al., mean circulating total IGF-I levels were significantly lower in patients with significant coronary artery disease than in those without, at all age groups studied. Whether these subnormal circulating IGF-I levels were due to abnormalities in the GH secretion or to other metabolic reasons (e.g., insulin resistance or fat distribution, or both) was unclear. In another cross-sectional study of healthy elderly people, we observed higher circulating free IGF-I concentrations in subjects without signs or symptoms of CVD than in those with angina pectoris or CVD (Janssen et al. 1998). In addition, in this study, higher free circulating IGF-I levels were associated with a decreased presence of athero-sclerotic plaques (Janssen et al. 1998). More recently Juul et al. (2002) reported the results of a 15-year prospective study among 231 cases and 374 age-and sex-matched controls, all without CVD at entry to the study .They observed that individuals with baseline circulatingIGF-I levels in the lowest quartile in the 15-year follow-up had a two-fold increased risk of CVD compared with the reference group, and this relationship remained constant when controlled for IGFBP-3-, the major circulating protein, BMI, diabetes, smoking, menopause and the use of antihypertensives. Conversely, individuals from the high IGFBP-3 quartile group also had an adjusted risk of more than 2 (2.16). The result was the identification of a high-risk population, i.e., those with low IGF-I levels and high IGFBP-3 levels, with a markedly higher risk for CVD, increased more than 4-fold compared with the index group, suggesting that IGF-I indeed may be involved in the pathogenesis of CVD.

Although the exact mechanisms by which IGF-I is involved in CVD are unknown at present, experimental studies have indicated that IGF-I may stimulate nitric oxide in the vessel wall, thereby inducing vasodilatation of the coronary and peripheral vessel wall (Walsh et al. 1996; Muniyappa et al. 1997). Furthermore, IGF-I has been shown to have important cardioprotective effects, by reducing myocardial apoptosis and injury in response to ischemia (Buerke et al. 1995; Li et al. 1999). All these data together suggest a role for IGF-I deficiency per se in increasing the risk for atherosclerosis and CVD.

Circulating IGF-1 levels and the IGF-1 gene

Circulating IGF-I levels are influenced by a number of interacting non-genetic factors, such as age, GH, and nutrition (Blum 2000). Genetic factors may also influence individual variation in serum IGF-I levels. Twin studies have shown that the inter-individual variability in circulating IGF-I levels is at least 38% genetically determined (Kao et al. 1994; Harrela et al. 1996), but the specific loci on the IGF-I gene have not yet been described.

Observations in the Rotterdam Study
about the 192-bp IGF-1 gene polymorphism

The IGF-I gene contains a region of multiple cytosine-adenosine nucleotides (so-called CA repeats). This CA repeat polymorphism is located approximately 1 kb upstream from the IGF-I gene promoter (Rosen et al. 1998; Takacs et al. 1999; Fig. 1). Studies of other genes (for example the androgen receptor),have shown that the number of CA repeats is inversely related to the transactivation of a gene (Westberg et al. 2001). Thus the CA repeat polymorphism in the IGF-I gene has the potential to influence directly the expression of IGF-I. As a consequence, circulating IGF-I levels may be influenced by CA repeat polymorphism variations (alleles) in the IGF-I gene.

In a case-control study, Vaessen et al. (2001) observed fewer subjects with type 2 diabetes or previous myocardial infarction in those homozygous for the 192-bp allele. Compared to those homozygous for the 192-bp allele, non-carriers of the 192 bp-allele had a relative risk of 1.7 for type 2 diabetes (95% CI 1.1-2.7) as well as for myocardial infarction (95% CI 1.1-2.5). Within the group of type 2 diabetes patients, the prevalence of myocardial infarction was 25 % in non-carriers of the 192-bp allele but only 7% in homozygotes for the 192-bp allele. The relative risk for myocardial infarction in non-carriers of the 192-bp allele (compared to homozygotes) was 3.4 (95% CI: 1.1-11.3). In addition, the 192-bp IGF-I genotypes were not associated with known cardiovascular risk factors, such as age, male gender, body mass index, waist-to-hip ratio, total cholesterol, HDL-cholesterol, and hypertension

To summarize the main findings of the study by Vaessen et al. (2001), the risk of both type 2 diabetes and myocardial infarction were significantly increased in non-carriers of the 192-bp allele when compared with carriers of the 192-bp allele. This finding suggests that a genetically determined exposure to relatively low IGF-I levels plays a role in the pathogenesis of both type 2 diabetes and myocardial infarction.

The role of interactions between IGF-1 genotype, life style and environment on phenotype

Stratification of the relationship between serum IGF-I level and age according to genotype in the Rotterdam Study showed that there was a highly significant relationship between IGF-I and age only in homozygous carriers of the 192-bp allele (Rietveld et al. 2003). This relationship was not significant in heterozygous carriers and in non-carriers. In addition, the circulating IGF-I levels were slightly higher in homozygous carriers of the 192-bp allele than in heterozygous and non-carriers.

The risk for diabetes mellitus increases with greater body mass index (Colditz et al. 1995). In the Rotterdam Study, obesity itself was associated with a 2.6-fold increased risk of diabetes mellitus (95% CI of odds ratio, 1.5 to 4.7; P=0.0003). In obese individuals (BMI>27 kg/m2), the risk for diabetes mellitus is also related to the number of 192-bp alleles. Using non-obese homozygous carriers for the 192-bp allele as a reference group, the odds ratio for diabetes mellitus was 2.9 in obese individuals heterozygous for the 192-bp allele (95% CI: 1.6-5.2; P=0.0003), whereas the odds ratio in obese non-carriers was 6.2 (95% CI 2.8-13.5, p<0.0001). In contrast, the risk for diabetes mellitus was independent from IGF-I genotype in non-obese subjects. These findings support the importance of maintaining a normal body weight throughout adult life and suggest that life style factors like obesity considerably amplify the risk for diabetes in heterozygotes and non-carriers of the 192-bp IGF-I allele.

In a substudy of the Rotterdam Study, the presence of atherosclerosis was evaluated at different sites by 1) a lateral X-ray of the lumbar spine, on which the presence of calcified deposits was determined, 2) measurement of the intima-media thickness of the carotid artery and the counting of atherosclerotic plaques in the carotid artery by ultrasound, and 3) measuring the ankle-arm index to assess the presence of atherosclerosis in the arteries.

The relative risks for a previous myocardial infarction and for a myocardial infarction during follow-up (i.e., after the baseline examination), respectively, were not significantly increased in heterozygous carriers and non-carriers of the 192-bp allele <u>without</u> evidence of atherosclerosis at the baseline examination. However, those subjects <u>with</u> atherosclerosis at the baseline examination who were also heterozygous for the 192-bp allele had increased relative risks: for a previous myocardial infarction the risk was 1.6 (95% CI 1.2-2.3) and the risk for a new myocardial infarction during follow-up was 2.7 (95% CI 1.5-4.9). In subjects <u>with</u> atherosclerosis who were non-carriers for the 192-bp allele of the IGF-I gene, the risk for a previous mycardial infarction was 3.7 (95% CI 2.2-6.3) and the risk for a new infarction during follow-up was 5.2 (95% CI 2.3-11.8).

These findings suggest that IGF-I has direct cardioprotective effects, possibly by reducing myocardial injury in response to ischemia.

Discussion and Future Perspectives

The genetic approach used in the Rotterdam Study overcomes the problem that cross-sectional studies cannot distinguish whether changes in IGF-I levels are causes or consequences of a disease. The association with low body height and low IGF-I serum levels in the Rotterdam Study suggests that subjects who are non-carriers of the 192-bp allele are chronically (i.e., life-long) exposed to lower IGF-I levels throughout the body. However, the population-based approach in the Rotterdam Study cannot distinguish whether this polymorphism is itself involved in regulation of IGF-I expression or merely flags another polymorphism in the promoter region that is functionally involved in the IGF-I expression. Further evaluation of sequence variation at this locus is needed to determine whether the observed effect is a direct consequence of IGF-I m-RNA expression or whether it is the result of linkage disequilibria with other polymorphisms. Molecular studies in vitro (transfection of this polymorphism into cells) or studies in transgenic animals (incorporation of the 192-bp polymorphism into a transgenic animal) may help to assess the effects of this 192-bp polymorphism on IGF-I expression.

The findings in the Rotterdam Study are in accordance with a recently reported case-control study conducted within the Nurses' Health Study (Missmer et al. 2002). Missmer et al. also reported that subjects homozygous for the 192-bp allele had significantly higher serum levels of IGF-I compared to subjects not carrying this allele. In contrast, Rosen et al. (1998) reported previously that homozygous carriers for the 192-bp allele had significantly lower serum levels of IGF-I compared to non-carriers of the 192-bp allele. However, the Rosen et al. study was based on a relatively small, highly selected study population, including males with idiopathic osteoporosis, participants of a calcium intervention trial, patients with chronic chest pain and participants in a study of hormonal determinants of

BMD. In addition, as already discussed above, actual circulating IGF-I levels might also be influenced by a number of interacting nongenetic factors. The inclusion of patients with putative IGF-I-related pathology in the Rosen et al. study might thus explain for a large part the discrepancy with the findings within the Rotterdam study.

From the findings in the Rotterdam Study we can estimate that the probability that type 2 diabetes or a myocardial infarction will develop in a subject who is a non-carrier of the 192-bp allele of the IGF-I gene polymorphism is only 16%. Thus genetic screening for variation in the IGF-I gene in the general (Dutch) population will not be very helpful as a diagnostic or predictive tool. Nevertheless, our observations in the Rotterdam Study demonstrated that genetically determined exposure to relatively low circulating IGF-I levels is a risk factor for the development of diabetes or myocardial infarction, and this finding may have an important impact on future clinical practice in specific subgroups. For example, we observed in the Rotterdam Study that the probability of developing myocardial infarction was 78% in non-carriers of the 192-bp allele with angina pectoris, whereas the probability of developing type 2 diabetes in obese non-carriers was as high as 75%. These findings provide a rationale for clinical studies comparing the effect of treatments that increase IGF-I levels (such as GH, GH-secretagogues, IGF-I/IGFBP-3 complex) in carriers and non-carriers of the 192-bp allele. Genetic variation at the IGF-I 192-bp allele could thus be among the factors responsible for the inter-individual differences observed in response to IGF-I-increasing treatments. Treatments that increase IGF-I levels may especially prevent the incidence of myocardial infarction and type 2 diabetes in non-carriers of the 192-bp allele. For instance, it could be that GH treatment of subjects with severe GH deficiency is more effective in reducing CVD in non-carriers than in carriers of the 192-bp allele. The effects of medical therapy may thus depend on IGF-I genotype background.

In a cross-sectional substudy we observed the well-known age-related decline in circulating total IGF-I levels only in homozygous carriers of the 192-bp alleles of the IGF-I gene, whereas this relationship was absent in heterozygotes and non-carriers of the 192-bp allele. In addition, the circulating IGF-I levels were slightly higher in homozygous carriers of the 192-bp allele than in heterozygous and non-carriers. We therefore hypothesize that the 192-bp allele of the IGF-I gene directly or indirectly influences GH-mediated regulation of IGF-I secretion with aging.

IGFBPs may also modify IGF-I activity. Therefore, it will also be important to study polymorphisms of the IGFBPs and the interactions of these IGFBP polymorphisms with the IGF-I genotype. A substantial genetic contribution for interindividual variations has already been reported for the circulating IGFBP-3 levels (Harrela et al. 1996; Deal et al. 2001).

In conclusion, our observations suggest that circulating (and presumably tissue expression of) IGF-I levels vary considerably between carriers and non-carriers of a 192-bp IGF-I gene polymorphism. Non-carriers of the 192-bp allele have a lower body height and are chronically (i.e., life-long exposed to lower IGF-I levels. In addition, the risks of both type 2 diabetes and myocardial infarction are significantly increased in non-carriers of the 192-bp allele when compared to carriers of this polymorphism, suggesting that this genetically determined exposure to relatively low IGF-I levels plays a role in the pathogenesis of both type 2 diabetes and myocardial infarction. Further study of the IGF-I promoter region may help to define subpopulations for whom IGF-I-increasing therapies are more or less likely to be effective. This process will help to optimize strategies for the use of (relatively) expensive drugs (such as GH) from a risk/benefit point of view.

References

Bartke A (2001) Mutations prolong life in flies; implication for aging in mammals. Trends I Endocrinol Metab 12: 233–234

Blum WF (2000) Chapter 3:Insulin-like growth factors (IGF) and IGF-binding proteins: their use for diagnosis of growth hormone deficiency. In: Juul A, Jorgensen (eds) Growth hormone in adults. Physiological and clinical aspects. 2nd edn. Cambridge: Cambridge University Press, pp. 54–86

Buerke M, Murohara T, Skurk C, Nuss C, Tomaselli K, Lefer AM (1995) Cardioprotective effect of insulin-like growth factor I in myocardial ischemia followed by reperfusion. Proc Natl Acad Sci USA 92: 8031–8035

Cerami A (1985) Hypothesis. Glucose as a mediator of aging. J Am Geriatr Soc 33(9):626–34

Cerami A, Vlassara H, Brownlee M. (1985) Protein glycosylation and the pathogenesis of atherosclerosis. Metabolism 34 (12 Suppl 1):37–42

Clauson PG, Brismar K, Hall K, Linnarsson R, Grill V (1998) Insulin-like growth factor-I and insulin-like growth factor binding protein-1 in a representative population of type 2 diabetic patients in Sweden. Scand J Clin Lab Invest 58:353–360

Clemmons D (1992) Age-related changes in IGF-I levels, p854–855. In: LeRoith D, Clemmons D, Nissley P, Rechler MM: NIH conference. Insulin-like growth factors in health and disease. Ann Intern Med 116: 854–862

Clemmons DR, Smith-Banks A, Underwood LE (1992) Reversal of diet-induced catabolism by infusion of recombinant insulin-like growth factor-I in humans. J Clin Endocrinol Metab 75: 234–238

Colditz GA, Willett WC, Rotnitzky A, Manson JE (1995) Weight gain as a risk factor for clinical diabetes mellitus in women. Ann Intern Med 122: 481–486

Coschigano KT, Clemmons D, Bellush LL, Kopchick JJ (2000) Assessment of growth parameters and life span of GHR/BP gene-disrupted mice. Endocrinology 141:2608–2613

Deal C, Ma J, Wilkin F, Paquette J, Rozen F, Ge B, Hudson T, Stampfer M, Pollak M. (2001) Novel promoter polymorphism in insulin-like growth factor-binding protein-3: correlation with serum levels and interaction with known regulators. J Clin Endocrinol Metab 86:1274–1280.

DeFronzo RA (1981) Glucose intolerance and aging. Diabetes Care 4: 493–501

Elahi D, Muller DC (2000) Carbohydrate metabolism in the elderly. Eur J Clin Nutr 54 Suppl 3: S112–120

Ferns GA, Motani AS, Anggard EE (1991) The insulin-like growth factors: their putative role in atherogenesis. Artery 18: 197–225

Froesch ER, Zapf J (1985) Insulin-like growth factors and insulin: comparative aspects. Diabetologia 28:485–493

Froesch ER, Schmid C, Schwander J, Zapf J (1985) Actions of insulin-like growth factors. Annu Rev Physiol 47:443–467

Hadsell DL, Abdel-Fattah G (2001) Regulation of cell apoptosis by insulin-like growth factor I.Adv Exp Med Biol 501:79–85

Harrela M, Koistinen H, Kaprio J, Lehtovirta M, Tuomilehto J, Eriksson J, Toivanen L, Koskenvuo M, Leinonen P, Koistinen R, Seppala M (1996) Genetic and environmental components of interindividual variation in circulating levels of IGF-I, IGF-II, IGFBP-1, and IGFBP-3. J Clin Invest 98: 2612–2615

Hochberg MC, Lethbridge-Cejku M, Scott WW Jr, Reichle R, Plato CC, Tobin JD (1994) Serum levels of insulin-like growth factor in subjects with osteoarthritis of the knee. Data from the Baltimore Longitudinal Study of Aging. Arthritis Rheum 37: 1177–1180

Hofman A, Grobbee DE, de Jong PT, van den Ouweland FA (1991) Determinants of disease and disability in the elderly: The Rotterdam Elderly Study. Eur J Epidemiol 1991 7:403–422

Holt RIG (2002) Fetal programming of the growth-hormone-insulin-like growth factor axis. Trends Endocrinol Metabol 13: 392–397

Janssen JAMJL, Stolk RP, Pols HAP, Grobbee DE, Lamberts SWJ (1998) Serum total IGF-I, free IGF-I, and IGFB-1 levels in an elderly population: relation to cardiovascular risk factors and disease. 18:277–282

Jones JI, Clemmons DR (1995) Insulin-like growth factors and their binding proteins: biological actions. Endocrinol Rev 16:3–34

Juul A, Scheike T, Davidsen M, Gyllenborg J, Jorgensen T (2002) Low serum insulin-like growth factor I is associated with increased risk of ischemic heart disease: a population-based case-control study. Circulation 106: 939–944

Kao PC, Matheny AP Jr, Lang CA (1994) Insulin-like growth factor-I comparisons in healthy twin children. J Clin Endocrinol Metab 78:310–312

Kiess W, Kessler U, Schmitt S, Funk B. (1993) Growth hormone and insulin-like growth factor-I: Basic aspects. In: Flyvbjerg A, Ørskov H, Alberti KGMM (eds) Growth hormone and insulin-like growth factor-I in human and experimental diabetes, John Wiley & Sons, Chicester, UK, pp. 1–21

Li B, Setoguchi M, Wang X, Andreoli AM, Leri A, Malhotra A, Kajstura J, Anversa P (1999) Insulin-like growth factor-1 attenuates the detrimental impact of nonocclusive coronary artery constriction on the heart. Circ Res 84: 1007–1019

Masoro EJ, Katz MS, McMahan CA(1989) Evidence for the glycation hypothesis of aging from the food-restricted rodent model. J Gerontol 44: B20–2

Missmer SA, Haiman CA, Hunter DJ, Willett WC, Colditz GA, Speizer FE, Pollak MN, Hankinson SE (2002) A sequence repeat in the insulin-like growth factor-1 gene and risk of breast cancer. Int J Cancer 100:332–336

Mobbs CV, Bray GA, Atkinson RL, Bartke A, Finch CE, Maratos-Flier E, Crawley JN, Nelson JF (2001) Neuroendocrine and pharmacological manipulations to assess how caloric restriction increases life span. J Gerontol A Biol Sci Med Sci 56:34–44

Moses AC, Young SC, Morrow LA, O'Brien M, Clemmons DR (1996) Recombinant human insulin-like growth factor I increases insulin sensitivity and improves glycemic control in type II diabetes. Diabetes 45: 91–100

Muniyappa R, Walsh MF, Rangi JS, Zayas RM, Standley PR, Ram JL, Sowers JR (1997) Insulin like growth factor 1 increases vascular smooth muscle nitric oxide production. Life Sci 161: 925–931

Paolisso G, Tagliamonte MR, Rizzo MR, Carella C, Gambardella A, Barbieri M, Varricchio M (1999) Low plasma insulin-like growth factor-1 concentrations predict worsening of insulin-mediated glucose uptake in older people. J Am Geriatr Soc 47:1312–1318

Reaven GM, Chen N, Hollenbeck C, Chen YD (1989) Effect of age on glucose tolerance and glucose uptake in healthy individuals. J Am Geriatr Soc 37: 735–740

Rietveld I, Janssen JAMJL, Hofman A, Pols HAP, van Duijn CM, Lamberts SWJ (2003). A polymorphism in the insulin-like growth factor I (IGF-I) gene influences the age-related decline in circulating total IGF-I levels. Eur J Endocrinol , 148: 171–175.

Rosen T, Bengtsson BA (1990) Premature mortality due to cardiovascular disease in hypopituitarism. Lancet 336: 285–288

Rosen CJ, Kurland ES, Vereault D, Adler RA, Rackoff PJ, Craig WY, Witte S, Rogers J, Bilezikian JP (1998) Association between serum insulin growth factor-I (IGF-I) and a simple sequence repeat in IGF-I gene: implications for genetic studies of bone mineral density. J Clin Endocrinol Metab 83: 2286–2290

Ruiz-Torres A, Soares de Melo Kirzner M (2002) Ageing and longevity are related to growth hormone/insulin-like growth factor-1 secretion. Gerontology 48:401–407

Sandhu MS, Heald AH, Gibson JM, Cruickshank JK, Dunger DB, Wareham NJ (2002) Circulating concentrations of insulin-like growth factor-I and development of glucose intolerance: a prospective observational study. Lancet 359:1740–1745

Spallarossa P, Brunelli C, Minuto F, Caruso D, Battistini M, Caponnetto S, Cordera R (1996) Insulin-like growth factor-I and angiographically documented coronary artery disease. Am J Cardiol 77: 200–202

Takacs I, Koller DL, Peacock M, Christian JC, Hui SL, Conneally PM, Johnston CC Jr, Foroud T, Econs MJ (1999) Sibling pair linkage and association studies between bone mineral densityand the insulin-like growth factor I gene locus. J Clin Endocrinol Metab 84: 4467–4471

Tan K, Baxter RC (1986) Serum insulin-like growth factor I levels in adult diabetic patients: the effect of age. J Clin Endocrinol Metab 63:651–655

Ruiz-Torres A, Soares De Melo Kirzner M. (2002) Ageing and longevity are related to growth hormone/insulin-like growth factor-1 secretion. Gerontology 48: 401–407

Vaessen N, Heutink P, Janssen JA, Witteman JC, Testers L, Hofman A, Lamberts SW, Oostra BA, Pols HA, van Duijn CM (2001) Polymorphism in the gene for IGF-I: functional properties and risk for type 2 diabetes and myocardial infarction. Diabetes 50:637–642

Walsh MF, Barazi M, Pete G, Muniyappa R, Dunbar JC, Sowers JR (1996) Insulin-like growth factor I diminishes in vivo and in vitro vascular contractility: role of vascular nitric oxide. Endocrinology 137:1798–1803

Westberg L, Baghaei F, Rosmond R, Hellstrand M, Landen M, Jansson M, Holm G, Bjorntorp P, Eriksson E. (2001) Polymorphisms of the androgen receptor gene and the estrogen receptor beta gene are associated with androgen levels in women. J Clin Endocrinol Metab 86: 2562–2568 dysfunction, insomnia, nervousness, depression, irritability, hot flushes, periodic sweating, and increase in fat mass (Vermeulen 2002). As regards the ageing of a male, certain gender-specific environmental and lifestyle factors (obesity, physical activity, smoking, alcohol consumption) are involved, but by far the most conspicuous gender-specific variable is the life-long exposure of a male to the androgenic sex hormones produced by the testis. Ageing of the human ovary starts with gradual diminution of steroid production, followed by an abrupt and almost complete cessation of ovarian sex hormone production at menopause. The impact of these hormonal alterations has been thoroughly studied in the female, and hormone replacement therapy of postmenopausal women is today widely used in clinical practise.

Unlike in women at menopause, the ageing-related alterations of testicular androgen production are gradual and occur with a large individual variability. The average decline of serum total T is 35%, and that of the biologically active free fraction is 50% between the ages of 20 and 80 (Vermeulen and Kaufman 1995). This decline is partly due to primary failure of Leydig cell function and is partly secondary to alterations in gonadotropin secretion at the hypothalamic-pituitary level. However, the serum levels of T decrease below the reference range only in a minority of elderly men; from 7% in the age group of 40-60 to 20% in the age group 60-80, and 35% in men aged over 80 years (Vermeulen and Kaufmann 1995). The factors influencing T levels in elderly men are multiple: heredity, environment (obesity, stress), and psychosocial (depression, smoking, drugs) or socioeconomic conditions (diet, hygiene). However, apparently the most important factor in the ageing-related decline in testicular endocrine function is the increased frequency of systemic diseases upon ageing. The term "andropause," denoting the male equivalent for female menopause, must be considered in many respects a misnomer, because testicular function shows only mild gradual decline with ageing and a more dramatic decline is often due to accompanying systemic diseases. Nevertheless, a recent study on the factors affecting the variability in individual circulating levels of sex steroids and their precursors identified age as the most important factor, followed by body mass index (BMI), race and lifestyle factors (Ukkola et al. 2001).

The impact of genetic factors on the male-specific features of ageing must therefore involue the genetic variability (polymorphisms) in the genes related to the regulation, production and actions of testicular hormones. In this review, we summarise the currently available information about polymorphisms affecting the hypothalamic-pituitary-testicular function, and some other hormones with anabolic effects, as explanatory parameters for the special features of normal male ageing and some ageing-related diseases.

Androgen receptor

The androgen receptor (AR) is a structurally conserved member of the nuclear receptor superfamily of ligand-activated transcription factors. Its gene has been localized to the q11-12 region of the X chromosome. T is the functionally most important AR ligand, but in some androgen target tissues, e.g., the prostate and hair follicles, T is converted to a biologically more active androgen, 5α-dihydrotestosterone (DHT) before activating the receptor. Androgens promote the growth and differentiation of the accessory sex organs in the male genital tract and maintain their normal function, including spermatogenesis. Androgens also have anabolic effects, promoting the development and maintenance of nongenital aspects of the male phenotype, including hair growth pattern, skeletal and muscle growth, and deepening of voice. Conspicuously, over 400 inactivating AR mutations have been detected (http://ww2.mcgill.ca/androgendb/), which are responsible for the wide phenotypic array of androgen insensitivity syndromes.

The transactivating function of AR resides in the N-terminal domain of the protein encoded by exon 1. This region also contains well-characterized polymorphic repeats and one of them is a CAG repeat encoding normally an 11-31 amino acid-long polyglutamine repeat (Edwards et al. 1992; Giovannucci et al. 1999). There is now considerable evidence that the lengths of the polyglutamine repeat correlate indirectly with the biological activity of AR (Nelson and Witte 2002), and a plethora of studies exists on correlates of this polymorphism with various conditions related to androgen action. Recent research suggests that men with shorter *AR* CAG repeat lengths (≤ 22) are at greater risk for developing prostate cancer than those with longer repeats (Edwards et al. 1992; Schoenberg et al. 1994; Irvine et al. 1995). The number of the CAG repeats is lowest in African-Americans, intermediate in non-Hispanic whites, and highest in Asians (Edwards et al. 1992; Irvine et al. 1995), and the frequency of prostatic cancer in the three racial groups is inversely proportional to the length of the repeat. A somatic mutation resulting in contraction of the CAG repeat from 24 to 18 has been found in an adenocarcinoma of the prostate, and the effect of the shorter allele was implicated in development of the tumour (Schoenberg et al. 1994). A significant correlation between the CAG repeat length and age at diagnosis was observed, whereas correlations with stage, level of prostate-specific antigen at diagnosis, and time to relapse were not significant. Shorter CAG repeat lengths may be associated with the development of prostate cancer in men at younger ages (Hardy et al. 1996).

The Chinese population is at low risk for prostate cancer. A population-based case-control study from China on the *AR* CAG and GGN (polyglycine, another repeat in exon 1) repeat polymorphisms and clinically significant prostate cancer confirmed longer CAG repeat lengths in Chinese than in Western men, and that shorter CAG repeats were also associated with increased prostate cancer risk in this low-risk population. Hence, the CAG repeat length is a potentially useful marker to identify individuals at higher risk for prostate cancer (Hsing et al. 2000). However, negative findings also exist on connections of the AR polymorphism and prostatic disease (Lange et al. 2000; Beilin et al. 2001).

The CAG repeat length has also been correlated with ageing-related endocrine and metabolic alterations. Several studies have now shown that short CAG repeats imply a greater chance for low levels of HDL-cholesterol and reduced endothelial response to ischemia, which are important risk factors for coronary heart disease (Zitzmann et al. 2001a).

A study on Asian men demonstrated that long CAG tracts of *AR* are associated with increased risk of defective spermatogenesis and undermasculinization (Loy and Yong 2001), and in patients from the USA, the mean *AR* CAG length was significantly longer in infertile men than in fertile controls (21.95 ± 0.31 vs. 20.72 ± 0.52; Mifsud et al. 2001). Tut et al. (1997) found that patients with ≥ 28 or more glutamines in their repeat had a greater than 4-fold increased risk of impaired spermatogenesis, and the more severe the spermatogenic defect, the higher the proportion of patients with longer repeats.

The number of CAG repeats in *AR* was determined in healthy younger males to investigate its potential impact on bone metabolism (Zitzmann et al. 2001b). In stepwise multiple regression models controlling for age, body fat content and lifestyle factors, the number of CAG repeats was an independent negative predictor of bone mineral density (BMD), whereas it was positively correlated with markers of bone turnover. Levels of free T and oestradiol showed an independent and positive association with BMD; age contributed significantly to lower BMD. The CAG repeat length thus correlates with increased age-dependent bone loss and appears to attenuate the positive T effect on bone density and metabolism, in keeping with its lower activity (Choong et al. 1996; Zitzmann 2001b). However, in another study there was no association of this AR polymorphism with any biochemical markers of bone turnover (Van Pottelbergh 2001).

Other AR gene polymorphisms (Ellis et al. 2001) have been studied in connection with cosmetically significant baldness. A *StuI* restriction site and the combination of shorter CAG and GGC triplet repeat lengths were found more prevalent in bald men, suggesting that these markers are very close to a functional variant that is a necessary component in the polygenic determination of male pattern baldness.

The serum T levels in healthy men decrease with ageing, although with considerable interindividual variability. There is a biologic relationship between the *AR* CAG repeat length, AR function and serum androgen levels. Men with shorter CAG repeats display lower circulating levels of total free T and albumin-bound T upon ageing (Krithivas et al. 1999). The association of the AR genotype with the variability of serum T suggests that multiple factors, e.g., serum androgen levels and AR function, should be taken into consideration when assessing the ageing-related changes in the androgenic/anabolic status of a man.

Oestrogen receptors α and β

The human oestrogen receptors (ER) α and β map to chromosomes 6q25.1 and 14q, respectively, and like AR they belong to the ligand-activated transcription factors. The human ER gene is more than 140 kb long, and it contains 8 exons with highly conserved positions of introns (Ponglikitmongkol et al. 1988). The two ERs are expressed with distinct tissue and cell-specific patterns, including the reproductive organs (Pelletier and El-Alfy 2000). ERβ is homologous to the previously identified ERα, with 96% conservation of nucleotides in the DNA-binding domain and 58% in the ligand-binding domain.

The physiological effects of oestrogens on bone in men were largely unanticipated until recently, when oestrogen deficiency in males with aromatase deficiency and oestrogen resistance was found to cause osteoporosis and delayed fusion of epiphyses despite sufficient serum T (Morishima et al. 1995; Carani et al. 1997; Deladoey et al. 1999; Smith et al. 1994). On the other hand, the importance of osteoporosis in the morbidity of ageing men has only recently been fully recognized (Stein and Ashok 2002). The age-related changes in bone mineral metabolism and the role of various factors in the pathogenesis of bone loss in men remain largely unknown. Nevertheless, besides genetics, the lifestyle and environmental factors contribute to bone mineral density (BMD). Greater muscle strength and physical activity are associated with higher bone mass, whereas radial bone loss is greater in cigarette smokers and those with a moderate alcohol intake (Huuskonen et al. 2000).

Sex hormone status also has important effects on bone physiology in men. As stated above, both serum total and free T levels show a gradual decline with age, and osteoporosis is common in men with hypogonadism. The majority of male oestrogens originate through peripheral aromatisation of androgens, and osteoblast-like cells also express aromatase. In men aged > 65 years, there is a positive correlation between BMD and greater serum oestradiol levels at all skeletal sites and a negative association between BMD and T at some sites (Ebeling 1998). The action of T on the male skeleton may be mediated in part by aromatisation to oestradiol (Anderson et al. 1998). It is possible that low-dose oestrogen therapy or specific estrogen receptor-modulating drugs might increase BMD in men as well as in women (Ebeling 1998).

On the basis of the above information it is likely that *ER* polymorphisms with functional significance could also have effects in males. There is evidence in women that *ER*α polymorphisms play a role in postmenopausal osteoporosis. The length of a (TA)-repeat in the *ER*α promoter region shows positive correlation with lumbar BMD (Becherini et al. 2000), and this polymorphism may prove useful in the prediction of vertebral fracture risk in postmenopausal osteoporosis.

To study the influence of *ER*α polymorphisms and oestradiol on height and bone density during and after puberty in males, the allelic variants in intron 1 (*PvuII* and *XbaI*), XX, Xx, xx, PP, Pp, and pp were determined in Caucasian boys (Lorentzon et al. 1999). The small letters represent the presence of restriction site. In a multivariate analysis including pubertal development, physical activity, and body weight, the X genotype independently predicted higher BMD parameters, and the P genotype predicted spine volumetric BMD and greater height. Thus *ER*α polymorphisms were related to bone density and height at puberty in young men (Lorentzon et al. 1999). In another study, the distributions of *BstUI* (exon 1), *PvuII* and *XbaI* (intron 1) RFLPs and the TA repeat polymorphism in the promoter region were examined in relation to osteoporosis. All four polymorphisms were in linkage disequilibrium. The TA repeat length in the *ER*α gene was inversely associated with increased risk of osteoporotic fractures and a modest reduction in bone mass. Polymorphisms in exon 1 and intron 1 (*PvuII* and *XbaI*) of *ER*α were not associated with osteoporotic fractures, bone mass, or bone turnover (Langdahl et al. 2000a).

No connection was found in a Japanese study between polymorphisms in *ERα* and the prevalence and severity of coronary arterial disease (CAD) and serum lipid levels in control subjects and patients (Matsubara et al. 1997). However, in middle-aged Finnish men with CAD, the length of the TA repeat polymorphism was directly related to the severity of CAD (Kunnas et al. 2000). In the Helsinki Sudden Death Study (Lehtimäki et al. 2002), 300 male autopsy cases were studied for histopathology of the coronary arteries and related to the *ERα PvuII* genotype. After adjusting for age and BMI, men ≥ 53 years of age with P/p and P/P genotypes had on average 2-5-fold larger coronary lesions than subjects with the p/p genotype. The finding persisted after additional adjustment for diabetes and hypertension.

The interaction of *ERα* (*XbaI/PvuII*, see above) and β (*AluI* in 3'-UTR) polymorphisms with the risk of Alzheimer's disease (AD) has recently been observed in a mixed male/female population (Lambert et al. 2001). If these first findings can be supported by other independent studies, the risk for AD may be shown to be modulated when both ERα and ERβ have particular variations in their expression and/or biological activities. However, the gender dependence of this finding is not yet known. Concerning prostatic cancer, in a study on the polymorphisms in *AR*, *ERα* and *aromatase*, homozygosity for the *ERα XbaI* restriction site together with long AR CAG repeat was found to be more frequent among controls than patients (Modugno et al. 2001). The study supported a multigene mode of prostatic cancer susceptibility, including those of *AR* and *ER*.

CYP17 (17α-hydroxylase/17,20-lyase)

Cytochrome P450c17α (*CYP17*), located on chromosome 10q24.3, encodes an enzyme with 17α-hydroxylase and 17,20-lyase activities. It is rate limiting for the normal production of adrenal and gonadal androgens, catalysing the conversion of pregnenolone to 17-hydroxypregnenolone and further to dehydroepiandrosterone, a compound with weak androgenic activity (Waterman and Keeney 1992). Because of the crucial role of CYP17 in androgen biosynthesis, sequence variations in the gene altering its catalytic activity have been hypothesized to associate with increased risk to prostate cancer, an androgen-dependent malignancy.

A common *CYP 17* polymorphism is a T (A1 allele)→C transition (A2 allele) in the 5'promoter region, which creates an additional Sp1 type (CCACCbox) transcription factor recognition site, and therefore the A2 allele may have increased rate of transcription (Feigelson et al. 1998). Several groups have studied the association between this polymorphism and prostate cancer, but the findings have remained negative or inconclusive (Chang et al. 2001; Haiman et al. 2001). Neither was there evidence for gene-gene interaction between *CYP17* and *SRD5A2* V89L polymorphisms on prostate cancer risk or endogenous steroid hormone levels. Several studies corroborate the association of the A2/A2 *CYP17* phenotype with higher prostatic cancer risk (Lunn et al. 1999; Gsur et al. 2000; Yamada et al. 2001; Haiman et al. 2001), and the *CYP17* genotype may confer a small increased susceptibility to prostate cancer, but it is not a strong predictor of endogenous steroid hormone levels in men. In contrast to prostatic cancer, no association between polymorphisms of *CYP17* and *vitamin D receptor (VDR)* to prostate volume/histology and endocrine patterns was found in elderly men with lower urinary tract symptoms (Schatzl et al. 2001).

Because androgens have powerful effects on bone growth and metabolism, the association of the T→C polymorphism in the *CYP17* promoter region with sex hormone levels, stature and femoral mass and size has been studied (Zmuda et al. 2001). Serum bioavailable T levels were 20% (0.5 SD) higher in men with C/C compared with the T/T genotype, whereas heterozygous men had intermediate hormone levels. Men with the C/C genotype were nearly 3 cm taller and had greater femoral neck cross-sectional areas than men with the T/T genotype. In contrast, the *CYP17* genotype was not associated with femoral neck bone mineral density, area or estimated volumetric BMD. These results suggest that allelic variation at the *CYP17* locus may contribute to the genetic influence on stature and femoral size in men.

CYP 19 (aromatase)

The *CYP19* gene encodes aromatase, a key steroidogenic enzyme involved in the conversion of androgens to estrogens. The human *CYP19* gene contains 10 exons and is located on chromosome 15q21 (Means et al. 1989; Toda et al. 1990). In men, T is the major source of plasma oestradiol and about 80% of it originates from peripheral aromatisation in extratesticular sites. Plasma oestrogen, 5% of which is converted to oestradiol, originates mainly from peripheral aromatisation. The plasma concentration of oestradiol in males is about 0.1 nmol/L and its production rate is about 0.1-0.2 micrograms/24 h; both of these values are significantly higher than in postmenopausal women. The age-associated decrease in T levels is scarcely reflected in plasma oestradiol levels, as a result of increasing aromatase activity with age and the age-associated increase in fat mass. Oestradiol levels are positively related to body fat mass and, more specifically, to subcutaneous abdominal fat. Oestrogens in males play an important role in the regulation of the gonadotropin feedback, several brain functions (Balthazart and Foidart 1993), bone maturation, regulation of bone resorption and lipid metabolism. They also affect skin metabolism and are an important factor in determining the sex interest of men (Vermeulen et al. 2002).

(*CYP19*) belongs to those genes that are potential candidates regulating bone metabolism and mass. Inactivating *CYP19* mutations, resulting in failure of oestrogen synthesis, are associated with osteopenia and decreased bone mineral density in both men and women (Morishima et al. 1995; Simpson 1998; Gennari and Brandi 2001; Khosla et al. 2001). A tetranucleotide simple tandem repeat (TTTA) polymorphism in intron 4 of *CYP19* has recently been described (Cheng and Zhou 2000). The genetic variations of *CYP19* and genes of some other steroid metabolic enzymes (e.g.,CYP1A2, CYP3A4, and *17β-HSD*) are potentially important factors affecting serum oestradiol levels and, indirectly, the risk of osteoporosis.

Determination of distribution of the tetranucleotide single tandem repeat $(TTTA)_n$ polymorphism in intron 4 of *CYP19* was recently combined with epidemiological studies on correlation of some other steroidogenic enzyme polymorphisms (*AR*, *SRD5A2* and *CYP17*) with the risk of prostatic cancer (Latil et al. 2001). The alleles yielding a 171 and 187 bp PCR products (8 and 12 repeats, respectively) over the polymorphic *CYP19* site significantly increased the prostate carcinoma risk. Conversely, and in contrast with some other studies (see above), no association was observed in this study between prostate carcinoma risk and the other polymorphisms. In prostate carcinoma patients, the CAG repeats of *AR*, and TA repeats of *SDR5A2*, were associated with the age of onset. The association with the 171-bp *CYP19* allele and prostate carcinoma risk suggests that aromatase could be a new factor in the prediction of risk for this malignancy.

SRD5A2 (5α-reductase)

Steroid 5α-reductase converts T to 5α-dihydrotestosterone (DHT). It occurs as two enzyme isoforms, types I and II, and the latter is the prostate-specific form. The *SRD5A2* gene is localized on chromosome 2p23. Due to its clinical importance in the regulation of benign and malignant prostatic growth, a number of competitive inhibitors have been developed for this enzyme (Makridakis et al. 2000). DHT is significantly more potent as androgen in comparison with T, having approximately 10-fold higher affinity for the AR (George and Noble 1984) and thus activating target genes at a lower concentration (Deslypere et al. 1992). Based on the evidence that intracellular DHT is the critical "carcinogen," the genetic polymorphisms in *SRD5A2* gene affecting T metabolism may relate to susceptibility to prostate cancer (Steers 2001).

The 5α-reductase activity varies in different ethnic populations, and there are polymorphisms in the *SRD5A2* gene. The population differences in this enzyme's activity may account for a part of the substantial racial/ethnic disparity in prostate cancer risk. In a population-based case-control study from China, a population with the lowest reported prostate cancer incidence in the world, the relationships of four polymorphic markers in *SRD5A2* [point mutations causing Ala49The, Val89Leu or Arg228Glu substitutions, or a (TA)n dinucleotide repeat in the 3'-UTR] were studied (Hsing et al. 2001). Men with the LL genotype at codon 89 had significantly higher serum levels of T and lower levels of 5α-androstane-3α,17β-diol glucuronide than men with other genotypes. The *SRD5A2* L genotype correlated with lower DHT levels and supported the hypothesis that genotypes associated with lower 5α-reductase activity are more common in low-risk populations for prostatic cancer. Although there was no statistically significant association of these *SRD5A2* polymorphisms with prostate cancer risk, a small effect of these markers cannot be ruled out because of the rarity of certain marker genotypes (Hsing et al. 2001). Hence, men who have the V allele of the *SRD5A2* gene have a two-fold increase in the risk of prostate cancer development and an additional two-fold increase in the risk of progression compared with men with the L/L genotype (Nam et al. 2001). Larger studies are needed to further clarify their role and to elucidate whether genetic diversity of the *SRD5A2* gene, alone or in combination with other susceptibility genes, can explain the large racial/ethnic differences in prostate cancer risk

In another study, African-American and Hispanic men with prostate cancer and healthy controls were screened for the A49T missense substitution in 5α-reductase. It increased the risk of clinically significant disease 7.2-fold in African-American men and 3.6-fold in Hispanic men. An increased conversion of testosterone to DHT catalysed by the variant enzyme may be the cause of the increased risk (Makridakis et al.1999). The presence of the same polymorphism was associated with a greater frequency of extracapsular disease and a higher pathological lymph node-metastasis stage, suggesting that the A49T mutation may influence the pathological characteristics of prostate cancers and thus the prognosis (Jaffe et al. 2000). The polymorphisms of the *SRD5A2* gene may be contributing factors to the striking racial/ethnic variation in the incidence of prostatic cancer.

Sex hormone binding globulin (SHBG)

SHBG is a plasma glycoprotein produced by hepatocytes. It is the specific human transporter protein for T, DHT and oestradiol in humans, thereby regulating the bioavailability of these steroids. The *SHBG* gene has eight exons separated by seven small introns, and it is located on chromosome 17p (Berube et al. 1990). Plasma SHBG levels are regulated by different physiological and pathological conditions as well as nutrition and body mass (Hammond and Bocchinfuso 1996; Longcope et al. 2000). Notably, in women with polycystic ovarian syndrome (PCOS), high insulin and androgen levels are often associated with low SHBG concentration (Wortsman et al. 1986; Pirwany et al. 2001). A low SHBG level indicates a state of hyperandrogenicity associated with a higher risk of developing non-insulin-dependent diabetes in women and is accepted as a marker of muscular insulin resistance (Kopp et al. 2001). Considerable individual variation exists in serum SHBG concentrations, irrespective of gender, body weight, thyroid, or androgen status.

There are genetic polymorphisms in *SHBG* with potential functional consequences. A variant *SHBG* has been identified (Power et al. 1992; Hardy et al. 1995), with a point mutation in exon 8 (GAC → AAC) encoding an amino acid substitution Asp327Asn and introducing an additional consensus site for N-glycosylation. This variant *SHBG* has been found to increase the half-life of SHBG in circulation (Cousin et al. 1998), but its steroid-binding affinity was equal to normal SHBG (Power et al. 1992). The frequency of this variant allele was very low in the population studied (0.083; Cousin et al. 1998). There is some evidence for a link between oestrogen-dependent breast cancer and the additionally glycosylated SHBG (Becchis et al. 1999; Fortunati et al. 1999).

A (TAAAA)(n) pentanucleotide repeat (normally n= 6-10), located within an Alu sequence at the 5' boundary of the human *SHBG* promoter, influences the transcriptional activity of the gene (Hogeveen et al. 2001) and could explain the individual differences in plasma SHBG levels and thereby influence the access of sex steroids to their target tissues. Very recently (Hogeveen et al. 2002), other *SHBG* variants (Pro156Leu) have been associated in women with low SHBG levels, hyperandrogenism and ovarian dysfunction. It remains to be shown whether there are associations of these polymorphisms with male physiology and pathophysiology.

Sex steroid hormones in both males and females have been closely related to the regulation of adiposity, either through direct or indirect physiological mechanisms. Evidence also suggests a direct relationship between sex hormones and risk factors for cardiovascular disease. A recent review (Tchernof and Despres 2000) discussed the complex interrelationships between sex hormones, SHBG, obesity and risk factors for cardiovascular disease. Male obesity and excess abdominal adipose tissue accumulation are associated with reduced gonadal and adrenal androgen levels. The alterations are also related to altered metabolic risk factor profile, including glucose intolerance and atherogenic dyslipidemic state. In both men and women, plasma levels of SHBG show strong correlation with obesity and risk factors for cardiovascular disease. More importantly, the relationships between low SHBG and altered plasma lipid levels appear to be independent of the concomitantly increased levels of visceral adipose tissue. In a study on the associations between CVD risk factors and sex hormones, *SHBG* was identified as the main predictive variable associated with atherogenic lipid profile in males, low T levels, and a high free androgen index (FAI; Gyllenborg et al. 2001). Males with high oestradiol levels may have a less atherogenic lipid profile and lower left ventricular mass (LVM). The SHBG concentration may, therefore, represent the most important and reliable marker of the sex hormone profile in the complex interrelation of sex steroid hormones, obesity, and cardiovascular disease risk. The role of the recently discovered *SHBG* polymorphisms (see above) in male endocrine functions is therefore worthy of exploring.

Luteinizing hormone β-subunit

The glycoprotein hormones, LH, FSH, hCG and TSH, are heterodimers consisting of two polypeptide subunits, α and β, that are associated through non-covalent interactions. The α-subunit is common for all glycoprotein hormones, whereas the β-subunit is hormone-specific and confers its biologic specificity. The luteinizing hormone β-subunit (LHβ), encoded by a gene on chromosome 19q13.32, is approximately 1.5 kb in length and consists of three exons and two introns (Fiddes and Talmadge 1984; Gharib et al. 1990).

Mutations in the *LHβ* are extremely rare; in fact, only one male with inactivating mutation has been described in the literature (Weiss et al. 1992). One *LHβ* polymorphism makes an exception; the variant allele has two point mutations leading to two amino acid substitutions, Trp8Arg and Ile15Thr. The first is mainly responsible for the altered immunoreactivity; the latter introduces an extra glycosylation site into Asn13 of the mutated LHβ peptide. The carrier frequency of this variant *LHβ* allele varies between 0 and >50% in various ethnic groups, being 10-20% in most Caucasian populations (Nilsson et al. 1997). The wide variability of frequency may imply that this polymorphism has offered an advantage in certain environments during human evolution (Nilsson et al. 1997, 1998; Huhtaniemi and Pettersson 1999; Huhtaniemi et al. 1999; Themmen and Huhtaniemi 2000). The variant form of LH possesses increased in vitro bioactivity, whereas its half-life in circulation is shorter in comparison to wild-type hormone, and the variant $LH\beta$ gene has additional changes in its promoter sequence (Jiang et al. 1999). Carriers of this variant gene are largely healthy, but certain mild differences in their gonadal function have been found, as reflected by alterations in gonadal steroidogenesis, pubertal development and predisposition to diseases such as infertility, PCOS, and breast cancer (Themmen and Huhtaniemi 2000; Lamminen and Huhtaniemi 2001). Pre- and postmenopausal women with variant LH had somewhat higher levels of serum androgens than wild-type controls (Rajkhowa et al. 1995; Hill et al. 2001).

A significant positive correlation between the type of LH, fat mass and serum leptin was observed in heterozygotes for the $LH\beta$ variant allele in an independently living population of elderly men, aged 73-94 (van den Beld et al. 1999). This finding may indicate that there is a difference in biological response between the two LH forms. T levels and the degrees of frailty were not different in the wild-type LH group compared with the heterozygotes LH variant group. The frailty was tightly related to LH, suggesting that LH levels reflect serum androgen activity in a different way than T, possibly reflecting more closely the combined feedback effect of estrogens and androgens.

Luteinizing hormone receptor (LHR)

LHR, together with the receptors of the other glycoprotein hormones (FSH and TSH), belongs to a subfamily of the seven transmembrane domain, G-protein-coupled receptors (Themmen and Huhtaniemi 2000). Human *FSHR* and *LHR* have been mapped to chromosome 2p21, and the *LHR* gene is encoded by 11 exons (Minegishi et al. 1990). The first ten exons encode the long, extracellular hormone-binding domain with a leucine-rich repeat structure, and the last (11th) exon encodes the heptahelical transmembrane domain, with intervening extra- and intracellular loops, and the intracellular tail. LHR function in men is necessary for the stimulation of Leydig cell androgen production and male genital differentiation, development and adult functions. Activating and inactivating *LHR* mutations have been identified in men. The former cause gonadotropin-independent, male-limited precocious puberty and the latter, in complete form, cause male pseudohermaphroditism (Themmen and Huhtaniemi 2000).

Several polymorphisms have been identified in the *LHR* gene. Base changes in intron 1 and exons 8 and 11 appear to be silent (Themmen and Huhtaniemi 2000; Richter-Unruh et al. 2002). The other three polymorphic sites cause a change in the receptor protein: an insertion of leucine-glutamine (LQ) at codon 18 of exon 1, Asn[291]Ser and Asn[312]Ser in exon 10 (Atger et al. 1995; Wu et al. 1998). The former of the two single amino acid substitutions also induces a loss of a

Vitamin D receptor (VDR)

The *VDR* belongs to the steroid hormone superfamily and its gene is located on chromosome 12q12-q14. There are some data that *VDR* polymorphisms affect the endocrine status of elderly men. Several lines of evidence suggest a potential role of vitamin D in prostatic growth (Taylor et al. 1996; Habuchi et al. 2000; Ingles et al. 1997a, 1998; Schatzl et al. 2001). There are several polymorphisms in the 3'-region of *VDR* that appear to be in linkage disequilibrium: specific intronic sites for *BsmI* (Morrison et al. 1992) and *ApaI* (Faraco et al. 1989), a silent *TaqI* site in exon 9 (Morrison et al. 1992), and a singlet (A) repeat in the portion of exon 9 encoding the 3'UTR (Ingles et al. 1997a). However, the strength of the linkage disequilibrium varies according to the ethnicity (Ingles et al. 1997b). The *VDR* polymorphisms have different effects on benign and malignant prostatic diseases (Taylor et al. 1996; Habuchi et al. 2000; Ingles et al. 1997a, 1998; Bousema et al. 2000). The *TaqI* and *ApaI* polymorphisms did not show significant association with either prostate cancer or benign prostatic hypertrophy (BPH), but absence of the *BsmI* restriction site reduced the risk of prostatic cancer to one-third (Habuchi et al. 2000).

The active metabolites of vitamin D play an important role in regulating bone cell function and the maintenance of serum calcium. Morrison et al. (1994) reported a significant association between polymorphisms in the 3' region of *VDR* and BMD in a population-based study and a twin study, and they concluded that the allelic variation of this gene may account for up to 75% of the genetic effect on BMD. However, a subsequent study showed that the effect of VDR on bone mass was much weaker than originally reported, due to genotyping errors (Gong et al. 1999). A large number of studies have subsequently been carried out on the relationships between VDR genotypes, bone density and other aspects of calcium metabolism (Stewart and Ralston 2000; Rizzoli et al. 2001). The evidence of haplotype-specific differences in transcription of *VDR* suggested that the *BsmI*, *ApaI* and *TaqI* polymorphisms might act as markers for other sequence variations in the 3'-UTR of *VDR* affecting RNA stability (Morrison et al. 1994). Another polymorphism in exon 2 of VDR, a T→C transition recognised by *FokI*, introduces an alternative translation start codon that results in a shorter isoform of the VDR protein (Langdahl et al. 2000b; Gross et al. 1998). There is a weak association between lumbar spine BMD and *FokI* restriction fragment length polymorphism at the translation initiation site of *VDR* of healthy Caucasian men (Kanan et al. 2000). The age, genetic background and gene-gene interactions may explain the inconsistent relationship between bone mass and VDR 3'- and 5'-genotypes. Significantly lower height was observed among women and men with VDR-3' BB compared with Bb or bb genotypes (Ferrari et al. 1999). An association was observed between the rate of bone loss at both the femoral neck and lumbar spine and the *TaqI* VDR polymorphism in dizygotic twin pairs and nuclear families (Brown et al. 2001). This association was strongest in those in the lowest tertile of calcium intake, also suggesting the presence of gene-environment interaction involving dietary calcium and VDR, influencing bone turnover. We can, at the moment, conclude that the allelic variation at the *VDR* gene locus has some role to play in the genetic regulation of bone mass. These effects appear to be modified by dietary calcium and vitamin D intake, and some studies show association with differences in intestinal calcium absorption (for reviews, see Stewart and Ralston 2000; Rizzoli et al. 2001). When examining the effects of calcium on BMD and bone modelling, *VDR* alleles could be one of the important factors explaining the variability observed in the population, but alone they do not provide clinically useful genetic markers for the risk of osteoporosis in the elderly.

Concluding remarks

The relevance of hormonal changes and ageing has been intensively studied in women, and more recently the same principles have been applied to men. The hormonal changes upon ageing contribute undoubtedly in both sexes to the common ageing-related complaints that impair the quality of life. Osteoporosis has only recently been recognised as a growing health problem, in men as well as in women. Low dietary calcium intake, weak muscle strength and low body weight are risk factors for low BMD in men. There is good evidence that the ageing-associated decrease in T levels is at least a co-determinant of these symptoms, and T supplementation has shown favourable effects on many of them. Side effects of this substitution therapy are minimal when care is taken to keep plasma T levels within the physiological range. However, it still remains unknown to what extent the declined T levels represent a physiological phenomenon and to what extent they represent a response to the stress caused by systemic diseases, a natural consequence of ageing. It also has to be kept in mind that testicular androgen production is not decreasing in isolation, but a similar downward trend occurs in most other endocrine systems, including the anterior pituitary, thyroid and pancreatic endocrine functions. It therefore sounds counterintuitive to concentrate our attention on only one endocrine system of the ageing male. When contemplating the need for hormonal replacement therapies, we also have to avoid the temptation to classify as a treatable and even curable "disease" something that represents the normal ageing phenomena of the human body.

One conspicuous feature of the ageing-related physiological and patho-physiological responses is their great individual variation. Besides environmental, life style and socio-economic factors, the genetic background of an individual undoubtedly plays a major role in ageing. There are also gender-specific features in the body's ageing response, and the most conspicuous factor in these differences is the different hormonal environments that the male and female bodies are exposed to during the life span. In the search for genetic components in the male-specific ageing phenomen, it is obvious that the endocrine regulatory systems related to testicular androgen production are being focussed on. As we have described above and summarised in Table 1, there are numerous polymorphisms in the key genes involved that outright alter the functions of the gene product or display an association with various phenomena of healthy or pathologic ageing of the male. Knowledge is still rather patchy and a great deal of new information is needed. However, it is possible that, with increasing knowledge

Table 1. A list of the gene polymorphisms that have been found to have association with the gender-specific normal or pathological ageing phenomena of men

Gene	Location	Polymorphisma	Phenotype	Key reference(s)
Androgen receptor	Exon 1	$(CAG)_n$	• Higher T with long repeats upon ageing	Krithivas et al. 1999
			• Repeat length correlates inversely with:	Edwards et al. 1992
			- risk of prostate cancer	
			- adverse lipid profile	
			- risk of coronary heart disease	Zitzmann et al. 2001a
			- spermatogenic failure	Tut et al. 1997
			- low bone mineral density	Zitzmann et al. 2001b
Oestrogen receptor α	Intron 1	PvuII	• Lower BMD in young men	Lorentzon et al. 1999
			• Smaller coronary artery lesions in autopsy	Lehtimäki et al. 2002
	Intron 1	XbaI	• Lower height in young men	Lorentzon et al. 1999
	Promoter	$(TA)_n$	• Reduces the risk of prostatic cancer	Modugno et al. 2001
			• Long repeats increase risk of:	Langdahl et al. 2000
			- osteoporotic fractures	Kunnas et al. 2000
			- risk of coronary artery disease	
17-Hydroxylase/ C17-20 lyase	Promoter	T→C transition	• C/C genotype increases:	Zmuda et al. 2001
			- serum bioavailable T	
			- the risk for prostatic cancer	Chang et al. 2001
			- stature	Haiman et al. 2001
Aromatase	Intron 4	(TTTA)n	• 8 and 12 repeats associated with increased prostatic cancer risk	Latil et al. 2001
5α-Reductase	Exon 1	Ala49Thr	• Risk of prostate cancer	Makridakis et al. 1999
	Exon 1	Val89Leu	• Leu[89] more common in low risk populations for	Hsing et al. 2001

Table 1. *Continued*

Gene	Location	Polymorphisma	Phenotype	Key reference(s)
LHβ Subunit	Promoter and Exon2	Multiple point mutations in promoter + Ttp8Arg/Ile15Thr	• Positive correlation of variant with obesity and serum leptin in ageing men	van den Beld et al. 1999
LH receptor	Exon1 Exon 10	LQ insertion Asn291Ser Asn312Ser	• Undermasculinisation with long *AR* CAG repeats • 291A/A + 312S/S genotype associated with under-masculinisation	Mongan et al. 2002
IGF-I	Promoter	CA repeat	• Absence of the wild-type (192 bp) allele increases risk of type II diabetes and myocardial infarction • 191/192 bp genotype associated with low serum IGF-I and osteoporosis	Vaessen et al. 2001 Rosen et al. 1998
Vitamin D receptor	3'-UTR Exon 2	BsmI FokI	• Increased risk of prostatic cancer • Lower height • Decreased BMD	Habuchi et al. 2000 Ferrari et al. 1999 Kanan et al. 2000

about genetic polymorphisms, we can explain the individual variability of certain aspects of the male gender-specific ageing phenomena at the genomic level. A major challenge will thereafter be how to use this information to promote healthy ageing of the male gender in practice.

References

Allen NE, Davey GK, Key TJ, Zhang S, Narod SA (2002) Serum insulin-like growth factor I (IGF-I) concentration in men is not associated with the cytosine-adenosine repeat polymorphism of the IGF-I gene. Cancer Epidemiol Biomarkers Prev 11: 319–320

Anderson FH, Francis RM, Selby PL, Cooper C (1998) Sex hormones and osteoporosis in men. Calcif Tissue Int 62:185–188

Asatiani K, Gromoll J, Eckardstein SV, Zitzmann M, Nieschlag E, Simoni M (2002) Distribution and function of FSH receptor genetic variants in normal men. Andrologia 34: 172–176

Atger M, Misrahi M, Sar S, Le Flem L, Dessen P and Milgrom E (1995) Structure of the human luteinizing hormone-choriogonadotropin receptor gene: unusual promoter and 5' non-coding regions. Mol Cell Endocrinol 111: 113–123

Balthazart J, Foidart A (1993) Brain aromatase and the control of male sexual behaviour. J Steroid Biochem Mol Biol 44: 521–540

Becchis M, Frairia R, Ferrera P, Fazzari A, Ondei S, Alfarano A, Coluccia C, Biglia N, Sismondi P, Fortunati N (1999) The additionally glycosylated variant of human sex hormone-binding globulin (SHBG) is linked to estrogen-dependence of breast cancer. Breast Cancer Res Treat 54: 101–107

Becherini L, Gennari L, Masi L, Mansani R, Massart F, Morelli A, Falchetti A, Gonnelli S. Fiorelli G, Tanini A, Brandi ML (2000) Evidence of a linkage disequilibrium between polymorphisms in the human estrogen receptor alpha gene and their relationship to bone mass variation in postmenopausal Italian women. Human Mol Genet 9: 2043–2050

Beilin J, Harewood L, Frydenberg M, Mameghan H, Martyres RF, Farish SJ, Yue C, Deam DR, Byron KA, Zajac JD (2001) A case-control study of the androgen receptor gene CAG repeat polymorphism in Australian prostate carcinoma subjects. Cancer 15: 941–949

Berube D, Seralini GE, Gagne R, Hammond GL (1990) Localization of the human sex hormone-binding globulin gene (SHBG) to the short arm of chromosome 17 (17p12-p13). Cytogenet Cell Genet 54: 65–67

Bousema JT, Bussemakers MJ, van Houwelingen KP, Debruyne FM, Verbeek AL, de La Rosette JJ, Kiemeney LA (2000) Polymorphisms in the vitamin D receptor gene and the androgen receptor gene and the risk of benign prostatic hyperplasia. Eur Urol 37: 234–238

Brown MA, Haughton MA, Grant SF, Gunnell AS, Henderson NK, Eisman JA (2001) Genetic control of bone density and turnover: role of the collagen 1alpha1, estrogen receptor, and vitamin D receptor genes. J Bone Miner Res 16: 758–764

Carani C, Qin K, Simoni M, Faustini-Fustini M, Serpente S, Boyd J, Korach KS, Simpson ER (1997) Effect of testosterone and estradiol in a man with aromatase deficiency. N Engl J Med 337: 91–95

Chang B, Zheng SL, Isaacs SD, Wiley KE, Carpten JD, Hawkins GA, Bleecker ER, Walsh PC, Trent JM, Meyers DA, Isaacs WB, Xu J (2001) Linkage and association of CYP17 gene in hereditary and sporadic prostate cancer. Int J Cancer 95: 354–359

Cheng ZN, Zhou HH (2000) Contribution of genetic variations in estradiol biosynthesis and metabolism enzymes to osteoporosis. Acta Pharmacol Sin 21: 587–590

Choong CS, Kemppainen JA, Zhou ZX, Wilson EM (1996) Reduced androgen receptor gene expression with first exon CAG repeat expansion. Mol Endocr 10: 1527–1535

Cousin P, Dechaud H, Grenot C, Lejeune H, Pugeat M (1998) Human variant sex hormone-binding globulin (SHBG) with an additional carbohydrate chain has a reduced clearance rate in rabbit. J Clin Endocrinol Metab 83: 235–240

Deladoey J, Fluck C, Bex M, Yoshimura N, Harada N, Mullis PE (1999) Aromatase deficiency caused by a novel P450arom gene mutation: impact of absent estrogen production on serum gonadotropin concentration in a boy. J Clin Endocrinol Metab 84:4050–4054

Deslypere JP, Young M, Wilson JD, McPhaul MJ (1992) Testosterone and 5 alpha-dihydro-testosterone interact differently with the androgen receptor to enhance transcription of the MMTV-CAT reporter gene. Mol Cell Endocrinol 88: 15–22

Ebeling PR (1998) Osteoporosis in men. New insights into aetiology, pathogenesis, prevention and management. Drugs Aging 13: 421–434

Edwards A, Hammond HA, Jin L, Caskey CT, Chakraborty R (1992) Genetic variation at five trimeric and tetrameric tandem repeat loci in four human population groups. Genomics 12: 241–253

Ellis JA, Stebbing M, Harrap SB (2001) Polymorphism of the androgen receptor gene is associated with male pattern baldness. J Invest Dermatol 116: 452–455

Faraco JH, Morrison NA, Baker A, Shine J, Frossard PM (1989) ApaI dimorphism at the human vitamin D receptor gene locus. Nucleic Acids Res 17: 2150

Feigelson HS, Shames LS, Pike MC, Coetzee GA, Stanczyk FZ, Henderson BE (1998) Cytochrome P450c17alpha gene (CYP17) polymorphism is associated with serum estrogen and progesterone concentrations. Cancer Res 58: 585–587

Ferrari S, Manen D, Bonjour JP, Slosman D, Rizzoli R (1999) Bone mineral mass and calcium and phosphate metabolism in young men: relationships with vitamin D receptor allelic polymorphisms. J Clin Endocrinol Metab 84: 2043–2048

Fiddes JC, Talmadge K (1984) Structure, expression, and evolution of the genes for the human glycoprotein hormones. Recent Prog Horm Res 40: 43–78

Fortunati N, Becchis M, Catalano MG, Comba A, Ferrera P, Raineri M, Berta L, Frairia R (1999) Sex hormone-binding globulin, its membrane receptor, and breast cancer: a new approach to the modulation of estradiol action in neoplastic cells. J Steroid Biochem Mol Biol 69 (1–6): 473–479

Frayling TM, Hattersley AT, McCarthy A, Holly J, Mitchell SM, Gloyn AL, Owen K, Davies D, Smith GD, Ben-Shlomo Y (2002) A putative functional polymorphism in the IGF-I gene: association studies with type 2 diabetes, adult height, glucose tolerance, and fetal growth in U.K. populations. Diabetes 51: 2313–2316

Gennari L, Brandi ML (2001) Genetics of male osteoporosis. Calcif Tissue Int 69: 200–204

George FW, Noble JF (1984) Androgen receptors are similar in fetal and adult rabbits. Endocrinology 115: 1451–1458

Gharib SD, Wierman ME, Shupnik MA and Chin WW (1990) Molecular biology of the pituitary gonadotropins. Endocr Rev 11: 177–199

Giovannucci E, Platz EA, Stampfer MJ, Chan A, Krithivas K, Kawachi I, Willett WC, Kantoff PW (1999) The CAG repeat within the androgen receptor gene and benign prostatic hyperplasia. Urology 53: 121–125

Gong G, Stern HS, Cheng SC, Fong N, Mordeson J, Deng HW, Recker RR (1999) The association of bone mineral density with vitamin D receptor gene polymorphisms. Osteoporos Int 9:55–64

Gross C, Krishnan AV, Malloy PJ, Eccleshall TR, Zhao XY, Feldman D (1998) The vitamin D receptor gene start codon polymorphism: a functional analysis of FokI variants. J Bone Miner Res 13: 1691–1699

Gsur A, Bernhofer G, Hinteregger S, Haidinger G, Schatzl G, Madersbacher S, Marberger M, Vutuc C, Micksche M (2000) A polymorphism in the CYP17 gene is associated with prostate cancer risk. Int J Cancer 87: 434–437

Gyllenborg J, Rasmussen SL, Borch-Johnsen K, Heitmann BL, Skakkebaek NE, Juul A (2001) Cardiovascular risk factors in men: The role of gonadal steroids and sex hormone-binding globulin. Metabolism 50: 882–888

Habuchi T, Suzuki T, Sasaki R, Wang L, Sato K, Satoh S, Akao T, Tsuchiya N, Shimoda N, Wada Y, Koizumi A, Chihara J, Ogawa O, Kato T (2000) Association of vitamin D receptor gene polymorphism with prostate cancer and benign prostatic hyperplasia in a Japanese population. Cancer Res 60: 305–308

Haiman CA, Stampfer MJ, Giovannucci E, Ma J, Decalo NE, Kantoff PW, Hunter DJ (2001) The relationship between a polymorphism in CYP17 with plasma hormone levels and prostate cancer. Cancer Epidemiol Biomarkers Prev 10: 743–748

Hammond GL, Bocchinfuso WP (1996) Sex hormone-binding globulin: gene organization and structure/function analyses. Horm Res 45: 197–201

Hardy DO, Carino C, Catterall JF, Larrea F (1995) Molecular characterization of a genetic variant of the steroid hormone-binding globulin gene in heterozygous subjects. J Clin Endocrinol Metab 80: 1253–1256

Hardy DO, Scher HI, Bogenreider T, Sabbatini P, Zhang ZF, Nanus DM, Catterall JF (1996) Androgen receptor CAG repeat lengths in prostate cancer: correlation with age of onset. J Clin Endocr Metab 81: 4400–4405

Hesse V, Jahreis G, Schambach H, Vogel H, Vilser C, Seewald HJ, Borner A, Deichl A (1994) Insulin-like growth factor I correlations to changes of the hormonal status in puberty and age. Exp Clin Endocrinol 102: 289–298

Hill M, Huhtaniemi IT, Hampl R, Starka L (2001) Genetic variant of luteinizing hormone: impact on gonadal steroid sex hormones in women. Physiol Res 50: 583–587

Hogeveen KN, Talikka M and Hammond GL (2001) Human sex hormone-binding globulin promoter activity is influenced by a (TAAAA)n repeat element within an Alu sequence. J Biol Chem 276: 36383–36390

Hogeveen KN, Cousin P, Pugeat M, Dewailly D, Soudan B, Hammond GL (2002) Human sex hormone-binding globulin variants associated with hyperandrogenism and ovarian dysfunction. J Clin Invest 109: 973–981

Hsing AW, Gao YT, Wu G, Wang X, Deng J, Chen YL, Sesterhenn IA, Mostofi FK, Benichou J, Chang C (2000) Polymorphic CAG and GGN repeat lengths in the androgen receptor gene and prostate cancer risk: a population-based case-control study in China. Cancer Res 15: 5111–5116

Hsing AW, Chen C, Chokkalingam AP, Gao YT, Dightman DA, Nguyen HT, Deng J, Cheng J, Sesterhenn IA (2001) Polymorphic markers in the SRD5A2 gene and prostate cancer risk: a population-based case-control study. Cancer Epidemiol Biomarkers Prev 10: 1077–1082

Huhtaniemi IT, Pettersson KS (1999) Alterations in gonadal steroidogenesis in individuals expressing a common genetic variant of luteinizing hormone. J Steroid Biochem Mol Biol 69: 281–285

Huhtaniemi I, Jiang M, Nilsson C, Pettersson K (1999) Mutations and polymorphisms in gonadotropin genes. Mol Cell Endocrinol 151 (1–2): 89–94

Huuskonen J, Vaisanen SB, Kroger H, Jurvelin C, Bouchard C, Alhava E, Rauramaa R (2000) Determinants of bone mineral density in middle aged men: a population-based study. Osteoporos Int 11: 702–708

Ingles SA, Ross RK, Yu MC, Irvine RA, La Pera G, Haile RW, Coetzee GA (1997a) Association of prostate cancer risk with genetic polymorphisms in vitamin D receptor and androgen receptor. J Natl Cancer Inst 89: 166–170

Ingles SA, Haile RW, Henderson BE, Kolonel LN, Nakaichi G, Shi CY, Yu MC, Ross RK, Coetzee GA (1997b) Strength of linkage disequilibrium between two vitamin D receptor markers in five ethnic groups: implications for association studies. Cancer Epidemiol Biomarkers Prev 6: 93–98

Ingles SA, Coetzee GA, Ross RK, Henderson BE, Kolonel LN, Crocitto L, Wang W, Haile RW (1998) Association of prostate cancer with vitamin D receptor haplotypes in African-Americans. Cancer Res 58: 1620–1623

Irvine RA, Yu MC, Ross RK, Coetzee GA (1995) The CAG and GGC microsatellites of the androgen receptor gene are in linkage disequilibrium in men with prostate cancer. Cancer Res 55: 1937–1940

Jaffe JM, Malkowicz SB, Walker AH, MacBride S, Peschel R, Tomaszewski J, Van Arsdalen K, Wein AJ, Rebbeck TR (2000) Association of SRD5A2 genotype and pathological characteristics of prostate tumors. Cancer Res 60: 1626–1630

Jiang M, Pakarinen P, Zhang FP, El-Hefnawy T, Koskimies P, Pettersson K, Huhtaniemi I (1999) A common polymorphic allele of the human luteinizing hormone beta-subunit gene: additional mutations and differential function of the promoter sequence. Hum Mol Genet 8: 2037–2046

Kanan RM, Varanasi SS, Francis RM, Parker L, Datta HK (2000) Vitamin D receptor gene start codon polymorphism (FokI) and bone mineral density in healthy male subjects. Clin Endocrinol (Oxf) 53: 93–98

Khosla S, Melton LJ 3rd, Riggs BL (2001) Estrogens and bone health in men. Calcif Tissue Int 69: 189–192

Kopp HP, Festa A, Krugluger W, Schernthaner G (2001) Low levels of Sex-Hormone-Binding Globulin predict insulin requirement in patients with gestational diabetes mellitus. Exp Clin Endocrinol Diabetes 109: 365–369

Krithivas K, Yurgalevitch SM, Mohr BA, Wilcox CJ, Batter SJ, Brown M, Longcope C, McKinlay JB, Kantoff PW (1999) Evidence that the CAG repeat in the androgen receptor gene is associated with the age-related decline in serum androgen levels in men. J Endocrinol 162: 137–142

Kunnas TA, Laippala P, Penttilä A, Lehtimäki T, Karhunen PJ (2000) Association of polymorphism of human alpha oestrogen receptor gene with coronary artery disease in men: a necropsy study. BMJ 29: 273–274

Kurland ES, Rosen CJ, Cosman F, McMahon D, Chan F, Shane E, Lindsay R, Dempster D, Bilezikian JP (1997) Insulin-like growth factor-I in men with idiopathic osteoporosis. J Clin Endocrinol Metab 82: 2799–2805

Kurland ES, Chan FK, Rosen CJ, Bilezikian JP (1998) Normal growth hormone secretory reserve in men with idiopathic osteoporosis and reduced circulating levels of insulin-like growth factor-I. J Clin Endocrinol Metab 83: 2576–2579

Lambert JC, Harris JM, Mann D, Lemmon H, Coates J, Cumming A, St-Clair D, Lendon C (2001) Are the estrogen receptors involved in Alzheimer's disease? Neurosci Lett 29: 193–197

Lamminen T, Huhtaniemi I (2001) A common genetic variant of luteinizing hormone; relation to normal and aberrant pituitary-gonadal function. Eur J Pharmacol 414: 1–7

Langdahl BL, Lokke E, Carstens M, Stenkjaer LL, Eriksen EF (2000a) A TA repeat polymorphism in the estrogen receptor gene is associated with osteoporotic fractures but polymorphisms in the first exon and intron are not. Bone Miner Res 5: 2222–2230

Langdahl BL, Gravholt CH, Brixen K, Eriksen EF (2000b) Polymorphisms in the vitamin D receptor gene and bone mass, bone turnover and osteoporotic fractures Eur J Clin Invest 30: 608–617

Lange EM, Chen H, Brierley K, Livermore H, Wojno KJ, Langefeld CD, Lange K, Cooney KA (2000) The polymorphic exon 1 androgen receptor CAG repeat in men with a potential inherited predisposition to prostate cancer. Cancer Epidemiol Biomarkers Prev 9: 439–442

Latil AG, Azzouzi R, Cancel GS, Guillaume EC, Cochan-Priollet B, Berthon PL, Cussenot O (2001) Prostate carcinoma risk and allelic variants of genes involved in androgen biosynthesis and metabolism pathways. Cancer 92: 1130–1137

Lehtimäki T, Kunnas TA, Mattila KM, Perola M, Penttila A, Koivula T, Karhunen PJ (2002) Coronary artery wall atherosclerosis in relation to the estrogen receptor 1 gene polymorphism: an autopsy study. J Mol Med 80: 176–180

Longcope C, Feldman HA, McKinlay JB, Araujo AB (2000) Diet and sex hormone-binding globulin. J Clin Endocrinol Metab 85: 293–296

Lorentzon M; Lorentzon R; Backstrom T; Nordstrom P (1999) Estrogen receptor gene polymorphism, but not estradiol levels, is related to bone density in healthy adolescent boys: a cross-sectional and longitudinal study. J Clin Endocr Metab 84: 4597–4601

Loy CJ, Yong EL (2001) Sex, infertility and the molecular biology of the androgen receptor. Curr Opin Obstet Gynecol 13: 315–321

Lunn RM, Bell DA, Mohler JL, Taylor JA (1999) Prostate cancer risk and polymorphism in 17 hydroxylase (CYP17) and steroid reductase (SRD5A2). Carcinogenesis 20: 1727–1731

Makridakis NM, Ross RK, Pike MC, Crocitto LE, Kolonel LN, Pearce CL, Henderson BE, Reichardt JK (1999) Association of mis-sense substitution in SRD5A2 gene with prostate cancer in African-American and Hispanic men. Lancet 354: 975–978

Makridakis NM, di Salle E, Reichardt JK (2000) Biochemical and pharmacogenetic dissection of human steroid 5 alpha-reductase type II. Pharmacogenetics 10: 407–413

Matsubara Y, Murata M, Kawano K, Zama T, Aoki N, Yoshino H, Watanabe G, Ishikawa K, Ikeda Y (1997) Genotype distribution of estrogen receptor polymorphisms in men and postmenopausal women from healthy and coronary populations and its relation to serum lipid levels. Arterioscler Thromb Vasc Biol 17: 3006–3012

Means GD, Mahendroo MS, Corbin CJ, Mathis JM, Powell FE, Mendelson CR, Simpson ER (1989) Structural analysis of the gene encoding human aromatase cytochrome P-450, the enzyme responsible for estrogen biosynthesis. J Biol Chem 264: 19385–19391

Mifsud A, Sim CK, Boettger-Tong H, Moreira S, Lamb DJ, Lipshultz LI, Yong EL (2001) Trinucleotide (CAG) repeat polymorphisms in the androgen receptor gene: molecular markers of risk for male infertility. Fertil Steril 75: 275–281

Minegishi T, Nakamura K, Takakura Y, Miyamoto K, Hasegawa Y, Ibuki Y, Igarashi M (1990) Cloning and sequencing of human LH/hCG receptor cDNA. Biochem Biophys Res Commun 172: 1049–1054

Miyao M, Hosoi T, Inoue S, Hoshino S, Shiraki M, Orimo H, Ouchi Y (1998) Polymorphism of insulin-like growth factor I gene and bone mineral density. Calcif Tissue Int 63: 306–311

Modugno F, Weissfeld JL, Trump DL, Zmuda JM, Shea P, Cauley JA, Ferrell RE (2001) Allelic variants of aromatase and the androgen and estrogen receptors: toward a multigenic model of prostate cancer risk. Clin Cancer Res 7: 3092-3096

Mongan NP, Hughes IA, Lim HN (2002) Evidence that luteinising hormone receptor polymorphisms may contribute to male undermasculinisation. Eur J Endocrinol 147: 103-107

Morishima A, Grumbach MM, Simpson ER, Fisher C, Qin K (1995) Aromatase deficiency in male and female siblings caused by a novel mutation and the physiological role of estrogens. J Clin Endocrinol Metab 80:3689-3698

Morrison NA, Yeoman R, Kelly PJ, Eisman JA (1992) Contribution of trans-acting factor alleles to normal physiological variability: vitamin D receptor gene polymorphism and circulating osteocalcin. Proc Natl Acad Sci USA 89: 6665–6669

Morrison NA, Qi JC, Tokita A, Kelly PJ, Crofts L, Nguyen TV, Sambrook PN, Eisman JA (1994) Prediction of bone density from vitamin D receptor alleles. Nature 367: 284–287

Nam RK, Toi A, Vesprini D, Ho M, Chu W, Harvie S, Sweet J, Trachtenberg J, Jewett MA, Narod SA (2001) V89L polymorphism of type-2, 5-alpha reductase enzyme gene predicts prostate cancer presence and progression. Urology 57: 199–204

Nelson KA, Witte JS (2002) Androgen receptor CAG repeats and prostate cancer. Am J Epidemiol 155: 883–890

Nilsson C, Pettersson K, Millar RP, Coerver KA, Matzuk MM, Huhtaniemi IT (1997) Worldwide frequency of a common genetic variant of luteinizing hormone: an international collaborative research. International Collaborative Research Group. Fertil Steril 67: 998–1004

Nilsson C, Jiang M, Pettersson K, Iitia A, Makela M, Simonsen H, Easteal S, Herrera RJ, Huhtaniemi I (1998) Determination of a common genetic variant of luteinizing hormone using DNA hybridization and immunoassays. Clin Endocrinol (Oxf) 49: 369–376

Pelletier G, El-Alfy M (2000) Immunocytochemical localization of estrogen receptors alpha and beta in the human reproductive organs. J Clin Endocr Metab 85: 4835–4840

Pirwany IR, Fleming R, Greer IA, Packard CJ, Sattar N (2001) Lipids and lipoprotein subfractions in women with PCOS: relationship to metabolic and endocrine parameters. Clin Endocrinol (Oxf) 54: 447–453

Ponglikitmongkol M; Green S; Chambon P (1988) Genomic organization of the human oestrogen receptor gene. EMBO J 7: 3385–3388

Power SG, Bocchinfuso WP, Pallesen M, Warmels-Rodenhiser S, Van Baelen H, Hammond GL (1992) Molecular analyses of a human sex hormone-binding globulin variant: evidence for an additional carbohydrate chain. J Clin Endocrinol Metab 75: 1066–1070

Rajkhowa M, Talbot JA, Jones PW, Pettersson K, Haavisto AM, Huhtaniemi I and Clayton RN (1995) Prevalence of an immunological LH beta-subunit variant in a UK population of healthy women and women with polycystic ovary syndrome. Clin Endocrinol (Oxf) 43: 297–303

Richter-Unruh A, Martens JW, Verhoef-Post M, Wessels HT, Kors WA, Sinnecker GH, Boehmer A, Drop SL, Toledo SP, Brunner HG, Themmen AP (2002) Leydig cell hypoplasia: cases with new mutations, new polymorphisms and cases without mutations in the luteinizing hormone receptor gene. Clin Endocrinol (Oxf) 56: 103–112

Rizzoli R, Bonjour JP, Ferrari SL (2001) Osteoporosis, genetics and hormones. J Mol Endocrinol 26: 79–94

Rodien P, Costagliola S, Tonacchera M, Duprez L, Minegishi T, Govaerts C, Vassart G (1998) Evidences for an allelic variant of the human LC/CG receptor rather than a gene duplication: functional comparison of wild-type and variant receptors. J Clin Endocrinol Metab 83: 4431–4434

Rosen CJ, Kurland ES, Vereault D, Adler RA, Rackoff PJ, Craig WY, Witte S, Rogers J, Bilezikian JP (1998) Association between serum insulin growth factor-I (IGF-I) and a simple sequence repeat in IGF-I gene: implications for genetic studies of bone mineral density. J Clin Endocrinol Metab 83: 2286–2290

Schatzl G, Gsur A, Bernhofer G, Haidinger G, Hinteregger S, Vutuc C, Haitel A, Micksche M, Marberger M, Madersbacher S (2001) Association of vitamin D receptor and 17 hydroxylase gene polymorphisms with benign prostatic hyperplasia and benign prostatic enlargement. Urology 57: 567–572

Schoenberg MP, Hakimi J M, Wang S, Bova GS, Epstein JI, Fischbeck KH, Isaacs WB, Walsh PC, Barrack ER (1994) Microsatellite mutation (CAG (24-to-18)) in the androgen receptor gene in human prostate cancer Biochem. Biophys Res Commun 198: 74–80

Simoni M, Gromoll J, Hoppner W, Kamischke A, Krafft T, Stahle D, Nieschlag E (1999) Mutational analysis of the follicle-stimulating hormone (FSH) receptor in normal and infertile men: identification and characterization of two discrete FSH receptor isoforms. J Clin Endocrinol Metab 84: 751–755

Simoni M, Nieschlag E, Gromoll J (2002) Isoforms and single nucleotide polymorphisms of the FSH receptor gene: implications for human reproduction. Hum Reprod Update 8: 413–421

Simpson ER (1998) Genetic mutations resulting in estrogen insufficiency in the male. Mol Cell Endocrinol 145: 55–59

Smith EP, Boyd J, Frank GR, Takahashi H, Cohen RM, Specker B, Williams TC, Lubahn DB, Korach KS (1994) Estrogen resistance caused by a mutation in the estrogen-receptor gene in a man. N Engl J Med 332:131

Steers WD (2001) 5alpha-reductase activity in the prostate. Urology 58 (6 Suppl 1): 17–24; discussion 24

Stein B, Ashok S (2002) Osteoporosis and the aging male. Med Health R I 85: 160–162

Stewart TL, Ralston SH (2000) Role of genetic factors in the pathogenesis of osteoporosis. J Endocrinol 166: 235–245

Takacs I, Koller DL, Peacock M, Christian JC, Hui SL, Conneally PM, Johnston CC Jr, Foroud T, Econs MJ (1999) Sibling pair linkage and association studies between bone mineral density and the insulin-like growth factor I gene locus. J Clin Endocrinol Metab 84: 4467–4471

Tapanainen JS, Aittomaki K, Jiang M, Vaskivuo T, Huhtaniemi I T (1997) Men homozygous for an inactivating mutation of the follicle-stimulating hormone (FSH) receptor gene present variable suppression of spermatogenesis and fertility. Nature Genet 15: 205–206

Taylor JA, Hirvonen A, Watson M, Pittman G, Mohler JL, Bell DA (1996) Association of prostate cancer with vitamin D receptor gene polymorphism. Cancer Res 56: 4108–4110

Tchernof A, Despres JP (2000) Sex steroid hormones, sex hormone-binding globulin, and obesity in men and women. Horm Metab Res 32: 526–536

Themmen AP, Huhtaniemi I (2000) Mutations of gonadotropins and gonadotropin receptors: elucidating the physiology and pathophysiology of pituitary-gonadal function. Endocr Rev 21: 551–583

Toda K, Terashima M, Kawamoto T, Sumimoto H, Yokoyama Y, Kuribayashi I, Mitsuuchi Y, Maeda T, Yamamoto Y, Sagara Y, et al. (1990) Structural and functional characterization of human aromatase P-450 gene. Eur J Biochem 193: 559–565

Tricoli JV, Rall LB, Scott J, Bell GI, Shows TB (1984) Localization of insulin-like growth factor genes to human chromosomes 11 and 12. Nature 310: 784–786

Tsai-Morris CH, Geng Y, Buczko E, Dehejia A, Dufau ML (1999) Genomic distribution and gonadal mRNA expression of two human luteinizing hormone receptor exon 1 sequences in random populations. Human Hered 49: 48–51

Tut TG, Ghadessy FJ, Trifiro MA, Pinsky L, Yong EL (1997) Long polyglutamine tracts in the androgen receptor are associated with reduced trans-activation, impaired sperm production, and male infertility. J Clin Endocr Metab 82: 3777–3782

Ukkola O, Gagnon J, Rankinen T, Thompson PA, Hong Y, Leon AS, Rao DC, Skinner JS, Wilmore JH, Bouchard C (2001) Age, body mass index, race and other determinants of steroid hormone variability: the HERITAGE Family Study. Eur J Endocrinol 145: 1–9

Vaessen N, Heutink P, Janssen JA, Witteman JC, Testers L, Hofman A, Lamberts SW, Oostra BA, Pols HA, van Duijn CM (2001) A polymorphism in the gene for IGF-I: functional properties and risk for type 2 diabetes and myocardial infarction. Diabetes 50: 637–642

Vaessen N, Janssen JA, Heutink P, Hofman A, Lamberts SW, Oostra BA, Pols HA, van Duijn CM (2002) Association between genetic variation in the gene for insulin-like growth factor-I and low birthweight. Lancet 359: 1036–1037

Van den Beld A, Huhtaniemi IT, Pettersson KS, Pols HA, Grobbee DE, de Jong FH, Lamberts SW (1999) Luteinizing hormone and different genetic variants, as indicators of frailty in healthy elderly men. J Clin Endocrinol Metab 84: 1334–1339

Van Pottelbergh I, Lumbroso S, Goemaere S, Sultan C, Kaufman JM (2001) Lack of influence of the androgen receptor gene CAG-repeat polymorphism on sex steroid status and bone metabolism in elderly men. Clin Endocrinol (Oxf) 55: 659–666

Vermeulen A (2002) Ageing, hormones, body composition, metabolic effects. World J Urol 20: 23–27

Vermeulen A, Kaufman JM (1995) Ageing of the hypothalamo-pituitary-testicular axis in men. Horm Res 43: 25–28

Vermeulen A, Kaufman JM, Goemaere S, van Pottelberg I (2002) Estradiol in elderly men. Aging Male 5: 98–102

Waterman MR, Keeney DS (1992) Genes involved in androgen biosynthesis and the male phenotype. Horm Res 38: 217–221

Weiss J, Axelrod L, Whitcomb RW, Harris PE, Crowley WF, Jameson JL (1992) Hypogonadism caused by a single amino acid substitution in the beta subunit of luteinizing hormone. N Engl J Med 326: 179–183

Wortsman J, Khan MS, Rosner W (1986) Suppression of testosterone-estradiol binding globulin by medroxyprogesterone acetate in polycystic ovary syndrome. Obstet Gynecol 67: 705–709

Wu SM, Jose M, Hallermeier K, Rennert OM, Chan WY (1998) Polymorphisms in the coding exons of the human luteinizing hormone receptor gene. Human Mutat 11: 333–334. Mutations in brief no. 124. Online

Yamada Y, Watanabe M, Murata M, Yamanaka M, Kubota Y, Ito H, Katoh T, Kawamura J, Yatani R, Shiraishi T (2001) Impact of genetic polymorphisms of 17-hydroxylase cytochrome P-450 (CYP17) and steroid 5alpha-reductase type II (SRD5A2) genes on prostate-cancer risk among the Japanese population. Int J Cancer 92: 683–686

Zitzmann M, Brune M, Kornmann B, Gromoll J, von Eckardstein S, von Eckardstein A, Nieschlag E (2001a) The CAG repeat polymorphism in the AR gene affects high density lipoprotein cholesterol and arterial vasoreactivity. J Clin Endocrinol Metab 86: 4867–4873

Zitzmann M, Brune M, Kornmann B, Gromoll J, Junker R, Nieschlag E (2001b) The CAG repeat polymorphism in the androgen receptor gene affects bone density and bone metabolism in healthy males. Clin Endocrinol (Oxf) 55: 649–657

Zmuda JM, Cauley JA, Kuller LH, Ferrell RE (2001) A common promotor variant in the cytochrome P450c17alpha (CYP17) gene is associated with bioavailability testosterone levels and bone size in men. J Bone Miner Res 16: 911–917

Age-related Changes in the Regulation of the Hypothalamic-Pituitary Adrenal Axis: The Role of Personality Variables

Jens C Pruessner[1,2], Catherine Lord[1,2], Robert Renwick[2], Michael Meaney[1] and Sonia Lupien[1]

Summary

The hypothalamic-pituitary adrenal (HPA) axis is one of the most important endocrine stress systems in humans. The HPA axis is activated upon the advent of a stressor, and as a consequence a cascade of hormones is released that serve different functions throughout the human organism, generally aimed at providing the necessary metabolic and immunomodulatory adjustments in response to a physiological or psychological stressor.

Basal secretion of the endproduct of the HPA axis, cortisol, follows a circadian rhythm, with the highest levels early in the morning and the lowest levels at night. Moreover, when released in response to stress, cortisol induces a negative feedback in the central nervous system (CNS) to terminate activity of the HPA axis when the stressor is no longer present. This normalization of activity is believed necessary to protect the organism from the long-term detrimental effects of chronic activation of the HPA axis.

Normal aging is accompanied by a number of changes in the regulation and activity of the HPA axis. Basal cortisol levels, especially at night around the time of the nadir, are increased, and feedback sensitivity to cortisol at different levels of the CNS is decreased.

The hippocampus is discussed as one of the structures involved in the changes of HPA regulation with aging. Receptors for glucocorticoids are primarily located in the hippocampus, and recent evidence suggests that basal cortisol and ACTH levels might be inversely associated with hippocampal volume, and thus might be at the origin of the age-related changes. Moreover, it has been shown that the inhibitory effect of glucocorticoid feedback on subsequent activity of the HPA axis is diminished in elderly subjects. Recently, we investigated cortisol levels during human aging together with CNS structures and personality variables. It appears that aging is not predictive of HPA axis regulation and structural CNS changes per se, but that specific personality types are less affected by age-related changes of the CNS and HPA axis regulation.

---

[1] Douglas Hospital Research Center, Brain Imaging Division, McGill University, Montreal, Canada

[2] McConnell Brain Imaging Center, Montreal Neurological Institute, McGill University, Montreal, Canada

Chanson et al.
Endocrine Aspects of Successful Aging
© Springer-Verlag Berlin Heidelberg 2004

The hypothalamic-pituitary adrenal axis

The hypothalamic-pituitary adrenal axis (HPA) is activated when the homeostasis of the organism is threatened. It is one of the endocrine systems that reacts to physical, pharmacological and psychosocial stressors. Besides the sympathetic nervous system, it is the most important system to guarantee adaptation and survival of the organism upon the advent of a stressor in both humans and rodents. The major components of the axis lie both within and outside of the brain: The hypothalamus releases corticotropin-releasing factor (CRF) upon perception of a stressor. CRF travels to the pituitary via the hypothalamus-median eminence pathway. In the pituitary, it triggers the release of adrenocorticotropic hormone (ACTH) into the portal circulation; ACTH uses the bloodstream to reach the adrenal cortex, where synthesis and release of cortisol are stimulated. These hormones have a variety of effects on the organism that can be differentiated into permissive, stimulatory, suppressive, and preparative actions (Sapolsky et al. 2000). The areas that are sensitive to glucocorticoid presence include immunity, inflammation, metabolism, neural function, behavior, and reproduction. For example, the glucose metabolism in non-essential peripheral tissue is inhibited, whereas the glucose supply to essential tissues is maintained. Gluconeogenesis and insulin resistance are augmented, whereas lipolysis, proteolysis and inflammation are inhibited. Whether glucocorticoids take stimulatory or suppressive actions in the organism depends on the concentration, the time course, and the target area.

Cortisol has the ability to cross the blood-brain barrier. Within the CNS, it reduces the activity of the HPA axis by occupying mineralcorticoid (MR) and glucocorticoid (GR) receptors in the hippocampus and frontal lobes, which then serve to inhibit subsequent hypothalamus activity and CRF release (De Kloet et al. 1998).

Besides the peak concentrations of cortisol, which are reached after stress, the secretion of cortisol follows a circadian rhythm. The highest levels of cortisol (the acrophase) are usually found in the morning around the time of awakening and immediately thereafter. Cortisol levels then gradually decrease until around noon, when a second peak can be observed around lunchtime. During the afternoon and evening, cortisol levels continually decline, with the lowest levels (the nadir) found around midnight. Besides this circadian rhythm, circavigintan, circatrigintan, and circaannual rhythms of cortisol have been described, reflecting seasonal effects and menstrual phase influences on HPA axis activity in women (Haus and Touitou 1994). Furthermore, the secretion of cortisol also follows a pulsatile pattern, with up to 15 distinct pulses per hour. These constant variations in hormone levels make exact measurement of HPA axis regulation difficult. Special strategies have thus been developed for precise determination, including repeated measurements of cortisol levels with up to 10-minute intervals throughout the 24-hour period, challenging the HPA axis with pharmacological agents or psychosocial stimuli to assess cortisol reactivity, or assessing activity of the axis at times with high reliability (early in the morning around the acrophase of the axis, or late in the evening, when the nadir is approached; Van Cauter et al. 1990; Kirschbaum et al. 1993; Pruessner et al. 1997).

HPA axis regulation and normal aging

Normal aging is accompanied by a number of subtle but consistent changes in the regulation and activity of the HPA axis. In older age, the amplitude of the circadian rhythm of basal cortisol appears to be reduced, caused by either lower levels in the morning during the time of the acrophase, or higher levels in the evening, around the time of the nadir (Van Cauter et al. 1996; van Coevorden et al. 1991). Furthermore, an interaction of gender with aging has been described: while in younger subjects, men usually show the strongest responses to psychosocial stress, recent studies demonstrated that women tend to show stronger responses in older age (Seeman and Robbins 1994). For basal levels, it has been reported that, with aging, women show stronger increases in the morning during the time of the acrophase (van Coevorden et al. 1991).

In addition, the feedback sensitivity of the HPA axis is reduced in older age, which might be directly related to the finding of higher basal cortisol levels. It can be speculated that, with compromised feedback, inhibition of subsequent HPA axis activity is less effective and thus higher cortisol levels might result (Wilkinson et al. 1997; Boscaro et al. 1998). Figure 1 shows the global changes associated with normal aging and the components of the HPA axis to be likely involved in these changes.

Effects of HPA axis regulation changes on the hippocampus

The hippocampus (HC), an important structure for memory and learning, is implicated in the changes of the regulation of the HPA axis that occur with aging. The HC normally exerts a regulatory function on HPA axis activity through MR and GR receptors, which inhibit the subsequent release of CRF from the hypothalamus.

Since glucocorticoids have been found to be neurotoxic in both rodents and humans, excessive activation of the HPA axis or cumulative activation of the axis throughout a lifetime can damage hippocampal tissue. In animals, hypersecretion of glucocorticoids leads to dendritic atrophy, especially in the CA3 region of the hippocampus (Magarinos and McEwen, 1995 a,b; Magarinos et al. 1996). The impaired integrity of the HC is then believed to result in decreased inhibition of CRF release from the hypothalamus and thus a less effective downregulation of HPA axis activity. This system of impairment that subsequently promotes further damage has been named the "glucocorticoid cascade hypothesis" and is one mechanism to explain the age-related changes of HPA axis regulation in humans (Sapolsky et al. 1986).

Direct evidence for the link between HPA axis regulation and hippocampal integrity in humans stems from recent studies showing that basal cortisol and ACTH levels are inversely associated with hippocampal volume (Wolf et al. 2002). Earlierstudies showed that acute or chronic increases in cortisol levels, either through psychosocial stress or pharmacological stimulation, lead to declined memory performance in cognitive tasks, suggesting that acute or chronic effects of occupation of GR receptors in the HC can impair memory processing in the HC (Kirschbaum, et al. 1995, 1996).

Individual differences in the association between HPA axis changes and aging and their consequence on HC volume and memory performance.

Recently, evidence emerged for a dynamic association between changes of the HPA axis regulation with aging and decline of hippocampal volume. First, it was shown that individual differences of HPA axis regulation changes with age exist, with subgroups in comparable age ranges demonstrating a progressive increase or decrease of cortisol levels. The subjects who exhibited a progressive increase could be further divided into those with already high baseline cortisol levels and those where baseline levels were in the moderate range, suggesting that the increase of basal levels might have started earlier or was progressing

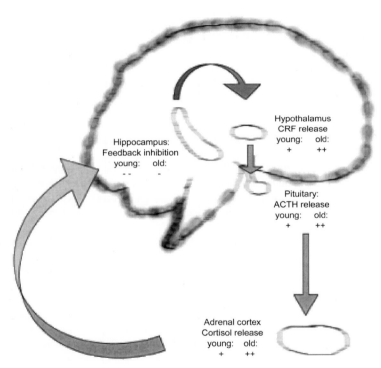

Fig. 1. Global changes of HPA axis functioning and regulation associated with normal aging. In general, aging is associated with a decrease of amplitude in basal cortisol levels and reductions in feedback sensitivity of the HPA axis. This combination leads to higher levels in the time of the nadir of the rhythm. The normal inhibitory action of glucocorticoids at the level of the hippocampus might be reduced in older age, thus leading to higher subsequent CRF release from the hypothalamus. This increased release in turn leads to a higher release of ACTH from the pituitary and higher release of cortisol from the adrenal cortex. Note that each of the components has its own feedback mechanisms and is probably involved in this changed regulation as well.

faster for part of the group. The existence of individuals with decreasing cortisol levels suggests that protective effects might exist that prevent the occurrence of the normally observed changes with aging. Alternatively, the results could also point to the existence of larger than circaannual rhythms of HPA axis regulation; however, a longitudinal study design is necessary to investigate this hypothesis. (Lupien et al. 1997).

Hippocampal volume in subjects with a progressive increase of cortisol levels turned out to be significantly smaller when compared to the group with decreasing cortisol levels and currently moderate cortisol levels, providing further evidence for a link between glucocorticoid exposure and structural integrity of HC (Lupien et al. 1998). However, it remains to be seen whether the acutely high or the chronically elevated cortisol levels are causally linked to the decrease in brain volume.

Interestingly, the individual differences in HPA axis regulation were also related to differences in cognitive functioning in these individuals. The subgroup of subjects who showed a progressive increase of cortisol levels with already high baseline levels showed significant impairments in HC-dependent forms of memory when comparing their cognitive levels with those of the other two groups, suggesting that the higher levels of cortisol also had an effect on cognitive functioning. This finding supports results from animal studies showing that persistent high levels of cortisol can lead to a reduction of hippocampal volume together with an impairment in cognitive functioning (McEwen 1997, 1998a). Variables determining individual differences of HPA axis regulation changes with aging.

Recent results from our group (Lupien et al. 1998) and other groups (Wolf et al. 2002) suggest that aging is not predictive of HPA axis regulation and structural CNS changes per se. In recent studies, we found that differences in locus of control seem to modulate HPA axis reactivity under conditions of acute (Pruessner et al. 1998) and chronic stress (Pruessner et al. 1999). First, we observed how, in young college students, external locus of control predicted the individual ability of subjects to habituate their cortisol response when repeatedly exposed to the same type of psychosocial stressor. In this study, one third of the subjects emerged with high external locus of control and low self-esteem, which demonstrated persistent high cortisol responses when exposed to the same psychosocial stressor for a total of five times. In comparison, the rest of the group, with average-to-low external locus of scores, habituated quickly and did not show significant cortisol responses to the stress after the second exposure (Kirschbaum et al. 1995).

We concluded at the time that one of the major characteristics of psychosocial stress – controllability of the situation – remained low in the subjects with high external locus of control, and thus the situation remained uncontrollable for them throughout the experiment. For the subjects with low-to-average external locus of control scores, however, the situation soon became predictable and thus was no longer perceived as stressful. We continued to investigate the impact of these individual differences in a study where we investigated the impact of experimentally induced failure on the individual stress response in a group experiment implementing a mental challenge task. Interestingly, the failure condition was not predictive of a higher cortisol response per se, but only in conjunction with an unfavorable set of stress-related personality factors, i.e., high external and low internal loci of control.

In a study with teachers suffering from burnout, the long-term effects of these personality factors were investigated. Although the endocrinological literature is sparse in this field, burnout seems to be associated with an endocrine profile similar to that seen in chronic fatigue syndrome: lower-than-normal cortisol levels combined with supersuppression of cortisol after an overnight, low-dose dexamethasone treatment.

In a recent study, we tested the potentially modulating effect of different levels of self-esteem on the effects of aging on endocrine, cognitive and brain volume variables. We examined a group of 20 healthy elderly subjects (mean age, 69.8 ± 7.8 years, range 60–84 years) living in the community, who were screened using sociodemographic and personality questionnaires. We used tests for global cognitive functioning and declarative memory (Alzheimer's disease assessment scale – cognitive subscale, ADAS-cog) that have been described in the literature as sensitive to pick up age-related cognitive decline (Molloy and Standish 1997; Teng et al. 1989; Rosen 1982). A medical record for all subjects ensured that no history of depression or other psychiatric illnesses was present.

For the investigation of volume of selected brain structures, we performed high-resolution 3D Magnetic Resonance (MR) Imaging scanning. All MR scans were standardized and coregistered using automatic segmentation protocols (Sled et al. 1998; Collins et al. 1994; Talairach and Tournoux 1988). Structures were quantified from the coregistered MR images using semi-automatic and manual segmentation protocols (Collins and Evans 1999; Pruessner et al. 2000, 2003). Temporal and frontal lobe structures for both left and right hemisphere were quantified, including HC and amygdala.

For assessment of the HPA axis, a monthly screening was performed with all subjects. Subjects were asked to provide saliva samples throughout the day for a period of 12 months at a specified day once a month. Cortisol assessment included the time immediately after awakening, which has been established as a marker of HPA axis regulation (Pruessner et al. 1997).

We found that, in the total group, age was negatively correlated with cognitive performance and brain volumes, as quantified from the structural MR. The correlation of age with volumes of brain structures and cognitive measures varied from $r = -0.52$ to $r = -0.68$ (all $p<0.05$). These correlations between age and reduction of global brain volume and age and cognitive performance are in line with previous studies demonstrating the effects of age on cognitive decline (Celsis 2000; O'Sullivan et al. 2001) and brain volume reduction (Jernigan et al. 1990; Ge et al. 2002).

To test the effects of self-esteem on the reported measures, subjects were split into two groups with high and low self-esteem (Wishart 1998). Effects of age on endocrine, brain and psychological variables were then investigated separately within the two groups. There was no difference in age between the two groups with high and low self-esteem, ensuring that subsequent findings were not confounded by general effects of age.

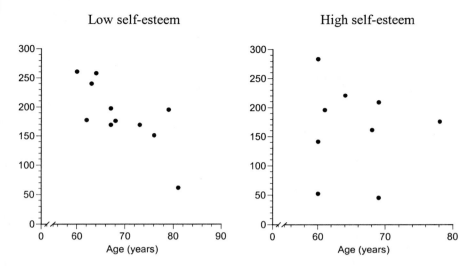

Fig. 2. Subjects with low and high self-esteem differed significantly with advancing age in their cortisol response to awakening. While a negative correlation with age was observed for the cortisol response to awakening in the low self-esteem group ($r = -0.75$ p >0.001), no such correlation could be seen in the high self-esteem group ($r = -0.20$, n.s.).

In the low self-esteem group, subjects showed a strong decline of cortisol levels after awakening with age, whereas this association was not present in the high self-esteem group. This result suggests that higher age was associated with lower cortisol responses to awakening and with a flattening of the circadian rhythm of HPA axis regulation only in the low-self esteem group. Figure 2 shows the scatterplot between age and the aggregated cortisol response to awakening over the observation period in the two groups of subjects with high and low self-esteem.

Furthermore, we observed that a reduction of cognitive function with age could no longer be observed in the high self-esteem group, whereas it was highly significant in the low self-esteem group. Figure 3 shows the scatterplot between the measure of cognitive assessment as used in this study and age for the two groups.

Finally, similar results emerged for the CNS variables, where correlations of age with total brain gray matter and left and right HC were highly significant for the low-self esteem group but failed to show significant associations in the high self-esteem group. The differences between the two groups were substantial, with age being correlated to $r = 0.65$ with total brain gray matter and $r = 0.76$ with the HC in the low self-esteem subjects (all $p < 0.01$), whereas the correlations of age with total brain gray matter ($r = 0.31$) and hippocampus ($r = 0.40$) in the high self-esteem group did not reach significance. Figure 4 shows the scatterplots between age and the hippocampal volume in the two groups.

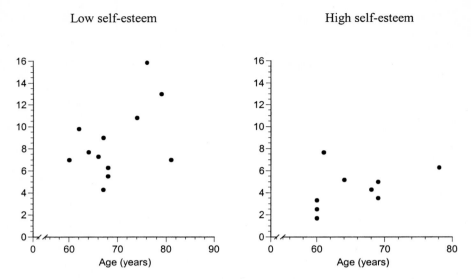

Fig. 3. Subjects with low and high self esteem differed significantly in the correlation of cognitive impairment with age (low self-esteem: r = 0.68, p > 0.01; high self esteem: r = 0.32, n.s.)

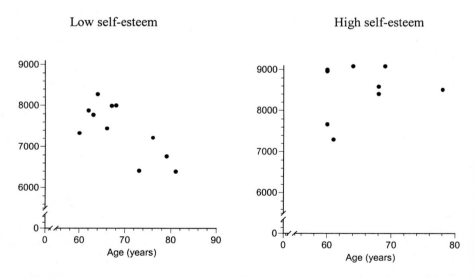

Fig. 4. Subjects with low and high self esteem differed significantly in the correlation of hippocampal volume with age (low self-esteem: r = 0.76, p > 0.01; high self esteem: r = 0.12, n.s.)

Discussion

In humans, age is associated with global changes on different levels. The HPA axis is one system that is affected by these changes. In general, it appears that advancing age is associated with a flattening of the circadian rhythm, as indicated by increased basal and ACTH levels in the evening and decreased levels in the morning (Van Cauter et al. 1996; Dodt et al. 1994). Moreover, the fast feedback inhibition of glucocorticoids on ACTH secretion is reduced with advancing age, suggesting that age might have an impact on HPA axis regulation at different levels (Boscaro et al. 1998).

Furthermore, there are several studies that have shown an association between age-related changes of HPA regulation and hippocampal volume and cognitive functioning, suggesting that the changes in the regulation of the HPA axis are not without consequences for the functioning and structure of the brain (Wolf et al. 2002; Lupien et al. 1998).

Investigations of age-related changes in humans need to take individual differences into consideration. The observation of cognitive decline and global deterioration with aging prompts the question of whether physical, psychological or environmental conditions exist where these changes are minimized or nonexistent. Endocrinologically, the recent studies investigating the effects of Dehydroepiandrosterone (DHEA) are a good example of the search for variables that potentially effect age-related changes (Wolf et al. 1997). In neurochemistry, the identification of risk genes that promote specific age-related diseases, like the APO-E4 gene for the development of Alzheimer's disease, is another good example of this line of research. Psychologically, it appears that personality variables like locus of control, self-concept, and self-esteem might contribute to individual differences in age-related changes in humans. In our group of healthy elderly people living in the community, the effects of age were clearly modulated by the aforementioned group of variables. This effect was quite strong, since age normally is one of the strongest predictors of reduction of gray matter and cognitive decline.

This considerable effect of a specific personality style allows speculation about the protective effect of some personality types against the effects of aging. First, the major concern of cause and effect needs to be addressed. If other factors are contributing to the observed cognitive decline with aging, then the perception of reduced cognitive abilities might have an effect on the personality of the individual, especially on self-esteem and locus of control. While this possibility cannot be excluded in the current study, the earlier observation of differences in stress responses based on differences in self-esteem in younger subjects suggests that this mechanism is not sufficient to explain all results (Pruessner et al. 1998; Kirschbaum et al. 1995).

It seems reasonable to propose that one possible mechanism by which self-esteem protects against the effects of age is through the perception of stress. With low self-esteem, subjects are prone to experience higher amounts of stress, independent of the specific type of stressor. Problems of comparable complexity will be experienced as more difficult in low self-esteem subjects due to a higher uncertainty about personal capabilities and potentials. The resulting increased stress load might lead to a higher frequency of HPA axis activation in the stressful situation, which – when accumulated over a lifetime – might have the effects discussed within the allostatic load model, i.e., increased wear and tear on the organism at different levels (McEwen 1998b, 2001). The findings of different regulation of the HPA axis after awakening in the low self-esteem subjects fits this hypothesis: similar observations of lower-than-average cortisol responses to awakening were recently made in teachers suffering from burnout and chronic stress. Interestingly, teachers with low self-esteem were more likely to be affected by burnout than teachers with high self-esteem.

Taken together, the observed effects of self-esteem could serve as the mechanism by which the effects of aging on cognition and brain integrity are either attenuated or augmented. In animal models, atrophy of the HC is mediated, at least in part, by toxic levels of glucocorticoids circulating in the CNS. Lifelong differences in the perception of stress, and discrepancies in coping styles due to differences in self-esteem, might lead to systematic variations in HPA axis regulation, which might have an effect on the integrity of the CNS.

References

Boscaro M, Paoletta A, Scarpa E, Barzon L, Fusaro P, Fallo F, Sonino N (1998) Age-related changes in glucocorticoid fast feedback inhibition of adrenocorticotropin in man. J Clin Endocrinol Metab 83: 1380–1383

Celsis P (2000) Age-related cognitive decline, mild cognitive impairment or preclinical Alzheimer's disease? Ann Med 32: 6–14

Collins L, Evans AC (1999) Animal: Automatic nonlinear image matching and anatomical labeling, Brain warping. Academic Press, San Diego

Collins DL, Neelin P, Peters TM, Evans AC (1994) Automatic 3D intrersubject registration of MR volumetric data in standardized Talairach space. J Computer Assisted Tomography 18: 192–205

De Kloet ER, Vreugdenhil E, Oitzl MS, Joels M (1998) Brain corticosteroid receptor balance in health and disease. Endocrinol Rev 19: 269–301

Dodt C, Theine KJ, Uthgenannt D, Born J, Fehm HL (1994) Basal secretory activity of the hypothalamo-pituitary-adrenocortical axis is enhanced in healthy elderly. An assessment during undisturbed night-time sleep. Eur J Endocrinol 131: 443–450

Ge Y, Grossman RI, Babb JS, Rabin ML, Mannon LJ, Kolson DL (2002) Age-related total gray matter and white matter changes in normal adult brain. Part II: Quantitative magnetization transfer ratio histogram analysis. AJNR Am J Neuroradiol 23: 1334–1341

Haus E, Touitou Y (1994) Principles of clinical chronobiology. In: Touitou Y, Haus E (eds) Biologic rhythms in clinical and laboratory medicine. Springer Verlag, Berlin, 6–33

Jernigan TL, Press GA, Hesselink JR (1990) Methods for measuring brain morphologic features on magnetic resonance images: validation and normal aging. Arch Neurol 47: 27–32

Kirschbaum C, Pirke KM, Hellhammer DH (1993) The 'Trier Social Stress Test'--a tool for investigating psychobiological stress responses in a laboratory setting. Neuropsychobiology 28: 76–81

Kirschbaum C, Prüssner JC, Stone AA, Federenko I, Gaab J, Lintz D, Schommer N, Hellhammer DH (1995) Persistent high cortisol responses to repeated psychological stress in a subpopulation of healthy men. Psychosomatic Med 57: 468–474

Kirschbaum C, Wolf OT, May M, Wippich W, Hellhammer DH (1996) Stress- and treatment-induced elevations of cortisol levels associated with impaired declarative memory in healthy adults. Life Sci 58: 1475–1483

Lupien S, Gaudeau S, Tchiteya BM, Maheu F, Sharma S, Nair NPV, Hauger RL, McEwen BS, Menaey MJ (1997) Stress-induced declarative memory impairment in healthy elderly subjects: relationship to cortisol reactivity. J Clin Endocrinol Metab 82: 2070–2075

Lupien SJ, de Leon M, de Santi S, Convit A, Tarshish C, Nair NP, Thakur M, McEwen BS, Hauger RL, Meaney MJ (1998) Cortisol levels during human aging predict hippocampal atrophy and memory deficits [see comments]. Nature Neurosci 1: 69–73

Magarinos AM, McEwen BS (1995a) Stress-induced atrophy of apical dendrites of hippocampal CA3c neurons: involvement of glucocorticoid secretion and excitatory amino acid receptors. Neuroscience 69: 89–98

Magarinos AM, McEwen BS (1995b) Stress-induced atrophy of apical dendrites of hippocampal CA3c neurons: comparison of stressors. Neuroscience 69: 83–88

Magarinos AM, McEwen BS, Flugge G, Fuchs E (1996) Chronic psychosocial stress causes apical dendritic atrophy of hippocampal CA3 pyramidal neurons in subordinate tree shrews. J Neurosci 16: 3534–3540

McEwen BS (1997) Possible mechanisms for atrophy of the human hippocampus. Mol Psychiatr 2: 255–262

McEwen BS (1998a) Protective and damaging effects of stress mediators. N Engl J Med 338: 171–179

McEwen BS (1998b) Stress, adaptation, and disease. Allostasis and allostatic load. Ann NY Acad Sci 840: 33–44

McEwen BS (2001) Plasticity of the hippocampus: adaptation to chronic stress and allostatic load. Ann NY Acad Sci 933: 265–277

Molloy DW, Standish TI (1997) A guide to the standardized Mini-Mental State Examination. Int Psychogeriatr 9: 87–94; discussion 143–50

O'Sullivan M, Jones DK, Summers PE, Morris RG, Williams SC, Markus HS (2001) Evidence for cortical "disconnection" as a mechanism of age-related cognitive decline. Neurology 57: 632–638

Pruessner JC, Wolf OT, Hellhammer DH, Buske-Kirschbaum AB, vonAuer K, Jobst S, Kaspers F, Kirschbaum C (1997) Free cortisol levels after awakening: a reliable biological marker for the assessment of adrenocortical acitvity. Life Sci 61: 2539–2549

Pruessner JC, Hellhammer DH, Kirschbaum C (1998) Low self-esteem, induced failure and the adrenocortical stress response. Personality Individual Differences 27: 477–489

Pruessner JC, Hellhammer DH, Kirschbaum C (1999) Burnout, perceived stress, and cortisol responses to awakening. Psychosom Med 61: 197–204

Pruessner JC, Kohler S, Crane J, Pruessner M, Lord C, Byrne A, Kabani N, Collins DL, Evans AC (2003) Volumetry of temporopolar, perirhinal, entorhinal and parahippocampal cortex from high-resolution MR images: considering the anatomical variability of the collateral sulcus. Cereb Cortex, in press

Pruessner JC, Li LM, Serles W, Pruessner M, Collins DL, Kabani N, Evans AC (2000) Volumetry of hippocampus and amygdala with high-resolution MRI and 3D analyzing software: minimizing the discrepancies between laboratories. Cereb Cortex 10: 433–442

Rosen G (1982) Alzheimer Disease Assessment Scale. Neuropsychologica 13: 34–43

Sapolsky RM, Krey LC, McEwen BS (1986) The neuroendocrinology of stress and aging: the glucocorticoid cascade hypothesis. Endocrinol Rev 7: 284–301

Sapolsky RM, Romero LM, Munck AU (2000) How do glucocorticoids influence stress responses? Integrating permissive, suppressive, stimulatory, and preparative actions. Endocrinol Rev 21: 55–89

Seeman TE, Robbins RJ (1994) Aging and hypothalamic-pituitary-adrenal response to challenge in humans. Endocrinol Rev 15: 233–260

Sled JG, Zijdenbos AP, Evans AC (1998) A nonparametric method for automatic correction of intensity nonuniformity in MRI data. IEEE Trans Med Imaging 17: 87–97

Talairach J, Tournoux P (1988) Co-planar stereotactic atlas of the human brain; 3-dimensional proportional system: an approach to cerebral imaging. Thieme, New York

Teng EL, Chui HC, Gong A (1989) Comparisons between the Mini-Mental State Exam (MMSE) and its modified version - the 3MS test. In: Hasegama K, Homma A (eds) Psychogeriatrics: Biomedical and social advances. Selected proceedings of the fourth congress of the International Psychogeriatrics Association. Excerpta Medica, Tokyo

Van Cauter E, Coevorden Av, Blackman J (1990) Modulation of neuroendocrine release by sleep and circadian rhythmicity. In: Yen SSC, Vale WW (eds) Advances in neuroendocrine regulation of reproduction. Serono Symposium, Norwell, 113–122

Van Cauter E, Leproult R, Kupfer DJ (1996) Effects of gender and age on the levels and circadian rhythmicity of plasma cortisol. J Clin Endocrinol Metab 81: 2468–2473

Van Coevorden A, Mockel J, Laurent E, Kerkhofs M, L'Hermite Baleriaux M, Decoster C, Neve P, Van Cauter E (1991) Neuroendocrine rhythms and sleep in aging men. Am –J Physiol 260: E651–61

Wilkinson CW, Peskind ER, Raskind MA (1997) Decreased hypothalamic-pituitary-adrenal axis sensitivity to cortisol feedback inhibition in human aging. Neuroendocrinology 65: 79–90

Wishart D (1998) Clustan graphics3: interactive graphics for cluster analysis. In: Gaul W, Locarek-Junge H (eds) Classification in the information age. Proceedings of the 22nd annual conference of the Society for Classification. . Springer, Berlin, pp. 268–275

Wolf OT, Neumann O, Hellhammer DH, Geiben AC, Strasburger CJ, Dressendörfer RA, Pirke KM, Kirschbaum C (1997) Effects of a two-week physiological dehydroepiandrosterone substitution on cognitive performance and well-being in healthy elderly women and men. J Clin Endocrinol Metab 82: 2363–2367

Wolf OT, Convit A, de Leon MJ, Caraos C, Qadri SF (2002) Basal hypothalamo-pituitary-adrenal axis activity and corticotropin feedback in young and older men: relationships to magnetic resonance imaging-derived hippocampus and cingulate gyrus volumes. Neuroendocrinology 75: 241–249

Aging Myelin and Cognitive Decline: a Role for Steroids

M. Schumacher[1], C. Ibanez[1], F. Robert[1], L.M. Garcia-Segura[2], R.J.M. Franklin[3], and R.C. Melcangi[4]

Summary

The functions of steroids go far beyond reproduction and adaptation to stress and, over the past few years, they have been shown to regulate a large number of vital neuronal and glial functions throughout the brain and in peripheral nerves. For example, progesterone exerts neuroprotective effects and plays an important role in myelination. This steroid, which is produced by the ovaries and adrenal glands and then reaches the nervous tissues via the bloodstream, can also be synthesized locally within the nervous system by neurons and glial cells. Age-associated alterations of the nervous system and cognitive decline have been related to decreased levels of steroid hormones and have been shown to be reversible by the systemic administration of steroids. It is indeed now recognized that age-related changes in the nervous system are less severe than previously thought and, most importantly, that they are partly reversible. Abnormalities, breakdown and loss of myelin sheaths are reliable markers of the aging nervous system, which correlate with both chronological age and cognitive decline. Prolonged administration of progestins over one month to old male rats has been shown to reverse the decrease in myelin protein gene expression as well as the age-related structural abnormalities of the peripheral myelin sheaths. In the brains of old rats, myelin repair is very much delayed when compared with young animals. In the cerebellar peduncle of old males, the systemic administration of progesterone for five weeks has been shown to stimulate slow remyelination after toxin-induced demyelination. Steroids that promote myelin repair and can reverse myelin sheath abnormalities thus offer a promising opportunity for preventing or treating age-dependent dysfunctions of the nervous system.

[1] INSERM U488, Kremlin-Bicêtre, France
[2] Instituto Cajal, C.S.I.C., 28002, Madrid, Spain
[3] Department of Clinical Veterinary Medicine and Cambridge Center for Brain Repair, University of Cambridge, UK
[4] Department of Endocrinology and Center of Excellence on Neurodegenerative Diseases, University of Milano, Italy

Chanson et al.
Endocrine Aspects of Successful Aging
© Springer-Verlag Berlin Heidelberg 2004

cognitive functions, protects against age-associated memory decline and lowers the risk of developing AD (Phillips and Sherwin 1992; Brenner et al. 1994; Paganini-Hill and Henderson 1994, 1996; Kawas et al. 1997; Jacobs et al. 1998; Resnick et al. 1998; Costa et al. 1999; Smith et al. 2001; Fillenbaum et al. 2001). Estrogens may not only protect against the onset of AD, they may also maintain cognitive functions in women who already have AD (Henderson et al. 1994; Asthana et al. 1999, 2001). However, some studies have questioned the impact of ERT on the risk of AD or on cognitive decline in women with AD (Brenner et al. 1994; Henderson et al. 2000; Mulnard et al. 2000; Wang et al. 2000).

The measure of estrogen levels in women with AD has provided conflicting results. Some studies have not shown significant differences in estradiol levels between healthy women and women suffering from AD (Cunningham et al. 2001). On the contrary, other studies have found decreased levels of estradiol in AD patients (Manly et al. 2000). A recent study has reported decreased estradiol levels in the cerebrospinal fluid of AD patients and a negative correlation with β-amyloid levels (Schonknecht et al. 2001).

The ovaries are also the main source of circulating PROG in women, except during pregnancy, when virtually all PROG is produced by the placenta (Csapo and Pulkkinen 1978). It is now standard practice to give combined replacement treatment with estrogens and progestins to postmenopausal women to reduce the risk of endometrial cancer (Sitruk-Ware 2000b). While progestins need to be given to protect the endometrium, their potential risks for the development of breast cancer and cardiovascular diseases are still a matter a debate (Pike and Ross 2000; Sitruk-Ware 2000a; Key 2000). The difficulty arises from the fact that different progestins with varying pharmacological profiles are used in HRT, some having androgenic potency, others being devoid of androgenic properties (natural PROG and the 19-norprogestins), some having antiandrogenic effects or bind to the mineralocorticoid receptor (Sitruk-Ware 2002; Pike and Ross 2000).

When discussing the risks and benefits of PROG administration, it should be kept in mind that progestins, like estrogens, are pleiotropic hormones with multiple actions in the central nervous system (CNS) and peripheral nervous system (PNS). Thus, PROG also exerts neuroprotective effects. In the rat spinal cord, the hormone promotes neurological and functional recovery after contusion injury (Thomas et al. 1999). After traumatic brain injury, PROG has remarkable protective effects. Male rats given bilateral contusions of the medial frontal cortex showed improved behavioral recovery, reduced edema and less secondary neuronal degeneration if the injury was followed by the systemic administration of PROG (Stein 2001). Elevated levels of circulating PROG explain why female rats have significantly less edema and show better cognitive recovery than males after cortical contusion injury and why brain edema is almost absent in pseudo-pregnant female rats (Roof et al. 1993, 1994). PROG has also been shown to offer neuroprotection after cerebral ischemia (Jiang et al. 1996) and to increase the survival of motoneurons following axotomy (Yu 1989). In addition to its protective effects on nerve cells, PROG plays an important role in the formation of new myelin sheaths, which are necessary for the efficient and rapid conduction of action potentials (see below).

The adrenal glands are another important source of circulating PROG (Feder et al. 1968; Holzbauer et al. 1969). Both synthesis and secretion of PROG by the adrenal glands can be stimulated by ACTH and have been shown to be very sensitive to stress in rats of both sexes (Fajer et al. 1971; Resko 1969; Schaeffer and Aron 1987). In men, circulating PROG is exclusively of adrenal origin and its levels can also be increased by the administration of ACTH and inhibited by dexamethasone, a synthetic glucocorticoid that exerts suppressive effects on pituitary and adrenal activity (Gutai et al. 1977).

Circulating levels of PROG do not significantly change with age in men (Vermeulen and Verdonck 1976; Belanger et al. 1994; Morley et al. 1997). In contrast, plasma levels of the PROG metabolite 3α,5α-tetrahydroprogesterone (3α,5α-TH PROG) significantly decease after the age of 40 in men, whereas they remain almost constant in women between the ages of 20 and 70 (Genazzani et al. 2002). Within target tissues, the formation of active PROG metabolites also decreases with age (see below).

The "andropause" is defined by the decline in serum testosterone. In healthy men, serum levels of total testosterone decrease by about 30% and serum levels of free testosterone decrease as much as 50% between ages 25 and 75 (Vermeulen 1991; Morley et al. 1997). Because testosterone has anabolic effects, the decreases in muscle strength and bone mass with age have been related to decreased androgen levels (van den Beld and Lamberts 2002). The limited number of studies concerning testosterone replacement therapy in older men have reported conflicting results (Sih et al. 1997; Tenover 1992; Snyder et al. 1999a,b) One possibility is that testosterone treatment only improves muscle and bone mass and mood in men with very low endogenous concentrations of testosterone.

Two hormones have attracted particular attention, namely, DHEA and its sulfated form DHEAS, which are the most abundant circulating steroids in adult humans and which show a marked gradual decline with progressing age (Orentreich et al. 1984; Ravaglia et al. 1996; Labrie et al. 1997; Nafziger et al. 1998; Mazat et al. 2001). In women, levels of DHEA and DHEAS are about 40% lower than in men, and their decrease is parallel between sexes until the age of 70 (Laughlin and Barrett-Connor 2000).

A wealth of studies in rodents, in which DHEA and DHEAS levels are very low, have documented beneficial effects of these steroids on obesity, diabetes, cancer, heart disease, and immune and nervous functions (Bellino et al. 1995; Kalimi and Regelson 1990). With respect to the latter, neurotrophic and neuroprotective effects of DHEA and its sulfate have been demonstrated both in cell culture and *in vivo*: 1) nanomolar concentrations of DHEA or DHEAS added to the culture medium of embryonic mouse brain neurons protected their survival and promoted their differentiation (Bologa et al. 1987); 2) DHEA and DHEAS protected hippocampal neurons from the toxic effects of glutamate and of the β-amyloid protein (Cardounel et al. 1999); 3) DHEA and DHEAS stimulated neurite growth in cultures of cortical neurons isolated from embryonic rat brains by modulating the activity of N-methyl-D-aspartate (NMDA) receptors (Compagnone and Mellon 1998).

When administered in vivo in mice, DHEAS significantly attenuated learning impairments induced by the administration of various molecules: the NMDA antagonist dizocilpine, the muscarinic acetylcholine receptor anatgonist scopolamine and the β25-35-amyloid peptide (Maurice et al. 1997, 1998; Urani et al. 1998). A recent study has shown that treatment of adult rats with DHEA stimulates neurogenesis and antagonizes the inhibitory effects of corticosterone on the proliferation of granule neurons within the hippocampal formation (Karishma and Herbert 2002).

Placebo-controlled studies support the concept that oral administration of DHEA has beneficial effects in the elderly. Daily treatment with DHEA of men and women of advancing age resulted in an increase in perceived physical and psychological well-being, increased lean body mass in both sexes and increased muscle strength in men (Morales et al. 1994, 1998). In a randomized, double-blind, placebo-controlled trial among 140 elderly men and 140 elderly women (60-79 years old), 50 mg of DHEA given daily for one year reestablished circulating levels of DHEAS and slightly increased levels of testosterone and estradiol. The treatment led to improved bone turnover and skin status (Baulieu et al. 2000).

However, in spite of the numerous animal studies documenting beneficial effects of DHEA or DHEAS on nervous functions and memory, most human trials have failed to demonstrate an effect of DHEA on cognitive performance in the elderly (Arlt et al. 2000; van Niekerk et al. 2001; Wolf et al. 1997), except for one study showing antidepressant and cognition-enhancing effects in major depression (Wolkowitz et al. 1995). Also, no study has revealed a relationship between circulating levels of DHEAS and cognitive performance in the elderly (Barrett-Connor and Edelstein 1994; Carlson and Sherwin 1999; Kalmijn et al. 1998; Mazat et al. 2001; Yaffe et al. 1998). Whether there is a link between reduced levels of DHEA or DHEAS and AD is still a controversial issue. Most studies have not found differences in DHEAS levels between AD patients and patients without dementia (Legrain et al. 1995; Yanase et al. 1996; Carlson et al. 1999; Ferrario et al. 1999), whereas two studies have reported decreased levels of DHEAS in AD patients (Leblhuber et al. 1993; Murialdo et al. 2000).

Not all adrenal steroid levels decrease with age. Thus, plasma levels of cortisol are maintained throughout life (Herbert 1995). Nevertheless, this stress hormone plays an important role in the aging process, and different glucocorticoid levels could underlie individual differences in cognitive impairment during aging (McEwen et al. 1999; Nichols et al. 2001). In addition, the aging brain may become more sensitive to circulating glucocorticoids. The marked decrease in levels of DHEA with progressing age may contribute to this increased sensitivity, as DHEA acts as an antiglucocorticoid (Kimonides et al. 1999; McIntosh et al. 1993).

It has not been proven that elevated levels of glucocorticoids are a risk factor for neurodegenerative diseases such as AD, although there are strong indications. Thus brain-imaging techniques have recently shown that aging subjects with increased cortisol levels show a reduction in hippocampal volume and decreased attention and memory performance, but it is unknown whether this finding predicts the development of dementia or whether it corresponds to a reversible change (Lupien et al. 1998, 1999). Nevertheless, damaging effects of chronically elevated levels of glucocorticoids and of stress have been demonstrated in animal experiments. In rats, elevated glucocorticoid levels alter hippocampal functions, produce the loss of hippocampal neurons and correlate with individual deficits in spatial learning (McEwen and Sapolsky 1995).

Origin of steroids present in nervous tissues

Steroids present in nervous tissues are either derived from the steroidogenic endocrine glands or from local synthesis. Steroid hormones produced by the gonads and adrenal glands reach the brain and peripheral nerves via the blood stream, and their free forms easily cross the blood-brain and the blood-nerve barriers. In addition, a local synthesis contributes to the pool of steroids present in the brain and in peripheral nerves. The term "neurosteroids" has been applied to steroids that are synthesized in the nervous system by neurons and glial cells (Baulieu 1981; Robel et al. 1999).

The cytochrome P450scc, which catalyzes the conversion of cholesterol to pregnenolone in the mitochondria and is characteristic of all steroidogenic cells, has been shown to be present in the nervous system of vertebrates (Le Goascogne et al. 1987; Robel et al. 1999; Mensah-Nyagan et al. 1999; Tsutsui et al. 2000; Mellon et al. 2001). Pregnenolone, either locally synthesized or derived from the circulation, is then converted by the 3β-hydroxysteroid dehydrogenase (3β-HSD) to PROG in the endoplasmic reticulum. The presence and activity of this enzyme have been demonstrated in both glial cells and neurons of the CNS and PNS (Jung-Testas et al. 1989; Guennoun et al. 1995, 1997; Ukena et al. 1999; Zwain and Yen 1999a; Robert et al. 2001).

In peripheral nerves, the 3β-HSD is present in Schwann cells and its expression and activity are induced by a diffusible neuronal factor (Robert et al. 2001). Schwann cells further metabolize the PROG formed from [³H]pregnenolone to 5α-dihydroprogesterone and 3α,5α-TH PROG (allopregnanolone; Guennoun et al. 1997). That rat Schwann cells possess 5α-reductase and 3α-hydroxysteroid oxidoreductase (3α-HSOR) activities was also shown by utilizing [³H]PROG as a substrate (Melcangi et al. 1998b). However, the synthesis of PROG in the PNS is not restricted to Schwann cells. The 3β-HSD is also expressed in dorsal root ganglia (DRG) sensory neurons, which convert [³H]pregnenolone to [³H]PROG and to [³H]5α-dihydroprogesterone (Guennoun et al. 1997).

Glial cells of the CNS also synthesize PROG. Mixed cultures of rat brain glial cells were found to form PROG from labelled precursors (Jung-Testas et al. 1989). In cultured astrocytes, PROG synthesis is dependent on cell density and is thus likely to be regulated by autocrine factors (Akwa et al. 1993). The synthesis of PROG has recently been investigated at three stages of maturation of the oligodendroglial cells, namely PSA-NCAM+ preprogenitors, oligodendrocyte progenitors and fully differentiated oligodendrocytes. Only the preprogenitors and progenitors, but not mature oligodendrocytes, expressed the 3β-HSD and synthesized [³H]PROG from [³H]pregnenolone (Gago et al. 2001). However, significant levels of 3β-HSD mRNA expression have been detected in adult white matter (Sanne and Krueger 1995).

Many neurons of the brain and spinal cord also express the 3β-HSD as shown by in situ hybridization (Mensah-Nyagan et al. 1994; Guennoun et al. 1995; Coirini et al. 2003).

Cultures of both brain glial cells (oligodendrocytes and astrocytes) and neurons further convert PROG to its 5α-reduced metabolites, with neurons possessing the highest 5α-reductase activity. On the contrary, 3α-HSOR, the enzyme that converts 5α-dihydroprogesterone to 3α,5α-TH PROG, is mainly present in astrocytes (Melcangi et al. 1994b). Neuronal factors were shown to stimulate the 5α-reductase and 3α-HSOR activities in astrocytes (Melcangi et al. 1994a). In a recent study of PROG metabolism in cells of the oligodendroglial lineage, PSA-NCAM+ preprogenitors, oligodendrocyte progenitors and fully differentiated oligodendrocytes were found to metabolize PROG into 5α-dihydroprogesterone, but only the preprogenitors further converted 5α-dihydroprogesterone to 3α,5α-TH PROG (Gago et al. 2001). In a previous study, oligodendrocytes were found to have significant 3α-HSOR activity (Melcangi et al. 1994b). The different results may be explained by different isolation procedures and culture conditions. Considerable 5α-reductase activity has been found associated with myelin membranes, strongly suggesting an important role of PROG metabolites in the formation and/or maintenance of myelin sheaths (Melcangi et al. 1988).

Whereas the synthesis of PROG and its 5α-reduced metabolites by neurons and glial cells is now well established, the possibility of a local synthesis of DHEA within the nervous system is still controversial. Although DHEA remains present in the rat brain after castration and adrenalectomy (Corpéchot et al. 1981), the demonstration of its synthesis has been difficult. DHEA is synthesized from pregnenolone by the cytochrome P450c17. The message for this enzyme has been detected by RT-PCR in the rodent brain and in cultured astrocytes and neurons (Strömstedt and Waterman 1995; Zwain and Yen 1999b). Recently, it has been shown that astrocytes in culture can convert pregnenolone to DHEA if they are grown in the absence of microglia (Zwain and Yen 1999b). In addition, an alternative pathway of DHEA formation in the brain involving the formation of hydroperoxydes has been proposed (Cascio et al. 1998). However, the significance of these observations needs to be examined.

Whereas andogens and estrogens can be formed in the amphibian brain (Mensah-Nyagan et al. 1999), they may not be synthesized de novo from cholesterol within the mammalian nervous system (Robel et al. 1999). However, they can be locally synthesized in the brain from circulating precursors, such as testosterone, which is converted to estradiol within the brain by the aromatase enzyme (Balthazart and Ball 1998). In response to injury, estrogen biosynthesis and estrogen receptor expression are increased in the adult rodent brain (Garcia-Segura et al. 2001).

Neurosteroid biosynthesis has been extensively studied in animal models, but it may also take place in the human CNS and PNS. The presence of cytochrome P450scc-immunoreactivity has been documented in human white matter (Le Goascogne et al. 1989), and elevated levels of pregnenolone have been measured in human sciatic nerves (Morfin et al. 1992). Cultured human Schwann cells isolated from peripheral nerve autopsies can convert [³H]pregnenolone to [³H]PROG and [³H]5α-dihydroprogesterone (F. Robert and M. Schumacher, unpublished observation).

Whether the formation of neurosteroids within the nervous system decreases with progressing age and whether decreased neurosteroid synthesis plays a role in age-dependent changes of nervous functions remains to be explored. So far, the activity of only the 5α-reductase has been shown to be considerably decreased in the sciatic nerve of old rats (Melcangi et al. 1990, 1992). For these experiments, [3H]testosterone has been used as a substrate, but the same 5α-reductase converts testosterone and PROG to their respective 5α-reduced metabolites, 5α-dihydrotestosterone and 5α-dihydroprogesterone. The content of 3α,5α-TH PROG decreased significantly with age in the cerebral cortex, whereas hypothalamic 3α,5α-TH PROG levels remained constant until 18 months and significantly increased thereafter (Bernardi et al. 1998). In the same study, adrenal 3α,5α-TH PROG content remained constant until 18 months, whereas testis and serum 3α,5α-TH PROG levels showed a significant age-related increase.

Progestins play an important role in myelination

The local synthesis of PROG in peripheral nerves plays an important role in the formation of new myelin sheaths (Schumacher et al. 2001). This was first demonstrated in the regenerating male mouse sciatic nerve after cryolesion. In response to this type of lesion, nerve fibers distal to the lesion site rapidly degenerate, but Schwann cells survive and subsequently form new myelin sheaths around the regenerating axons. Blocking the local synthesis or the local actions of PROG during the process of regeneration, by administering either the PROG synthesis inhibitor trilostane or the PR antagonist mifepristone (RU486), strongly inhibited the formation of new myelin sheaths. Conversely, myelination was promoted by the repeated local administration of a high dose of PROG (Koenig et al. 1995). Another observation supports a role of locally synthesized PROG in peripheral myelin formation. After lesion of the male rat sciatic nerve, changes in 3β-HSD mRNA levels paralleled those of mRNA coding for the major peripheral myelin proteins, protein zero (P0) and peripheral myelin protein 22 (PMP22; Robert et al. 2001).

A stimulation of myelin formation by PROG has also been shown in explant cultures of embryonic rat DRG, which mainly contain Schwann cells and sensory neurons, the fibroblasts having been eliminated by treatment with an antimitotic drug. Adding PROG to the culture medium of these cocultures dramatically increased the number of myelinated axons without affecting the density of neurites, or the number of Schwann cells (Koenig et al. 1995). It was then shown that PROG accelerated the initiation and enhanced the rate of myelin synthesis in this culture system. In the same study, it was reported that levels of mRNAs coding for the enzymes involved in PROG synthesis (cytochrome P450scc and 3β-HSD) and for the PROG receptor (PR) were markedly increased during peak myelin formation, further supporting an important role for the local synthesis and action of PROG in myelin formation (Chan et al. 1998).

One mechanism by which PROG may promote myelination in the PNS is by stimulating the expression of myelin protein genes. In transient transfection experiments, it was indeed shown that PROG could activate the promoters of the genes coding for the peripheral myelin proteins P0 and PMP22 in a promoter-, hormone-, and cell-specific manner (Désarnaud et al. 1998; Fig. 1). P0 and PMP22 are two proteins that are tightly coupled to myelin formation, and their mutations or altered expression are at the origin of peripheral neuropathies (Suter and Snipes 1998). Increases in P0, PMP22 and myelin basic protein (MBP) levels by PROG have been shown by immunocytochemistry in cocultures of sensory neurons and Schwann cells (Notterpek et al. 1999). In cultured Schwann cells, PROG and its metabolites, 5α-dihydroprogesterone and 3α,5α-TH PROG, increase endogenous P0 gene expression, whereas only 3α,5α-TH PROG increases PMP22 expression (Melcangi et al. 1999).

Locally synthesized progestins regulate myelination in peripheral nerves by autocrine signaling, either through the classical intracellular PR or through a membrane $GABA_A$ receptor, both of which are expressed by Schwann cells (Jung-Testas et al. 1996a; Magnaghi et al. 1999, 2001; Melcangi et al. 1999). These two receptor systems are involved in the expression of distinct myelin proteins: PROG and 5α-dihydroprogesterone, both of which bind with high affinity to the intracellular PR, increase P0 expression via this receptor; 3α,5α-TH PROG, a positive allosteric modulator of $GABA_A$ receptors, increases PMP22 expression via Schwann cell $GABA_A$ receptors (Melcangi et al. 1999; Magnaghi et al. 2001). This has been demonstrated by pharmacological experiments. Thus, the increase in P0 mRNA levels in cultured rat Schwann cells by either PROG or 5α-dihydroprogesterone could be blocked by the PR antagonist mifepristone. On the other hand, mifepristone was ineffective in blocking the effect of 3α,5α-TH PROG on PMP22 expression, but the activity of this neurosteroid could be mimicked by the $GABA_A$ receptor agonist muscimol and inhibited by the $GABA_A$ receptor antagonist bicuculline (Magnaghi et al. 2001). It has previously been reported that mifepristone can activate the promoters of the P0 and PMP22 genes when they are transiently transfected into rat Schwann cells (Désarnaud et al. 1998). However, in this particular study, Schwann cells were cultured in the presence of forskolin, a specific adenylate cyclase activator, and it is known that mifepristone can act as an agonist in cells that have been cultured in the presence of elevated levels of cAMP (Beck et al. 1993; Nordeen et al. 1993). The importance of a PR-mediated action of

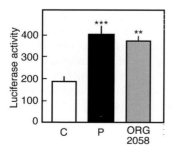

Fig. 1. Progesterone (P) and the selective progesterone agonist ORG2058 activate the promoter of the peripheral myelin protein gene *P0*. Cultured rat Schwann cells, purified from neonatal sciatic nerves, were transiently transfected with a gene construct in which 1 kb of the 5'-flanking sequence of the *P0* gene was linked to the luciferase reporter gene. After transfection, cells were cultured for 24h in the presence of 1 μM of steroid (modified from Désarnaud et al. 1998).

PROG in myelination is further supported by the observation that mifepristone inhibits myelin sheath formation in the mouse sciatic nerve after lesion (Koenig et al. 1995).

The finding that progestins regulate myelination in the PNS via intracellular PRs and via membrane $GABA_A$ receptors is striking for two reasons: 1) it shows that steroids can regulate long-term gene expression in glial cells and regulate slow processes such as myelination by acting on glial membrane receptors for neurotransmitters; and 2) it implies that progestins can activate different signaling pathways involved in myelination in a well-coordinated manner. In fact, P0 and PMP22 are dosage-sensitive genes that need to be expressed in a very precise ratio to preserve the integrity of the peripheral myelin sheaths (Suter and Nave 1999)

The process of myelination differs between peripheral nerves and the CNS: axons are myelinated in the PNS by Schwann cells and in the CNS by oligodendrocytes, the protein composition of peripheral and central myelin is different, and distinct transcription factors activate and coordinate the expression of myelin genes in Schwann cells and oligodendrocytes (Lemke 1993; Messing et al. 1992; Goujet-Zalc et al. 1993; Topilko et al. 1994). There is now evidence that progestins also regulate myelination in the brain. Glial cells isolated from neonatal rat brain express an intracellular, estrogen-inducible PR (Jung-Testas et al. 1991) and, when added to the medium, PROG increases the number of MBP-immunoreactive oligodendrocytes in these cultures (Jung-Testas et al. 1996b). A recent study showed that spontaneous remyelination is promoted in old rats by systematically administered PROG (see below).

Age-related changes in myelin

Peripheral nerves undergo a variety of changes with normal aging, some of which are qualitatively similar to those observed in the main peripheral neuropathies. As a consequence, the distinction between the "normally" and "pathologically" aging PNS can be difficult, in particular in very old patients (Maisonobe and Hauw 1997). Detailed examinations of peripheral nerves in old rats and cats have revealed that, in particular, the large-diameter nerve fibers undergo atrophy and their myelin sheaths become thicker and show many abnormalities, including retraction at the nodes of Ranvier, vacuolation, ballooning, fragmentation, infolding and reduplication. In addition, the number of myelinated fibers is significantly decreased (Adinolfi et al. 1991; Grover-Johnson and Spencer 1981; Knox et al. 1989; Thomas et al. 1980; for review, see Melcangi et al. 2000). The aging human peripheral nerves also undergo structural changes, resulting from segmental demyelination and remyelination and from axonal regeneration after degeneration (Maisonobe and Hauw 1997). These changes correspond to the shortening and increased variability of internodal length and to severe morphological alterations of myelinated fibers (Stevens et al. 1973; Hildebrand et al. 1994; Lascelles and Thomas 1966).

Age-dependent deterioration of myelinated fibers may result from altered neuronal or glial functions. In fact, there are complex reciprocal interactions between axons and myelinating glial cells in both PNS (Dewaegh et al. 1992; Reynolds and Woolf 1993; Snipes and Suter 1994) and CNS (Demerens et al. 1996; Marchionni et al. 1999; Fernandez et al. 2000). In humans, changes in white matter structure may also be partly dependent on neuronal changes, but myelin degeneration can also be primary and independent of axonal atrophy, and it can occur with relative sparing of the axons (Maisonobe and Hauw 1997).

Aging also affects functional parameters of peripheral nerves. Age-associated neurophysiological changes include decreased sensory and motor nerve conduction. A decline in velocity and especially in amplitude of action potentials in aged individuals has been documented by many studies, and these changes appear to accelerate with advancing age (Buchthal et al. 1984; Maisonobe and Hauw 1997). It is worth mentioning that age-related changes in nerves mainly affect the myelinated fibers, with the unmyelinated ones being relatively spared. Thus, a study in rats has shown that the conduction velocity of myelinated fibers decreases with age, whereas it remains quite constant for unmyelinated fibers (Sato et al. 1985). However, morphological changes due to aging have been reported in unmyelinated nerve fibers (Kanda et al. 1991). In addition to functional alterations, the capacity of peripheral nerve regeneration decreases with progressing age, as has been documented in human and animal models (for review, Melcangi et al. 2000).

The white matter of the brain, formed by myelinated nerve fibers, glial cells and blood vessels, also undergoes important changes during aging. In individuals aged over 60, there in a significant decrease in cerebral white matter, which may in part result from the loss or shrinkage of neurons. In addition to the reduction in mass, other changes occur in central white matter with aging, such as the formation of lacunes, astrogliosis and the accumulation of various substances (Pittella 1997). Structural changes in cerebral white matter have also been observed by magnetic resonance imaging (MRI) and, in a few cases, have been related to cognitive and motor deficits (Pittella 1997).

The effect of age on brain myelin has been extensively studied in rhesus monkeys. Age-dependent changes include loss of white matter, myelin abnormalities, increased thickness of the myelin sheaths, breakdown of myelin sheaths and alterations in oligodendrocytes (Peters 1996; Peters et al. 2001, 2000; Sandell and Peters 2001). Based on these observations, it has been proposed that myelin changes may significantly contribute to the age-related cognitive decline by altering conduction velocities along axons (Peters 2002).

In the CNS, age is an important factor influencing remyelination after demyelination induced by gliotoxins such as lysolecithin or ethidium bromide. It was first shown that remyelination after lysolecithin injection into the dorsal funiculus of the rat spinal cord is very much reduced in old rats (> 12 months) in comparison with young animals (< 3 months) (Gilson and Blakemore 1993). The gliotoxin lesions in the CNS undergo extensive remyelination even in old rats, but the process takes much longer than in young animals and may require as much as several months (Shields et al. 1999). This finding was made using a new model of demyelination/remyelination based on the stereotaxic injection of ethidium bromide into the caudal cerebellar peduncle of adult male rats. Infusion of this toxin produces a large area of demyelination with minimal axonal damage. The lesion site can be easily sampled in a highly reproducible way and spontaneous remyelination can be easily quantified (Woodruff and Franklin 1999).

The reasons for the age-associated decline in myelin repair are not well understood. A recent study has shown that impaired recruitement of oligodendrocyte progenitors and their delayed differentiation into myelinating oligodendrocytes both contribute to the slowing down of remyelination with age (Sim et al. 2002). This may be related to the delayed expression of signalling molecules such as insulin growth factor-1 (IGF-I) and transforming growth factor-1 (TGF-β1) (Hinks and Franklin 2000). An interesting possibility is that the age-related impairment in remyelination and growth factor expression may be in part a consequence of neuronal deficiency, with axons in the nervous system of old animals being less supportive for myelinating glial cells.

In humans, differences in the speed of remyelination could explain the much slower functional recovery in older patients after diseases such as optic neuritis (Jones 1993). The age-dependent decrease in the efficiency of CNS remyelination may also have implications for the evolution of a demyelinating disease like multiple sclerosis.

Only a few studies have dealt with biochemical changes in myelin during aging. A decrease in cholesterol and an increase in the white matter content of water have been described (Pittella 1997). Two studies have reported decreased protein P0 levels in peripheral nerves of aged rats and humans (Uchida et al. 1986; Koski and Max 1980). More recently, it has been shown that mRNA levels of the major myelin proteins P0, PMP22 and MBP in the sciatic nerve are significantly decreased in 22- to 24-month-old rats when compared to 3-month-old animals (Fig. 2; Melcangi et al. 1998a, 2000). P0 protein levels were also found to be decreased (Melcangi et al. 1998b).

Reversal of age-related myelin abnormalities by progestins

As described above, progestins play an important role in myelination and the age-dependent decrease in peripheral myelin gene expression is associated with a significant decrease in myelin-associated 5α-reductase activity, an enzyme which converts PROG to 5α-dihydroprogesterone or testosterone to 5α-dihydrotestosterone. It was thus worth trying to reverse the age-dependent

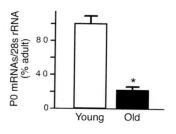

Fig. 2. Effect of aging on peripheral myelin protein P0 gene expression in the male rat sciatic nerve analyzed by Northern blot and normalized for 28s rRNA. Young rats were three months old and old rats were 22-24 months old (* : p ≤ 0.01; modified from Melcangi et al. 1998b)

decline in myelin protein gene expression by the administration of steroids. When old rats were injected every four days for one month with 1 mg of PROG, 3α,5α-TH PROG or 5α-dihydroprogesterone, the latter was found to significantly increase P0 mRNA levels (Fig. 3). Administration of the androgens testosterone or 5α-dihydrotestosterone did not affect P0 gene expression (Melcangi et al. 1998a,b). In contrast to P0, the low levels of PMP22 mRNA present in the sciatic nerve of old rats could not be restored by progestin treatment (Melcangi et al. 1999).

The prolonged administration of progestins not only counteracted the drop in P0 mRNA, it also allowed the reversal of age-related structural abnormalities of the peripheral myelin sheaths. The systemic treatment of old male rats with PROG, 5α-dihydroprogesterone or 3α,5α-TH PROG significantly decreased the percentage of fibers with myelin abnormalities and the number of fibers with irregular shapes, and it increased the number of small (< 5μm) myelinated fibers. Again, the administration of androgens was found to be inefficient in reversing the myelin abnormalities (Fig. 4; Azcoitia et al. 2003).

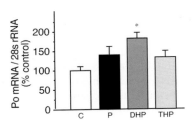

Fig. 3. Effect of *in vivo* treatment with progesterone (P), 5α-dihydroprogesterone (DHP) and 3α,5α-tetrahydroprogesterone (THP) on P0 mRNA expression in the sciatic nerve of aged (22-24 months old) male rats (c = control). Data were obtained by Northern blot analysis and were normalized for 28s rRNA. Rats were treated eight times with 1 mg of steroid over 32 days (every four days; * : p ≤ 0.01 versus control; modified from Melcangi et al. 2000)

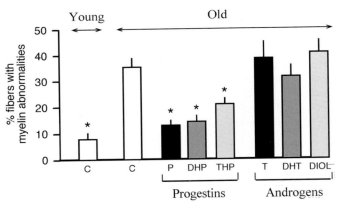

Fig. 4. Percentage of fibers presenting abnormalities of their myelin sheaths in the sciatic nerves of young (three months old) and old (22-24 months old) male rats. Rats were treated eight times with 1 mg of steroid over 32 days (every four days). C = vehicle, P = progesterone, DHP = 5α-dihydroprogesterone, THP = 3α,5α-terahydroprogesterone, T = testosterone, DHT = 5α-dihydrotestosterone, DIOL = 3α,5α- androstanediol (* : p ≤ 0.01 versus control; modified from Azcoitia et al. 2003).

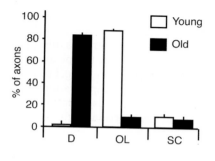

Fig. 5. Extent of spontaneous remyelination in the cerebellar peduncle of young (10 weeks old) and old (9 months old) male rats five weeks after infusion of the gliotoxin ethidium bromide (D = demyelinated axons, OL = axons remyelinated by oligodendrocytes, SC = axons remyelinated by Schwann cells of unknown origin; modified from Ibanez et al., submitted).

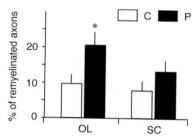

Fig. 6. Proportion of axons remyelinated by oligodendrocytes (OL) or by Schwann cells (SC) in control (C) versus progesterone-treated (P) nine-month-old male rats five weeks after gliotoxin-induced lesion. Two subcutaneous implants of PROG produced constant high physiological levels of circulating progesterone in the treated males (*: $p \leq 0.051$ versus control; modified from Ibanez et al., submitted).

As already mentioned, spontaneous remyelination after gliotoxin-induced demyelination is rapid in the CNS of young rats, but it is very much delayed in old rats (Fig. 5). The administration of subcutaneous implants of PROG, which produced persistent high physiological levels of circulating PROG, promoted the slow remyelination after toxin-induced demyelination in the cerebellar peduncle of old male rats. Five weeks after the lesion, the number of axons remyelinated by oligodendrocytes was slightly but significantly increased by the PROG treatment (Fig. 6). In young males, no effect of PROG could be detected because spontaneous remyelination was very rapid and nearly completed after only three weeks (Ibanez et al., 2003a; 2003b).

Conclusions

The findings that age-related changes in the nervous system are not as important as previously thought and that the aging nervous system retains capacity for regeneration are two important new concepts, as they signify that the treatment of age-related dysfunctions of the nervous system becomes possible. Steroids offer an attractive opportunity for reversing age-dependent dysfunctions of the brain and peripheral nerves for several reasons: 1) they easily cross the blood-brain and the blood-nerve barriers and they rapidly distribute and accumulate within the different parts the nervous system; 2) their administration can transiently restore age-associated learning- and memory deficits; and 3) they have been shown to reverse age-related decrease in myelin protein gene expression and structural abnormalities of myelin sheaths and also to accelerate myelin repair in old rats.

It is likely that steroids will take an increasingly important place in the field of research on aging. Indeed, it is now well recognized that they are not only sex or stress hormones, but that they also regulate many important nervous and glial functions throughout the nervous systems. On the other hand, the pleiotropic actions of natural steroids, in the nervous system and in peripheral target tissues, raise the problem of the selectivity of their potential therapeutic applications. For example, PROG may be useful to promote myelin repair, but it also affects many neurotransmitter systems and interferes with reproductive functions (Schumacher and Robert 2002). One strategy for overcoming the problem of the multiple side effects of natural steroids is to design synthetic analogues with selective actions on specific nervous functions. This could be achieved by taking advantage of the variety of molecular mechanisms involved in the actions of steroids that have recently been discovered: 1) there has been enormous progress in our understanding of the mechanisms by which ligand-activated intracellular steroid receptors regulate gene transcription in a cell-specific manner, in particular by the discovery of nuclear coregulator proteins (McKenna et al. 1999; Mani and O'Malley 2002); 2) steroids directly act on the cellular membrane and regulate the activity of specific neurotransmitter receptors (Schumacher et al. 1999; Lambert et al. 1999; Schmidt et al. 2000; Rupprecht et al. 2001; Razandi et al. 2002); and 3) steroids regulate intracellular signaling pathways (Boonyaratanakornkit et al. 2001; Beyer et al. 2002; Kousteni et al. 2001).

Neurosteroids are synthesized by neurons and glial cells in the CNS and PNS (Baulieu et al. 1999). Therefore, age-related changes in circulating steroid levels do not necessarily reflect changes of steroid levels within different parts of the nervous system. It is indeed possible that the local synthesis of neurosteroids compensates for the decrease in circulating levels. The concept of neurosteroids also offers the interesting therapeutic possibility of selectively increasing steroid synthesis within nervous tissues. Unfortunately, the regulation of neurosteroid synthesis within the nervous system is only poorly understood. Ligands of the mitochondrial benzodiazepine receptor, which increase the transport of cholesterol into the mitochondria, a rate-limiting step in steroid synthesis, could be used to locally increase the synthesis of neurosteroids (Papadopoulos et al. 1992; Papadopoulos and Brown 1995).

Acknowledgments

This work was supported by the Commission of the European Communities, specific RTD program "Quality of life and Management of Living Resources," QLK6-CT-2000-00179, "The role of neurosteroids in healthy aging: therapeutical perspectives." We also acknowledge support by the Projet Myéline (France) and the Myelin Project (USA).

References

Adinolfi AM, Yamuy J, Morales FR, Chase MH (1991) Segmental demyelination in peripheral nerves of old cats. Neurobiol Aging 12: 175–179

Akwa Y, Sananès NG, Robel P, Baulieu EE, Le Goascogne C (1993) Astrocytes and neurosteroids: metabolism of pregnenolone and dehydroepiandrosterone. Regulation by cell density. J Cell Biol 121: 135–143

Arlt W, Callies F, Allolio B (2000) DHEA replacement in women with adrenal insufficiency: pharmacokinetics, bioconversion and clinical effects on well-being, sexuality and cognition. Endocrinol Res 26: 505–511

Asthana S, Craft S, Baker LD, Raskind MA, Birnbaum RS, Lofgreen CP, Veith RC, Plymate SR (1999) Cognitive and neuroendocrine response to transdermal estrogen in postmenopausal women with Alzheimer's disease: results of a placebo-controlled, double-blind, pilot study. Psychoneuroendocrinology 24: 657–677

Asthana S, Baker LD, Craft S, Stanczyk FZ, Veith RC, Raskind MA, Plymate SR (2001) High-dose estradiol improves cognition for women with AD: results of a randomized study. Neurology 57: 605–612

Azcoitia I, Leonelli E, Magnaghi V, Veiga S, Garcia-Segura LM, Melcangi RC (2003) Progesterone and its derivatives dihydroprogesterone and tetrahydroprogesterone reduce myelin fiber morphological abnormalities and myelin fiber loss in the sciatic nerve of aged rats. Neurobiol Aging, 24: 853–860.

Balthazart J, Ball GF (1998) New insights into the regulation and function of brain estrogen synthase (aromatase). Trends Neurosci 21: 243–249

Barrett-Connor E, Edelstein SL (1994) A prospective study of dehydroepiandrosterone sulfate and cognitive function in an older population : the Rancho Bernardo Study. J Am Geriatr Soc 42: 420–423

Baulieu EE (1981) Steroid hormones in the brain: several mechanisms? In: Fuxe K, Gustafsson JA, Wetterberg L (eds), Steroid hormone regulation of the brain. (Oxford, Pergamon Press, pp 3–14

Baulieu EE, Robel P, Schumacher M (1999) Neurosteroids. A new regulatory function in the nervous system. Totowa, New Jersey, Humana Press.

Baulieu EE, Thomas G, Legrain S, Lahlou N, Roger M, Debuire B, Faucounau V, Girard L, Hervy MP, Latour F, Leaud MC, Mokrane A, Pitti F, Trivalle C, de Lacharriere O, Nouveau S, Rakoto A, Souberbielle JC, Raison J, Le Bouc Y, Raynaud A, Girerd X, Forette F (2000) Dehydroepiandrosterone (DHEA), DHEA sulfate, and aging: contribution of the DHEAge Study to a sociobiomedical issue. Proc Natl Acad Sci USA 97: 4279–4284

Beck CA, Weigel NL, Moyer ML, Nordeen SK, Edwards DP (1993) The progesterone antagonist RU486 acquires agonist activity upon stimulation of cAMP signaling pathways. Proc Natl Acad Sci USA 90: 4441–4445

Behl C, Skutella T, Lezoualc'h F, Post A, Widmann M, Newton CJ, Holsboer F (1997) Neuroprotection against oxidative stress by estrogens: structure-activity relationship. Mol Pharmacol 51: 535–541

Belanger A, Candas B, DuPont A, Cusan L, Diamond P, Gomez JL, Labrie F (1994) Changes in serum concentrations of conjugated and unconjugated steroids in 40- to 80-year-old men. J Clin Endocrinol Metab 79: 1086–1090

Bellino FL, Daynes RA, Hornsby PJ, Lavrin DH, Nestler JE (1995) Dehydroepiandrosterone (DHEA) and aging. New York, New York Academy of Sciences, vol. 774

Bernardi F, Salvestroni C, Casarosa E, Nappi RE, Lanzone A, Luisi S, Purdy RH, Petraglia F, Genazzani AR (1998) Aging is associated with changes in allopregnanolone concentrations in brain, endocrine glands and serum in male rats. Eur J Endocrinol 138: 316–321

Beyer C, Ivanova T, Karolczak M, Kuppers E (2002) Cell type-specificity of nonclassical estrogen signaling in the developing midbrain. J Steroid Biochem Mol Biol 81: 319

Bologa L, Sharma J, Roberts E (1987) Dehydroepiandrosterone and its sulfated derivative reduce neuronal death and enhance astrocytic differentiation in brain cell cultures. J Neurosci Res 17: 225–234

Boonyaratanakornkit V, Scott MP, Ribon V, Sherman L, Anderson SM, Maller JL, Miller WT, Edwards DP (2001) Progesterone receptor contains a proline-rich motif that directly interacts with SH3 domains and activates c-Src family tyrosine kinases. Mol Cell 8: 269–280

Brenner DE, Kukull WA, Stergachis A, van Belle G, Bowen JD, McCormick WC, Teri L, Larson EB (1994) Postmenopausal estrogen replacement therapy and the risk of Alzheimer's disease: a population-based case-control study. Am J Epidemiol 140: 262–267

Buchthal F, Rosenfalck A, Behse F (1984) Sensory potentials of normal and diseased nerves. In: Dyck PJ, Thomas PK, Lambert EH (eds) Peripheral neuropathy. Philadelphia: Saunders, pp 981–1105

Burger HG, Dudley EC, Robertson DM, Dennerstein L (2002) Hormonal changes in the menopause transition. Recent Prog Horm Res 57: 257–275

Callier S, Morissette M, Grandbois M, Di Paolo T (2000) Stereospecific prevention by 17beta-estradiol of MPTP-induced dopamine depletion in mice. Synapse 37: 245–251

Cardounel A, Regelson W, Kalimi M (1999) Dehydroepiandrosterone protects hippocampal neurons against neurotoxin-induced cell death: mechanism of action. Soc Exp Biol Med 222: 145–149

Carlson LE, Sherwin BB (1999) Relationships among cortisol (CRT), dehydroepiandrosterone-sulfate (DHEAS), and memory in a longitudinal study of healthy elderly men and women. Neurobiol Aging 20: 315–324

Carlson LE, Sherwin BB, Chertkow MH (1999) Relationship between dehydroepiandrosterone sulfate (DHEAS) and cortisol (CRT) plasma levels and everyday memory in Alzheimer's disease patients compared to healthy controls. Horm Behav 35: 254–263

Cascio C, Prasad VV, Lin YY, Lieberman S, Papadopoulos V (1998) Detection of P450c17-independent pathways for dehydroepiandrosterone (DHEA) biosynthesis in brain glial tumor cells. Proc Natl Acad Sci USA 95: 2862–2867

Chan JR, Phillips LJ, Glaser M (1998) Glucocorticoids and progestins signal the initiation and enhance the rate of myelin formation. Proc Natl Acad Sci USA 95: 10459–10464

Coirini H, Gouézou M, Liere P, Delespierre B, Pianos A, Eychenne B, Schumacher M, Guennoun R (2003) 3beta-hydroxysteroid dehydrogenase expression in rat spinal cord. Neuroscience, 113: 883–891

Compagnone NA, Mellon SH (1998) Dehydroepiandrosterone: a potential signalling molecule for neocortical organization during development. Proc Natl Acad Sci USA 95: 4678–4683

Corpéchot C, Robel P, Axelson M, Sjövall J, Baulieu EE (1981) Characterization and measurement of dehydroepiandrosterone sulfate in the rat brain. Proc Natl Acad Sci USA 78: 4704–4707

Costa MM, Reus VI, Wolkowitz OM, Manfredi F, Lieberman M (1999) Estrogen replacement therapy and cognitive decline in memory-impaired post-menopausal women. Biol Psychiat 46: 182–188

Csapo AI, Pulkkinen M (1978) Indispensability of the human corpus luteum in the maintenance of early pregnancy. Luteectomy evidence. Obstet Gynecol Surv 33: 69–81

Cunningham CJ, Sinnott M, Denihan A, Rowan M, Walsh JB, O'Moore R, Coakley D, Coen RF, Lawler BA, O'Neill DD (2001) Endogenous sex hormone levels in postmenopausal women with Alzheimer's disease. J Clin Endocrinol Metab 86: 1099–1103

Demerens C, Stankoff B, Logak M, Anglade P, Allinquant B, Couraud F, Zalc B, Lubetzki C (1996) Induction of myelination in the central nervous system by electrical activity. Proc Natl Acad Sci USA 93: 9887–9892

Désarnaud F, Do T, Brown AM, Lemke G, Suter U, Baulieu EE, Schumacher M (1998) Progesterone stimulates the activity of the promoters of peripheral myelin protein-22 and protein zero genes in Schwann cells. J Neurochem 71: 1765–1768

Dewaegh SM, Lee VMY, Brady ST (1992) Local modulation of neurofilament phosphorylation, axonal caliber, and slow axonal transport by myelinating Schwann cells. Cell 68: 451–463

Fajer AB, Holzbauer M, Newport HM (1971) The contribution of the adrenal gland to the total amount of progesterone produced in the female rat. J Physiol (Lond) 214: 115–126

Feder HH, Resko JA, Goy RW (1968) Progesterone levels in the arterial plasma of pre-ovulatory and ovariectomized rats. J Endocrinol 41: 563–569

Fernandez PA, Tang DG, Cheng L, Prochiantz A, Mudge AW, Raff MC (2000) Evidence that axon-derived neuregulin promotes oligodendrocyte survival in the developing rat optic nerve. Neuron 28: 81–90

Ferrario E, Massaia M, Aimo G, di Ceva PA, Fabris F (1999) Dehydroepiandrosterone sulfate serum levels: no significance in diagnosing Alzheimer's disease. J Endocrinol Invest 22: 81

Ferreira A, Caceres A (1991) Estrogen-enhanced neurite growth: evidence for a selective induction of Tau and stable microtubules. J Neurosci 11: 392–400

Fillenbaum GG, Hanlon JT, Landerman LR, Schmader KE (2001) Impact of estrogen use on decline in cognitive function in a representative sample of older community-resident women. Am J Epidemiol 153: 137–144

Gago N, Akwa Y, Sananes N, Guennoun R, Baulieu EE, El-Etr M, Schumacher M (2001) Progesterone and the oligodendroglial lineage: stage-dependent biosynthesis and metabolism. Glia 36: 295–308

Garcia-Segura LM, Azcoitia I, Doncarlos LL (2001) Neuroprotection by estradiol. Prog Neurobiol 63: 29–60

Genazzani AD, Petraglia F, Bernardi F, Casarosa E, Salvestroni C, Tonetti A, Nappi RE, Luisi S, Palumbo M, Purdy RH, Luisi M (2002) Circulating levels of alloprenanolone in humans: gender, age and endocrine influences. J Clin Endocrinol Metab 83: 2099–2103

Gilson J, Blakemore WF (1993) Failure of remyelination in areas of demyelination produced in the spinal cord of old rats. Neuropathol Appl Neurobiol 19: 173–181

Gomez-Isla T, Price JL, McKeel DW, Morris JC, Growdon JH, Hyman BT (1996) Profound loss of layer II entorhinal cortex neurons occurs in very mild Alzheimer's disease. J Neurosci 16: 4491–4500

Goodman Y, Bruce AJ, Cheng B, Mattson MP (1996) Estrogens attenuate and corticosterone exacerbates excitotoxicity, oxidative injury, and amyloid beta-peptide toxicity in hippocampal neurons. J Neurochem 66: 1836–1844

Goujet-Zalc C, Babinet C, Monge M, Timsit S, Cabon F, Gansmuller A, Miura M, Sanchez M, Pournin S, Mikoshiba K, Zalc B (1993) The proximal region of the MBP gene promoter is sufficient to induce oligodendroglial-specific expression in transgenic mice. Eur J Neurosci 5: 624–632

Gould E, Tanapat P, Rydel T, Hastings N (2000) Regulation of hippocampal neurogenesis in adulthood. Biol Psychiat 48: 715–720

Green PS, Perez EJ, Calloway T, Simpkins JW (2000) Estradiol attenuation of beta-amyloid-induced toxicity: a comparison of MTT and calcein AM assays. J Neurocytol 29: 419–423

Grover-Johnson N, Spencer PS (1981) Peripheral nerve abnormalities in aging rats. J Neuropathol Exp Neurol 40: 155–165

Guennoun R, Fiddes RJ, Gouézou M, Lombès M, Baulieu EE (1995) A key enzyme in the biosynthesis of neurosteroids, 3β-hydroxysteroid dehydrogenase/Δ5-Δ4-isomerase (3β-HSD), is expressed in rat brain. Mol Brain Res 30: 287–300

Guennoun R, Schumacher M, Robert F, Delespierre B, Gouézou M, Eychenne B, Akwa Y, Robel P, Baulieu EE (1997) Neurosteroids: expression of functional 3β-hydroxysteroid dehydrogenase by rat sensory neurons and Schwann cells. Eur J Neurosci 9: 2236–2247

Gutai JP, Meyer WJ, Kowarski AA, Migeon CJ (1977) Twenty-four hour integrated concentrations of progesterone, 17-hydroxyprogesterone and cortisol in normal male subjects. J Clin Endocrinol Metab 44: 116–120

Henderson VW, Paganini-Hill A, Emanuel CK, Dunn ME, Buckwalter JG (1994) Estrogen replacement therapy in older women. Comparisons between Alzheimer's disease cases and nondemented control subjects. Arch Neurol 51: 896–900

Henderson VW, Paganini-Hill A, Miller BL, Elbe RJ, Reyes PF, Shoupe D, McCleary CA, Klein RA, Hake AM, Farlow MR (2000) Estrogen for Alzheimer's disease in women: randomized, double-blind, placebo-controlled trial. Neurology 54: 295–301

Herbert J (1995) The age of dehydroepiandrosterone. Lancet 345: 1193–1194

Hildebrand C, Bowe CM, Remahl IN (1994) Myelination and myelin sheath remodelling in normal and pathological PNS nerve fibers. Prog Neurobiol 43: 85–141

Hinks GL, Franklin RJM (2000) Delayed changes in growth factor gene expression during slow remyelination in the CNS of aged rats. Mol Cell Neurosci 16: 542–556

Holzbauer M, Newport HM, Birmingham MK, Traikov H (1969) Secretion of pregn-4-ene-3,20-dione (progesterone) in vivo by the adrenal gland of the rat. Nature 221: 572–573

Ibanez C, Shields SA, El Etr M, Leonelli E, Magnaghi V, Li WW, Sim FJ, Baulieu EE, Melcangi RC, Schumacher M, Franklin RJ (2003a) Steroids and the reversal of age-associated changes in myelination and remyelination. Prog Neurobiol, in press.

Ibanez C, Shields SA, Liere P, el-Etr M, Baulieu EE, Schumacher M, Franklin RJM (2003b) Systemic progesterone administration results in a partial reversal of the age-associated decline in CNS remyelination following toxin-induced demyelination in male rats. Neuropathol Appl Neurobiol, in press.

Jacobs DM, Tang MX, Stern Y, Sano M, Marder K, Bell KL, Schofield P, Dooneief G, Gurland B, Mayeux R (1998) Cognitive function in nondemented older women who took estrogen after menopause. Neurology 50: 368–373

Jiang N, Chopp M, Stein DG, Feldblum S (1996) Progesterone is neuroprotective after transient middle cerebral artery occlusion in male rats. Brain Res 735: 101–107

Jones SJ (1993) Visual evoked potentials after optic neuritis. J Neurol 240: 489–494.

Jung-Testas I, Hu ZY, Baulieu EE, Robel P (1989) Neurosteroids: Biosynthesis of pregnenolone and progesterone in primary cultures of rat glial cells. Endocrinology 125: 2083–2091

Jung-Testas I, Renoir JM, Gasc JM, Baulieu EE (1991) Estrogen-inducible progesterone receptor in primary cultures of rat glial cells. Exp Cell Res 193: 12–19

Jung-Testas I, Schumacher M, Robel P, Baulieu EE (1996a) Demonstration of progesterone receptors in rat Schwann cells. J Steroid Biochem Mol Biol 58: 77–82

Jung-Testas I, Schumacher M, Robel P, Baulieu EE (1996b) The neurosteroid progesterone increases the expression of myelin proteins (MBP and CNPase) in rat oligodendrocytes in primary culture. Cell Mol Neurobiol 16: 439–443

Kalimi M, Regelson W (1990) The biological role of dehydroepiandrosterone. Berlin, Walter de Gruyter

Kalmijn S, Launer LJ, Stolk RP, De Jong FH, Pols HA, Hofman A, Breteler MM, Lamberts SW (1998) A prospective study on cortisol, dehydroepiandrosterone sulfate, and cognitive function in the elderly. J Clin Endocrinol Metab 83: 3487–3492

Kanda T, Tsukagoshi H, Oda M, Miyamoto K, Tanabe H (1991) Morphological changes in unmyelinated fibers in the sural nerve with age. Brain 114: 585–599

Karishma KK, Herbert J (2002) Dehydroepiandrosterone (DHEA) stimulates neurogenesis in the hippocampus of the rat, promotes survival of newly formed neurons and prevents corticosterone-induced suppression. Eur J Neurosci 16: 445–453

Kawas C, Resnick S, Morrison A, Brookmeyer R, Corrada M, Zonderman A, Bacal C, Lingle DD, Metter E (1997) A prospective study of estrogen replacement therapy and the risk of developing Alzheimer's disease: the Baltimore Longitudinal Study of Aging. Neurology 48: 1517–1521

Key TJ (2000) Progestins in postmenopausal women: epidemiological data on relationships with endometrial and breast cancer risk. In: Sitruk-Ware R, Mishell DR (eds) Progestins and antiprogestins in clinical practice New York: Marcel Dekker, pp 279–287

Khaw KT (1992) Epidemiology of the menopause. Br Med Bull 48: 249–261

Kimonides VG, Spilantini MG, Sofroniew MV, Fawcett JW, Herbert J (1999) Dehydroepiandrosterone antagonizes the neurotoxic effects of corticosterone and translocation of stress-activated protein kinase 3 in hippocampal primary cultures. Neuroscience 89: 429–436

Knox CA, Kokmen E, Dyck PJ (1989) Morphometric alteration of rat myelinated fibers with aging. J Neuropathol Exp Neurol 48: 119–139

Koenig H, Schumacher M, Ferzaz B, Do Thi AN, Ressouches A, Guennoun R, Jung-Testas I, Robel P, Akwa Y, Baulieu EE (1995) Progesterone synthesis and myelin formation by Schwann cells. Science 268: 1500–1503

Koski CL, Max SR (1980) Comparison of the protein composition of myelin of motor and sensory nerves. J Neurochem 34: 449–452

Kousteni S, Bellido T, Plotkin LI, Brien CA, Bodenner DL, Han L, Han K, DiGregorio GB, Katzenellenbogen JA, Katzenellenbogen BS, Roberson PK, Weinstein RS, Jilka RL, Manolagas SC (2001) Nongenotropic, sex-nonspecific signaling through the estrogen or androgen receptors: dissociation from transcriptional activity. Cell 104: 719–730

Labrie F, Bélanger A, Cusan L, Candas B (1997) Physiological changes in dehydroepiandrosterone are not reflected by serum levels of active androgens and estrogens but of their metabolites: intracrinology. J Clin Endocrinol Metab 82: 2403–2409

Lambert JJ, Belleli D, Shepherd SE, Pistis M, Peters JA (1999) The selective interaction of neurosteroids with the GABA$_A$ receptor. In: Baulieu EE, Robel P, Schumacher M (eds), Neurosteroids. A new regulatory function in the nervous system. (Totowa, New Jersey, Humana Press, pp 125–142

Lamberts SW, van den Beld AW, van der Lely AJ (1997) The endocrinology of aging. Science 278: 419–424

Lascelles RG, Thomas PK (1966) Changes due to age in internodal length in the sural nerve in man. J Neurol Neurosurg Psychiat 29: 40–44

Laughlin GA, Barrett-Connor E (2000) Sexual dimorphism in the influence of advanced aging on adrenal hormone levels: the Rancho Bernardo Study. J Clin Endocrinol Metab 85: 3561–3568

Leblhuber F, Neubauer C, Peichl M, Reisecker F, Steinparz FX, Windhager E, Dienstl E (1993) Age and sex differences of dehydroepiandrosterone sulfate (DHEAS) and cortisol (CRT) plasma levels in normal controls and Alzheimer's disease (AD). Psychopharmacology 111: 23–26

Le Goascogne C, Robel P, Gouézou M, Sananès N, Baulieu EE, Waterman M (1987) Neurosteroids: cytochrome P450scc in rat brain. Science 237: 1212-1215

Le Goascogne C, Gouézou M, Robel P, Defaye G, Chambaz E, Waterman MR, Baulieu EE (1989) The cholesterol side-chain cleavage complex in human brain white matter. J Neuroendocrinol 1: 153–156

Lee SJ, McEwen BS (2001) Neurotrophic and neuroprotective actions of estrogens and their therapeutic implications. Annu Rev Pharmacol Toxicol 41: 569–591

Legrain S, Berr C, Frenoy N, Gourlet V, Debuire B, Baulieu EE (1995) Dehydroepiandrosterone sulfate in a long-term care aged population. Gerontology 41: 343–351

Lemke G (1993) The molecular genetics of myelination: an update. Glia 7: 263–271

Lorenzo A, Diaz H, Carrer H, Caceres A (1992) Amygdala neurons in vitro – neurite growth and effects of estradiol. J Neurosci Res 33: 418–435

Lupien SJ, De Leon M, de Santi S, Convit A, Tarshish C, Nair NP, Thakur M, McEwen BS, Hauger RL, Meaney MJ (1998) Cortisol levels during human aging predict hippocampal atrophy and memory deficits. Nature Neurosci 1: 69–73

Lupien SJ, Nair NP, Briere S, Maheu F, Tu MT, Lemay M, McEwen BS, Meaney MJ (1999) Increased cortisol levels and impaired cognition in human aging: implication for depression and dementia in later life. Rev Neurosci 10: 117–139

Magnaghi V, Cavarretta I, Zucchi I, Susani L, Rupprecht R, Hermann B, Martini L, Melcangi RC (1999) Po gene expression is modulated by androgens in the sciatic nerve of adult male rats. Mol Brain Res 70: 36–44

Magnaghi V, Cavarretta I, Galbiati M, Martini L, Melcangi RC (2001) Neuroactive steroids and peripheral myelin proteins. Brain Res Rev 37: 360–371

Maisonobe T, Hauw JJ (1997) Changes in the peripheral nervous system. In: Dani SU, Hori A, Walter GF (eds) Principles of neural aging (Amsterdam, Elsevier, pp 304–316

Mani SK, O'Malley BW (2002) Mechanisms of progesterone receptor action in the brain. In: Pfaff DW, Arnold AP, Etgen AM, Fahrbach SE, Rubin RT (eds) Hormones, brain and behavior. Volume 3. Amsterdam, Academic Press, pp 643–682

Manly JJ, Merchant CA, Jacobs DM, Small SA, Bell K, Ferin M, Mayeux R (2000) Endogenous estrogen levels and Alzheimer's disease among postmenopausal women. Neurology 54: 833–837.

Marchionni MA, Cannella B, Hoban C, Gao YL, Garcia A, Lawson D, Happel E, Noel F, Tofilon P, Gwynne D, Raine CS (1999) Neuregulin in neuron/glial interactions in the central nervous system. GGF2 diminishes autoimmune demyelination, promotes oligodendrocyte progenitor expansion, and enhances remyelination. Adv Exp Med Biol 468: 283–295

Maurice T, Junien JL, Privat A (1997) Dehydroepiandrosterone sulfate attenuates dizocilpine-induced learning impairment in mice via sigma 1-receptors. Behav Brain Res 83: 159–164

Maurice T, Su TP, Privat A (1998) Sigma1 (sigma 1) receptor agonists and neurosteroids attenuate B25-35-amyloid peptide-induced amnesia in mice through a common mechanism. Neuroscience 83: 413–428

Mayo W, Vallée M, Darnaudéry M, Le Moal M (1999) Neurosteroids: behavioral studies. In: Baulieu EE, Robel P, Schumacher M (eds) Neurosteroids. A new regulatory function in the nervous system. (Totowa, New Jersey, Humana Press, pp 317–336

Mazat L, Lafont S, Debuire B, Tessier JF, Dartigues JF, Baulieu EE (2001) Prospective measurements of dehydroepiandrosterone sulfate in a cohort of elderly subjects: relationship, to gender, subjective health, smoking habits, and 10-year mortality. Proc Natl Acad Sci USA 98: 8145–8150

McEwen BS, Sapolsky RM (1995) Stress and cognitive function. Curr Opin Neurobiol 5: 205–216

McEwen BS, Alves SE (1999) Estrogen actions in the central nervous system. Endocrinol Rev 20: 279–307

McEwen BS, De Leon MJ, Lupien SJ, Meaney MJ (1999) Corticosteroids, the aging brain and cognition. Trends Endocrinol Metab 10: 92–96

McIntosh MK, Pan JS, Berdanier CD (1993) In vitro studies on the effects of dehydro-epiandrosterone and corticosterone on hepatic-steroid receptor-binding and mitochondrial respiration. Comp Biochem Physiol 104: 147–153

McKenna NJ, Lanz RB, O'Malley BW (1999) Nuclear receptor coregulators: cellular and molecular biology. Endocrinol Rev 20: 321–344

Melcangi RC, Celotti F, Ballabio M, Castano P, Poletti A, Milani S, Martini L (1988) Ontogenic development of the 5α-reductase in the rat brain: cerebral cortex, hypothalamus, purified myelin and isolated oligodendrocytes. Dev Brain Res 44: 181–188

Melcangi RC, Celotti F, Ballabio M, Poletti A, Martini L (1990) Testosterone metabolism in peripheral nerves: presence of the 5α-reductase-3β-hydroxysteroid-dehydrogenase enzymatic system in the sciatic nerve of adult and aged rats. J Steroid Biochem 35: 145–148

Melcangi RC, Celotti F, Castano P, Martini L (1992) Is the 5α-reductase-3α-hydroxysteroid dehydrogenase complex associated with the myelin in the peripheral nervous system of young and old male rats ? Endocrine Res 26: 119–125

Melcangi RC, Celotti F, Martini L (1994a) Neurons influence the metabolism of testosterone in cultured astrocytes via hormonal signals. Endocrine J 2: 709–713

Melcangi RC, Celotti F, Martini L (1994b) Progesterone 5α-reduction in neuronal and in different types of glial cell cultures: type 1 and type 2 astrocytes and oligodendrocytes. Brain Res 639: 202–206

Melcangi RC, Magnaghi V, Cavarretta I, Riva MA, Piva F, Martini L (1998a) Effects of steroid hormones on gene expression of glial markers in the central and peripheral nervous system: variations induced by aging. Exp Gerontol 33: 827–836

Melcangi RC, Magnaghi V, Cavarretta I, Martini L, Piva F (1998b) Age-induced decrease of glycoprotein Po and myelin basic protein gene expression in the rat sciatic nerve. Repair by steroid derivatives. Neuroscience 85: 569–578

Melcangi RC, Magnaghi V, Cavarretta I, Zucchi I, Bovolin P, D'Urso D, Martini L (1999) Progesterone derivatives are able to influence peripheral myelin protein 22 and P0 gene expression: possible mechanisms of action. J Neurosci Res 56: 349–357

Melcangi RC, Magnaghi V, Martini L (2000) Aging in peripheral nerves: regulation of myelin protein genes by steroid hormones. Prog Neurobiol 60: 291–308.

Mellon SH, Griffin LD, Compagnone NA (2001) Biosynthesis and action of neurosteroids. Brain Res Rev 37: 3–12

Mensah-Nyagan AG, Feuilloley M, Dupont E, Do-Rego JL, Leboulenger F, Pelletier G, Vaudry H (1994) Immunocytochemical localization and biological activity of 3β-hydroxysteroid dehydrogenase in the central nervous system of the frog. J Neurosci 14: 7306–7318

Mensah-Nyagan AG, Do-Rego JL, Beaujean D, Luu-The V, Pelletier G, Vaudry H (1999) Neurosteroids: expression of steroidogenic enzymes and regulation of steroid biosynthesis in the central nervous system. Pharmacol Rev 51: 63–81

Messing A, Behringer RR, Hammang JP, Palmiter RD, Brinster RL, Lemke G (1992) Po promoter directs expression of reporter and toxin genes to Schwann cells of transgenic mice. Neuron 8: 507–520

Morales AJ, Nolan JJ, Nelson JC, Yen SSC (1994) Effects of replacement dose of dehydro-epiandrosterone in men and women of advancing age. J Clin Endocrinol Metab 78: 1360–1367

Morales AJ, Haubrich RH, Hwang JY, Asakura H, Yen SS (1998) The effect of six months treatment with 100 mg daily dose of dehydroepiandrosterone (DHEA) on circulating sex steroids, body composition and muscle strength in age-advanced men and women. Clin Endocrinol 49: 421–432

Morfin R, Young J, Corpéchot C, Egestad B, Sjövall J, Baulieu EE (1992) Neurosteroids: pregnenolone in human sciatic nerves. Proc Natl Acad Sci USA 89: 6790–6793

Morley JE, Kaiser F, Raum WJ, Perry HM, Flood JF, Jensen J, Silver AJ, Roberts E (1997) Potentially predictive and manipulable blood serum correlates of aging in the healthy human male: progressive decreases in bioavailable testosterone, dehydroepiandrosterone sulfate, and the ratio of insulin-like growth factor 1 to growth hormone. Proc Natl Acad Sci USA 94: 7537–7542

Mulnard RA, Cotman CW, Kawas C, van Dyck CH, Sano M, Doody R, Koss E, Pfeiffer E, Jin S, Gamst A, Grundman M, Thomas R, Thal LJ (2000) Estrogen replacement therapy for treatment of mild to moderate Alzheimer disease: a randomized controlled trial. JAMA 283: 1007–1015

Murialdo G, Nobili F, Rollero A, Gianelli MV, Copello F, Rodriguez G, Polleri A (2000) Hippocampal perfusion and pituitary-adrenal axis in Alzheimer's disease. Neuropsychobiology 42: 51–57

Nafziger AN, Bowlin SJ, Jenkins PL, Pearson TA, Melcangi RC, Celotti F, Ballabio M, Poletti A, Castano P, Martini L, Biegon A, Fischette CT, Rainbow TC, McEwen BS (1998) Longitudinal changes in dehydroepiandrosterone concentrations in men and women. J Lab Clin Med 131: 316–323

Notterpek L, Snipes GJ, Shooter EM (1999) Temporal expression pattern of peripheral myelin protein 22 during in vivo and in vitro myelination. Glia 25: 358–369

Nichols NR, Zieba M, Bye N (2001) Do glucocorticoids contribute to brain aging? Brain Res Rev 37: 273–286

Nordeen SK, Bona BJ, Moyer ML (1993) Latent agonist activity of the steroid antagonist, RU486, is unmasked in cells treated with activators of protein kinase A. Mol Endocrinol 7: 731–742

Orentreich N, Brind JL, Rizer RL, Vogelman JH (1984) Age changes and sex differences in serum dehydroepiandrosterone sulfate concentrations throughout adulthood. J Clin Endocrinol Metab 59: 551–555

Paganini-Hill A, Henderson VW (1994) Estrogen deficiency and risk of Alzheimer's disease in women. Am J Epidemiol 140: 256–261

Paganini-Hill A, Henderson VW (1996) Estrogen replacement therapy and risk of Alzheimer's disease. Arch Intern Med 156: 2213–2217.

Papadopoulos V, Brown AS (1995) Role of the peripheral-type benzodiazepine receptor and the polypeptide diazepam binding inhibitor in steroidogenesis. J Steroid Biochem Mol Biol 53: 103–110

Papadopoulos V, Guarneri P, Krueger KE, Guidotti A, Costa E (1992) Pregnenolone biosynthesis in C6-2B glioma cell mitochondria – regulation by a mitochondrial diazepam binding inhibitor receptor. Proc Natl Acad Sci USA 89: 5113–5117

Peters A (1996) Age-related changes in oligodendrocytes in monkey cerebral cortex. J Comp Neurol 371: 153–163

Peters A (2002) Structural changes in the normally aging cerebral cortex of primates. Prog Brain Res 136: 455–465

Peters A, Rosene DL, Moss MB, Kemper TL, Abraham CR, Tigges J, Albert MS (1996) Neurobiological bases of age-related cognitive decline in the rhesus monkey. J Neuropathol Exp Neurol 55: 861–874

Peters A, Morrison JH, Rosene DL, Hyman BT (1998) Feature article: are neurons lost from the primate cerebral cortex during normal aging? Cereb Cortex 8: 295–300

Peters A, Moss MB, Sethares C (2000) Effects of aging on myelinated nerve fibers in monkey primary visual cortex. J Comp Neurol 419: 364–376

Peters A, Sethares C, Killiany RJ (2001) Effects of age on the thickness of myelin sheaths in monkey primary visual cortex. J Comp Neurol 435: 241–248

Phillips SM, Sherwin BB (1992) Effects of estrogen on memory function in surgically menopausal women. Psychoneuroendocrinology 17: 485–495

Pike MC, Ross RK (2000) Progestins and menopause: epidemiological studies of risks of endometrial and breast cancer. Steroids 65: 659–664

Pittella JEH (1997) Changes in white matter. In: Dani SU, Hori A, Walter GF (eds) Principles of neural aging. Amsterdam, Elsevier, pp 285–295

Ravaglia G, Forti P, Maioli F, Boschi F, Bernardi M, Pratelli L, Pizzoferrato A, Gasbarrini G (1996) The relationship of dehydroepiandrosterone sulfate (DHEAS) to endocrine-metabolic parameters and functional status in the oldest-old. Results from an Italian study on healthy free-living over-ninety-year-olds. J Clin Endocrinol Metab 81: 1173–1178

Razandi M, Oh P, Pedram A, Schnitzer J, Levin ER (2002) ERs associate with and regulate the production of caveolin: implications for signaling and cellular actions. Mol Endocrinol 16: 100–115

Resko JA (1969) Endocrine control of adrenal progesterone secretion in the ovariectomized rat. Science 164: 70–71

Resnick SM, Maki PM, Golski S, Kraut MA, Zonderman AB (1998) Effects of estrogen replacement therapy on PET cerebral blood flow and neuropsychological performance. Horm Behav 34: 171–182

Reynolds ML, Woolf CJ (1993) Reciprocal Schwann cell-axon interactions. Curr Opin Neurobiol 3: 683–693

Robel P, Schumacher M, Baulieu EE (1999) Neurosteroids: from definition and biochemistry to physiological function. In: Baulieu EE, Robel P, Schumacher M)eds) Neurosteroids. A new regulatory function in the nervous system. (Totowa, Humana Press, pp 1–25

Robert F, Guennoun R, Desarnaud F, Do-Thi A, Benmessahel Y, Baulieu EE, Schumacher M (2001) Synthesis of progesterone in Schwann cells: regulation by sensory neurons. Eur J Neurosci 13: 916–924

Roof RL, Duvdevani R, Stein DG (1993) Gender influences outcome of brain injury - progesterone plays a protective role. Brain Res 607: 333–336

Roof RL, Duvdevani R, Braswell L, Stein DG (1994) Progesterone facilitates cognitive recovery and reduces secondary neuronal loss caused by cortical contusion injury in male rats. Exp Neurol 129: 64–69

Rowe JW, Kahn RL (1997) Successful aging. Gerontology 37: 433–440

Rupprecht R, di M, Hermann B, Strohle A, Lancel M, Romeo E, Holsboer F (2001) Neuroactive steroids: molecular mechanisms of action and implications for neuropsychopharmacology. Brain Res Rev 37: 59–67

Sandell JH, Peters A (2001) Effects of age on nerve fibers in the rhesus monkey optic nerve. J Comp Neurol 429: 541–553

Sanne JL, Krueger KE (1995) Expression of cytochrome P450 side-chain cleavage enzyme and 3β-hydroxysteroid dehydrogenase in the rat central nervous system: a study by polymerase chain reaction and in situ hybridization. J Neurochem 65: 528–536

Sato A, Sato Y, Suzuki H (1985) Aging effects on conduction velocities of myelinated and un-myelinated fibers of peripheral nerves. Neurosci Lett 53: 15–20.

Schaeffer C, Aron C (1987) Stress-related effects on the secretion of progesterone by the adrenals in castrated male rats presented to stimulus males. Involvement of oestrogen. Acta Endocrinol 114: 440–445

Schmidt BM, Gerdes D, Feuring M, Falkenstein E, Christ M, Wehling M (2000) Rapid, nongenomic steroid actions: A new age? Front Neuroendocrinol 21: 57–94

Schonknecht P, Pantel J, Klinga K, Jensen M, Hartmann T, von Bergmann K, Beyreuther K, Schroder J (2001) Reduced cerebrospinal fluid estradiol levels are associated with increased beta-amyloid levels in female patients with Alzheimer's disease. Neurosci Lett 307: 83–85

Schumacher M, Robert F (2002) Progesterone: synthesis, metabolism, mechanisms of action, and effects in the nervous system. In: Pfaff DW, Arnold AP, Etgen AM, Fahrbach SE, Rubin RT (eds) Hormones, brain and behavior. Volume 3. Amsterdam, Academic Press, pp 683–745

Schumacher M, Coirini H, Robert F, Guennoun R, el-Etr M (1999) Genomic and membrane actions of progesterone: implications for reproductive physiology and behavior. Behav Brain Res 105: 37–52

Schumacher M, Guennoun R, Mercier G, Desarnaud F, Lacor P, Benavides J, Ferzaz B, Robert F, Baulieu EE (2001) Progesterone synthesis and myelin formation in peripheral nerves. Brain Res Rev 37: 343–359

Shields SA, Gilson JM, Blakemore WF, Franklin RJ (1999) Remyelination occurs as extensively but more slowly in old rats compared to young rats following gliotoxin-induced CNS demyelination. Glia 28: 77–83

Shors TJ, Miesegaes G, Beylin A, Zhao M, Rydel T, Gould E (2001) Neurogenesis in the adult is involved in the formation of trace memories. Nature 410: 372–376

Sih R, Morley JE, Kaiser FE, Perry HM, Patrick P, Ross C (1997) Testosterone replacement in older hypogonadal men: a 12-month randomized controlled trial. J Clin Endocrinol Metab 82: 1661–1667

Sim FJ, Zhao C, Penderis J, Franklin RJM (2002) The age-related decrease in CNS remyelination efficiency is attributable to an impairment of both oligodendrocyte progenitor recruitment and differentiation. J Neurosci 22: 2451–2459

Sitruk-Ware R (2000a) Progestins in hormonal replacement therapy and cardiovascular risk. In: (Sitruk-Ware R, Mishell DR (eds) Progestins and antiprogestins in clinical practice New York, Marcel Dekker, pp 289–304

Sitruk-Ware R (2000b) Progestins in hormonal replacement therapy and prevention of endometrial disease. In: Sitruk-Ware R, Mishell DR (eds) Progestins and antiprogestins in clinical practice (New York, Marcel Dekker, pp 269–277

Sitruk-Ware R (2002) Progestogens in hormonal replacement therapy: new molecules, risks, and benefits. Menopause 9: 6–15

Smith YR, Giordani B, Lajiness O, Zubieta JK (2001) Long-term estrogen replacement is associated with improved nonverbal memory and attentional measures in postmenopausal women. Fertil Steril 76: 1101–1107

How do Changes in the GH/IGF-1 Status of the Elderly Occurring Naturally, Pathologically or Therapeutically-Induced Impact on their Lives?

S.K. Abdul Shakoor[1], Andrew A. Toogood[2], and Stephen M. Shalet[1]

Introduction

There is a progressive failure of numerous organ systems with increasing age in humans. The reduction in lean body mass, increased adiposity, and reduced bone mineral density associated with aging, contribute to the increasing lack of physical strength, poor mobility, fractures, and increased cardiovascular risk profile. Similar changes are also observed in adults with growth hormone deficiency (GHD), some of which have been shown to improve with growth hormone replacement. This has led to the theory that the relative reduction in GH and IGF-1 levels with increasing age (somatopause) may be causal with regard to these changes. In this review, we will consider changes in the GH/IGF-1 axis with increasing age and their implications, the effect of GH use in healthy elderly subjects, the impact of GHD in the elderly with hypothalamic pituitary disease and the response to GH replacement.

GH Status in normal elderly

The activity of the growth hormone (GH)- insulin-like growth factor-1 (IGF-1) axis undergoes marked variation across the human life span. GH secretion is transiently elevated at birth, markedly increases at puberty, and decreases progressively to very low levels in old age. The biological role of GH in adults has only recently been explored; it has wide ranging effects on carbohydrate, lipid and protein metabolism thereby effecting changes in body composition, physical performance and quality of life.

The amount of GH released by the pituitary gland is reduced in healthy elderly compared to healthy young adults (15,20,22,52). Iranmanesh et al (22) evaluated GH secretion by 24 hour profiling in 21 healthy men aged 21-71 yrs; compared to younger men, older individuals had significant reductions in GH secretory burst frequency, and daily GH secretion, but there was no change in the duration and amplitude of GH secretory bursts; GH secretion declined with increasing age at a

[1] Department of Endocrinology, Christie Hospital, Wilmslow Road, Manchester, UK
[2] Department of Medicine, Division of Medical Sciences, Queen Elizabeth Hospital, Edgbaston, Birmingham, UK

Chanson et al.
Endocrine Aspects of Successful Aging
© Springer-Verlag Berlin Heidelberg 2004

rate of 14% per decade of adult life. However, Ho et al (20) reported that the GH secretory burst frequency was not affected by age and also that the mean pulse amplitude, duration, and fraction of GH secreted in pulses (FGHP) were greater in young adults compared with older subjects. The sensitivity of the GH assays used in these early studies was poor. Using modern assays with a sensitivity of 0.005µgs/l, it has been shown that GH secretion continues throughout adult life (23).

GH secretion is increased by physiological stimulation such as exercise and fasting. The GH response (50) to resistance exercise is grossly diminished in normal elderly subjects compared with young adults (peak mean GH value 14.9 µgs/L in the young vs. 3.5 µgs/L in old). The effect of calorie deprivation on GH secretion in 6 older subjects (55-81 years) revealed that two days of fasting induced a 4-fold increase in the 24-hour GH production rate (38+/-25 vs 166+/-42 µgs/L) and a 2-fold increase in the amount of GH secreted in pulses (2.4+/-1.4 vs 5.5+/-1.2µgs/L) compared with the control (fed) state. The fold increase in GH secretion with fasting was similar to that previously observed in young men, although absolute levels of GH secretion were approximately 50 % lower in both fed and fasted conditions. The increase in GH secretion was not related to slow wave sleep, as fasting did not increase the duration of time spent in slow wave sleep (19).

The impact of age on the GH response to a variety of GH secretagogues is dependent on the nature of the secretagogue. Studies of the GH response to an insulin tolerance test (ITT) in normal elderly subjects have produced conflicting results. Kalk et al (30) showed no change in the GH response in elderly subjects compared with young adults, whereas Muggeo et al (42) reported that the GH response was diminished in older subjects. The GH response to arginine stimulation (AST) appears unaffected by age (17), whereas the GH response to growth hormone releasing hormone (GHRH) appears to be diminished in elderly individuals (17,54), although Ghigo et al (17) has shown that arginine potentiates the GH response to GHRH in older subjects; the GH response to the latter combined stimulation is not age-dependent.

A new class of synthetic peptides called GH releasing peptides (GHRPs) possesses strong GH releasing activity. Hexarelin has been the most widely studied GHRP as it is more stable. The effect of hexarelin on the GH response in normal elderly subjects is reduced compared with young subjects (1). Furthermore, arginine potentiates the GH response to hexarelin in elderly subjects, but not in young adults (Fig. 1).

The reason for the age related fall in GH secretion might be due to changes in GHRH and somatostatin input from the hypothalamus. GHRH is thought to determine the amplitude of a GH pulse as it stimulates the synthesis and release of GH from the pituitary gland. Somatostatin inhibits the release of GH from the pituitary gland without affecting the synthesis of GH. The combination of declining GHRH action and increasing somatostatin tone is likely to explain the reduction in GH secretion with increasing age. Hypothalamic GHRH synthesis and release are reduced in the aged hypothalamus (17). Prolonged treatment with GHRH has been shown to increase 24-hour GH secretion and IGF-1 levels in elderly men (10,11). It is generally accepted although not by all authors that

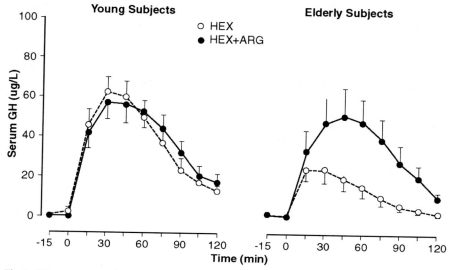

Fig 1. GH responses to hexarelin (2μg/kg, iv), administered alone or combined with arginine (0.5g/kg infused over 30 minutes from 0-30 minutes), in six young (left panel) and eight elderly (right panel) males. [Reproduced with permission from Arvat E, Gianotti L, Grottoli S, Imbimbo BP, Lenaerts V, Deghehghi R, Camanni F, and Ghigo E. J Clin Endocrinol Metab 79: 1440-1443,1994.]

arginine inhibits the secretion of somatostatin from the hypothalamus thereby inducing a GH response. The GH response to arginine in healthy elderly subjects is not impaired (17,61). Furthermore arginine, potentiates the GH response to GHRH in elderly subjects showing that the GH releasable pool in the pituitary is preserved and that a state of somatostatin hyperactivity may exist. Other factors that may contribute to the reduced GH secretion in elderly subjects are hypothalamic cholinergic hypoactivity, changes in catecholamine and galanin activity, age related variations in the activity of the natural GH secretagogue receptor ligand in the hypothalamus, and decline in the duration of slow wave sleep with increasing age (64).

IGF-1 and IGFBPs in the normal elderly:

The serum levels of IGF-1 and IGFBP-3 fall with increasing age. Several cross sectional studies have reported low serum IGF-1 levels in elderly subjects (52,11,24); Rudman et al (52) showed that the prevalence of a low IGF-1 level increases progressively from the fourth through the ninth decades. However, IGF-1 measured in serum is the total extractable IGF-1, which offers only a crude estimate of the biologically active IGF-1 due to the wide inter-individual variation in circulating IGFBPs. The molar ratio of IGF-1/IGFBP-3, which has been claimed to represent free or biologically active IGF-1 was also found to be low in healthy elderly subjects (28). However, in a different study, Janssen et al (24), measuring free IGF-1 directly, showed that the free IGF-1 levels in serum did not decline with age, unlike total IGF-1and IGFBP-3 levels.

The serum levels of IGF-1 correlate strongly with 24-hour GH secretion in children and young adults. However, this relationship does not hold in older subjects (11,20,52), indicating that IGF-1 levels are affected by factors other than GH secretion. Recently, a polymorphism in the IGF-1 gene has been associated with a change in serum IGF-1 levels in adults; IGF-1 levels being lower in those who did not carry the 192-bp allele (63). This genetic variation may have implications in terms of subsequent morbidity due to malignancy or vascular disease in elderly subjects.

The serum level of IGFBP-3, the major IGF-1 binding protein in the plasma, also decreases with increasing age (24,28). The synthesis of IGFBP-3 is GH dependent. Corpas et al (11) showed that there was a strong correlation between levels of IGF-1 and IGFBP-3 irrespective of age.

Growth hormone binding protein (GHBP) is a soluble circulating ectodomain of the GH receptor (GHR). Its plasma level is thought to reflect GHR levels. Maheshwari et al (40), observed that the serum levels of GHBP in subjects more than 80 years of age was about half that of persons aged 60-65 years. This might suggest the possibility of GH resistance in elderly subjects, which may contribute to the changes associated with diminished activity of the GH/IGF-1 axis. However, the acute generation of IGF-1 in healthy volunteer groups of 3 different ages (mean of 3 age groups 26, 49, and 74.9 years) studied using 3 doses of GH (0.8, 2.0, and 21 units) revealed that the increment in IGF-1 and IGFBP-3 levels in response to GH does not decline with increasing age (38). These findings suggest that peripheral responsiveness to GH is not attenuated with increasing age and therefore does not contribute to the fall in GH dependent peptide levels (IGF-1 and IGFBP-3).

Age related changes in GH/IGF-1 axis and somatic change: GH/IGF-1 status and body composition

Normal aging is associated with reduced muscle mass and increased total body fat mass, and in particular intra-abdominal fat mass. There is a significant age-independent inverse correlation between measures of adiposity and basal GH secretion (13). This suggests that the age -associated increase in fat mass is not mediated by reduced GH secretion. Increased adiposity in men is associated with reduced frequency of GH secretory episodes (22) and increased GH clearance (65). GHRH induced GH secretion is also reduced in overweight men (48). Thus there is a reciprocal relationship between adiposity and GH secretion, with more fat leading to less GH secretion, which theoretically may cause a further increase in body fat.

Kiel et al (33) assessed the relationship between body composition and functional status in elderly individuals and the influence of GH status. There was no association between IGF-1 levels and indices of body composition even though IGF-1 levels declined with age. O' Connor et al (44) showed similar results; advanced age rather than serum IGF-1 levels was a major determinant of changes in body composition.

GH/IGF-1 status and skeletal aging

GH exerts its action on the skeleton mainly through IGF-1; IGF-1 is an osteotropic agent. In normal subjects and individuals with osteoporosis, positive associations between circulating IGF-1 and bone mineral density (BMD) have been reported (49). Furthermore, GHD in childhood and young adults is associated with reduced BMD. However, studies of the relationship between serum IGF-1 and BMD in healthy elderly subjects have shown variable results (35,25).

Langlois et al (35) reported a significant association between serum IGF-1 levels and BMD at all sites in women aged between 72-94 years, but no association in male subjects. In another study (25), free and total IGF-1 levels were positively related to lumbar BMD in men, but not in women.

Various explanations have been suggested for the rather weak associations between serum IGF-1 levels and bone mass with age; gradual blunting of the anabolic effect of IGF-1 with age, possible variations between skeletal IGF-1 concentrations and circulating IGF-1, and other unknown factors (49).

GH/IGF-1 status and physical performance

Poor muscle strength and physical performance in elderly subjects has been attributed to diminished activity of the GH/IGF-1 axis. Kiel et al (33) assessed muscle strength by isokinetic dynamometry and functional performance by timed performance measures and self- report in 155 elderly subjects; there was no significant association between serum IGF-1 levels and muscle strength or physical functioning. Papakadis et al (46) reported similar results in 104 ambulatory community-dwelling men. However, in another study by Cappola et al (3), which included frail older women (70-79 years), low serum IGF-1 levels were associated with poor knee extensor muscle strength, slow walking speed, and self-reported difficulty with mobility tasks.

In a cross sectional population based study of 218 healthy elderly subjects (55-80 years) by Janssen et al (26) low serum IGF-1 levels were associated with decreased self-reported quality of health, but were not related to physical disability. The same group also evaluated the relationship between IGF-1 and IGFBP-3 levels and cognitive function (31); higher total IGF-1 levels and IGF-1/IGFBP3 ratios were associated with less cognitive decline over a 2year period; however, there was no correlation between free IGF-1 and cognitive decline.

In summary, there is no overwhelmingly conclusive evidence that with increasing age, the reduction of GH and IGF-1 levels is responsible for the physical and mental decline that is seen.

Growth hormone therapy in the elderly

There has been a significant interest in the potential for growth hormone use in the normal elderly to reverse some of the changes associated with aging even though a causal relationship between the decline in the GH secretion and the physical changes of the somatopause has not been established. The pioneering study in this field is that of Rudman et al (53), who reported that GH treatment in the normal elderly with a low IGF-1 level, induced favourable changes in body composition and lumbar spine BMD.

Body composition

Rudman et al (53) studied 21 healthy elderly men (61-81years) who had low IGF-1 levels; This was a 6 month trial in which 12 subjects received GH in a dose of 0.03mg/kg three times a week and 9 men received no treatment; in the treatment group, IGF-1 levels increased accompanied by an 8.8% increase in lean body mass, and a 14.4% decrease in fat mass. Other studies have also reported improvements in body composition with GH treatment, either alone or in combination with exercise with the exception of one study by Munzer et al (43). The effects of 6 months of therapy in 110 healthy aged subjects (65-88 years) with GH alone (20μg/kg three times a week), sex steroids (testosterone enanthate 100 mg every 2 weeks in men, and 100μg/day estraderm patch and 2.5 mg medroxyprogesterone for the first 10 days of each month in women), or GH and sex steroids combined was assessed in a randomised, double blind placebo controlled, non cross over study. In women, there was no significant change in the total abdominal area, or subcutaneous fat or visceral fat with GH, or combination of GH and HRT. In contrast, there was a significant decrease in total, subcutaneous and visceral fat in men after GH and also combined GH and testosterone treatment, but the distribution of the changes are proportionate in subcutaneous and visceral areas. Taaffe et al (57) assessed the effect of GH and or IGF-1 treatment on regional fat loss in 27 postmenopausal women (59-70 years) undergoing a regimen of diet plus exercise; GH at a dose of 0.025mg/kg/day, in combination with a diet and exercise programme, reduced truncal fat in post-menopausal overweight women after 12 weeks. There was no significant change in body fat distribution with IGF-1 treatment (0.015mg/kg/day) either alone or combined with GH. Furthermore, there was no association between the change in fat distribution, serum lipoprotein levels and maximal aerobic capacity.

Skeletal changes

Rudman et al (53) reported an increase of 1.6% in lumbar spine BMD after 6 months of GH therapy in 12 healthy elderly men (61-81years), but no significant changes in BMD at other skeletal sites. Sugimoto et al (55) assessed the effect of GH in 8 elderly osteoporotic women (68-75years); GH treatment at a dose of 0.125U/kg/wk for the first 4 weeks followed by 0.25U/kg/wk for 48 weeks increased markers of bone formation and resorption at 24 weeks. The markers of bone formation (serum bone alkaline phosphatase and osteocalcin) remained high during GH therapy, but urinary deoxypyridinoline, a bone resorption marker, returned to baseline after 24 weeks. BMD changes were not significant at 48 weeks, but became so 48 weeks after discontinuation of GH therapy (8.1+/- 2.1% at mid radius and 3.8+/-1.4% at lumbar spine).

Christmas et al (6), investigated the effects of GH and sex steroids on bone in 125 healthy older subjects (> 65 years) in a 6 month double blind placebo controlled study; GH therapy (20µg/kg three times a week) alone increased markers of bone formation (osteocalcin and type1 procollagen peptide) and resorption (urinary deoxypyridinoline), but did not increase BMD in females. There was a significant increase in BMD following HRT and combination of GH and HRT. In men, GH alone increased serum osteocalcin and type1 procollagen peptide, but there was no change in BMD.

Ghiron et al (18) assessed the effects of GH (25mcg/kg/day), and IGF-1 at low (15 mcg/kg twice daily) and high doses (60 mcg/kg twice daily) on bone turnover in elderly women. GH and high-dose IGF-1 increased both markers of bone formation and bone resorption, whereas low dose IGF-1 increased only markers of bone formation, suggesting that low dose IGF-1 increases osteoblastic activity directly.

The impact of GH and IGF-1therapy has also been assessed in healthy elderly subjects following a recent hip fracture. In a randomised placebo controlled design, Van der Lely et al (65) studied the effect of GH in 111 elderly subjects older than 60 years with hip fracture; GH at a dose of 20 mcg/kg/day for 6 weeks significantly increased the rate of return to the pre-fracture living condition compared with the placebo treated subjects (for those over 75 years of age).

In summary, short- term studies have shown some beneficial effect on bone markers, but the changes in BMD are neither significant nor consistent. There are no data on long- term effects nor any solid evidence of reduction in fracture rate. Furthermore, there are no compelling comparative studies against less expensive and more convenient orally taken compounds such as bisphosphonates, which have been shown to be effective in increasing BMD and also reducing fracture rates.

Physical performance and functional ability

GH therapy can improve the adverse body composition changes associated with aging; however, whether these changes will result in improved functional performance is not established. Papadakis et al (47) showed that in healthy aged men (70-85 years), GH treatment in a dose of 0.03mg/kg three times a week for 6 months improved lean body mass (4.3%), and decreased fat mass by 13% compared with placebo. However, there was no significant change in muscle strength at the knee or handgrip. Taaffe et al (56), in a double blind placebo controlled study, evaluated the effect of GH therapy in 18 healthy elderly subjects

(65-82 years) after a period of progressive training for 14 weeks; GH treatment at a dose of 0.02mg/kg/day did not improve muscle strength in any muscle group, even though the expected positive changes occured in lean body mass and fat mass.

Welle et al (68), however, have reported that 3 months GH treatment (0.03 mg/kg 3 times a week) improved muscle strength measured by isokinetic dynamometry in the thigh compared with placebo in healthy elderly subjects (62-74 years). There was no effect of GH on whole body protein synthesis, or on myofibrillar protein synthesis in the quadriceps muscle.

Lange et al (34) evaluated the effect of GH therapy, alone or in combination with resistance exercise training in 31 healthy elderly men (mean age 74 years) in a placebo controlled double blind design; GH (1.77 +/-0.18 IU/day) alone for12 weeks had no effect on isokinetic quadriceps strength, muscle power, cross sectional area or fibre size, whereas resistance exercise and placebo combination caused significant improvements in quadriceps isokinetic muscle strength, muscle power, and an increase in cross sectional area. The addition of GH with resistance exercise however, did not improve the above parameters. There was an increase in myosin heavy chain (MHC) 2X isoform with GH treatment alone, which can be explained as a change into a more youthful MHC composition (with increasing age, there is a trend toward a shift in MHC composition from 2X to 2A and 1). However, GH and exercise combination did increase MHC 2A and decreased MHC 2X, suggesting that the resistance exercise seems to overrule the changes in MHC composition induced by GH alone.

The effect of GH and or sex steroids was assessed by Blackman et al (2) in healthy ambulatory aged men and women (65-88 years) in a 26 week randomised placebo controlled study; participants were randomised to receive GH in a dose of 30 µg/kg, reduced to 20 µg/kg three times a week and sex steroids (transdermal estradiol 100 µg/day, plus oral medroxyprogesterone, 10 mg/day, during the last 10 days of each cycle for women, and testosterone enanthate, biweekly intramuscular injections of 100 mg for men). GH treatment with or without sex steroids increased lean body mass significantly in both men and women. Muscle strength did not increase with both GH and sex steroids in women. In men, there was a marginally significant increase in muscle strength with GH and testosterone treatment, but no significant improvement with GH alone. Maximal oxygen uptake (VO2 max) during treadmill test increased after GH and combined GH and sex steroids in both men and women. The changes in muscle strength and VO2 max was directly related to changes in lean body mass.

In summary, the few short- term studies of elderly subjects receiving GH therapy fail to show significant improvement in muscle strength and functional performance.

Growth hormone therapy in malnourished elderly patients

Malnutrition is very common in elderly subjects and is often unrecognised. They are at increased risk of morbidity as well as mortality. Kaiser et al (29) evaluated the effect of GH treatment in 10 elderly subjects (64-99years), who were more than

20% below average body weight and had serum albumin levels less than 3.8 gm/dl; GH (0.1 mg/kg/day) therapy for 21 days increased mid-arm muscle circumference, weight (average of 2.2 kg) and urinary nitrogen retention compared with the placebo group. Recently, Chu et al (7) reported similar benefit with GH at a low dose of 0.09U/kg three times a week given for 4 weeks in 19 malnourished elderly subjects (mean age 83years). There was a significant improvement in body weight, haemoglobin, serum albumin, and 5 metre walking time in the GH treated group compared with placebo.

Safety issues

Elderly subjects receiving GH treatment experienced significant side effects such as fluid retention, carpal tunnel syndrome, and gynaecomastia (2,8), and diabetes / glucose intolerance (2) thereby limiting the potential use of GH in this age group. However, the major theoretical issue arising from the potential long-term use of GH in the elderly is the association between IGF-1 and cancer risk. An increased risk of prostate and colon cancer has been reported to be associated with the upper normal range quartile/tertile of serum IGF-1 levels in various studies. Chan et al (4) demonstrated that among a cohort of normal men (40-82 years) in the Physician's health study, the highest quartile of serum IGF-1 levels was associated with a 4.3 fold relative risk of prostate cancer compared with the lowest quartile. This relationship is particularly pronounced in men over 60 years of age. Men over age of 60 years and in the highest quartile of IGF-I had a relative risk (RR) of 7.9 (95% CI 2.1 to 30.7) with adjustment for IGFBP-3, compared with men of similar age and in the lowest quartile; the comparable RR among men age 60 or less was 1.6 (95% CI 0.4 to 6.1). A similar association between serum IGF-1 and colon cancers has also been reported in another study with a cohort of men aged between 40 and 84 years (39).

Normally both IGF-1 and IGFBP-3 are primarily regulated by GH and therefore these two peptides exhibit a direct correlation in the serum. This is the case in normal elderly subjects as well as in patients with acromegaly. The risk of future malignancy in the normal population is maximal in those subjects with high normal IGF-1 and low IGFBP-3 levels; thus GH therapy might be considered safe as it will elevate both IGF-1 and IGFBP-3 levels, but this is not established. Thus there are important safety issues to be considered before long-term GH therapy is offered to elderly subjects.

Use of GHRH and GH secretagogues in the elderly

GH therapy is associated with side effects in the elderly population; hence, there have been attempts to correct the hyposomatotropism with the use of GHRH and GH secretagogues rather than GH itself. GHRH therapy has been shown to increase GH secretion and also normalise IGF-1 levels. However, the effect of GHRH appears to vary depending on the mode of administration.

Body composition

GHD in young adults results in changes in body composition with an increase in fat mass and reduced lean body mass. Evaluation of body composition in the elderly with GHD by dual energy X-ray absorptiometry (DEXA) demonstrated a significant increase in fat mass (median of 27.76 kg compared with 21.23 kg in the age matched controls) (59); there was no significant difference in fat-free mass however. Furthermore, there was no regional difference in fat distribution between the patients and controls, but this could be explained by the limitations of the technique, as DEXA cannot differentiate between intra-abdominal visceral fat from subcutaneous fat. Li Voon Chong et al (36) confirmed that fat mass is increased in elderly patients with GHD compared with controls, but only in females. Patients and controls were followed for a further 2 years and reassessed (37). Body composition in elderly patients with GHD did not deteriorate during this time; in fact, fat mass fell slightly (31.7+/- 11.2 vs. 28.5+/-10.9%). Colao et al (9) demonstrated a significant increase in fat mass (37.4+/-2.2 vs. 28.0+/-1.0%, P<0.001) and a decrease in lean mass (62.6+/-2.2vs 72.0+/-1%, P<0.001) in 18 elderly GHD subjects (60-72years) compared with controls.

Obesity is known to cause diminished GH secretion; this was illustrated by the significant negative correlation between fat mass and GH secretion in the controls in the study of Toogood (58). However, a similar relationship did not exist in the elderly patients with GHD suggesting that the increased fat mass was not responsible for the reduction in GH secretion.

In summary, GHD in elderly subjects is associated with changes in body composition, namely increased fat mass, but the changes in fat free mass seem to be attenuated compared with those seen in younger patients with GHD.

Skeletal effects

Studies in GHD adults have demonstrated that BMD is reduced compared with age- matched controls. BMD results in GHD adults reveal a greater degree of osteopaenia in adults with childhood onset GHD rather than adult onset GHD (45). The severity of osteopenia appears to be related to the age of onset of GHD. The majority of bone mineral acquisition is completed by the third or early part of the fourth decade. Hence, those who develop GHD after the age of 30 years are less osteopenic (21). Furthermore, BMD determined by DEXA in elderly GHD adults is not significantly different from age-matched controls at hip and lumbar spine (Fig. 3); however, there is evidence of reduced bone turnover as markers of bone formation (serum osteocalcin) and bone resorption (urinary deoxypyridinoline) are reduced in elderly patients with GHD. Similar findings were observed in another study (27); BMD in lumbar spine was normal in16 older (>55 years) GHD patients at baseline before receiving GH replacement. Garnero et al (16) has shown that in healthy elderly adults, reduction in bone turnover may actually protect against fractures. Thus elderly subjects with GHD may be at less rather than more risk of fractures unlike younger GHD adults.

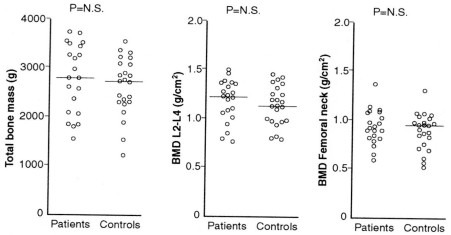

Fig 3. Total bone mass and BMD in the lumbar spine and at the hip in patients and controls. The median values are indicated by the bars. [Reproduced with permission from Toogood AA, Adams JE, O'Neill P, and Shalet SM. J Clin Endocrinol Metab 82: 1462-1466, 1997.]

Quality of life

GHD adults experience impairment in various aspects of quality of life (QOL), including lower energy levels, emotional lability, increased social isolation, low self-esteem, and a greater level of perceived health problems (51,67).

Li voon Chong et al (36) assessed QOL in elderly patients with GHD by five different questionnaires and also disease specific scores. The 27 patients with GHD reported significantly less energy, mobility and personal life fulfilment compared with age -matched controls. There were more problems with emotional reaction, social isolation and mental fatigue, social functioning, general health and mental health. In terms of disease impact scale, the elderly patients with GHD showed a mean score of 14.1, which reflects modest impairment compared with younger patients with GHD who had a mean score of 24.8. In contrast, Monson et al (41) reported similar QOL scores measured by disease specific questionnaire (QOL-AGHDA) in younger (<65yr) and older (>65yr) subjects with GHD although the overall degree of impairment was extremely modest in both cohorts.

In conclusion impairment in QOL beyond that seen in the normal elderly is present in the elderly GHD population.

Growth hormone treatment in elderly patients with GHD

GH replacement therapy in young GHD adults has been shown to improve the adverse changes in body composition, physical performance, quality of life and cardiovascular profile. However, the changes in biological end points associated with GHD in young adults are severe compared with that seen in elderly subjects with GHD. Only a few reports have been published specifically examining the effects of GH replacement in elderly GHD patients.

The replacement dose of GH required in elderly patients with GHD is considerably lower than that in their younger counterparts. Toogood et al (62) evaluated 3 different doses of GH (0.17, 0.33 and 0.5mg per day) each administrated for 12 weeks in 12 elderly GHD subjects. A dose of 0.33 mg /day maintained the IGF-1 level in the upper part of the normal reference range in 83% of patients, whereas a dose of 0.5 mg/day dose was associated with supra-physiological IGF-1 levels in 50% of subjects. In the same study, there was a significant increase in lean body mass and a decrease in fat mass with GH replacement; the change in lean body mass being a surprise as the previous study (59) failed to demonstrate a significant reduction in lean mass at baseline in elderly subjects with GHD. There was a significant, but small improvement in the quality of life measured by AGHDA score. However, this change should be interpreted with caution, as the baseline values in this group were low (mean score of 4.5, cf: maximum of25) suggesting that the quality of life of this cohort was not severely affected by GHD. In spite of this, 75% of patients expressed a wish to continue GH therapy at the end of the study, having discontinued for 12 weeks. In fairness, however, the latter study was a dose finding trial, which did not select patients by virtue of their QOL at baseline.

Monson et al (41) evaluated the effect of GH replacement therapy in 109 elderly patients with GHD (>65 years) comparing with younger GHD patients; baseline characteristics were not different between the two groups. After 6 months of GH treatment (initial dose of 0.125 U/kg/week, titrated to the maximum dose of 0.25 U/kg/week), there was a significant reduction in total and LDL- cholesterol in both young and elderly groups. In addition, there was a reduction in diastolic blood pressure and quality of life scores (AGHDA) in males. The changes in female subjects were not significant probably due to fewer numbers of patients studied. However, AGHDA scores at baseline in both groups were only moderately abnormal (7.0-10.6, cf maximum score 25) as in the other study (62), which suggests that the impairment in quality of life was not severe.

Fernholm et al (14) studied the effect of GH in 31 elderly patients with GHD (60-79 years); there was a significant increase in lean body mass, and reduction in fat mass after 6 and 12 months of GH therapy (0.75-1.25IU/day). Markers for bone formation (bone specific alkaline phosphatase, osteocalcin and procollagen type1 carboxy terminal peptide) and bone resorption (urinary pyridinoline) increased following GH treatment. There was no improvement in bone mineral density, however an observation that may reflect the lack of difference in BMD values between patient and healthy groups at baseline.

In summary, a few studies demonstrate a beneficial effect of GH replacement in elderly subjects with GHD. However, further studies are required to evaluate the long-term benefit.

Conclusion

There is a reduction in the GH/IGF-1 axis activity with increasing age, but there is evidence that the pool of GH available for release is not diminished in elderly subjects. Furthermore, this reduction in GH secretion is not solely responsible for the physical changes associated with aging. There is a clear distinction between the normal elderly subjects and elderly subjects with GHD due to hypothalamic pituitary disease, in whom, GH secretion is reduced by more than 90%. GH replacement therapy may be useful in elderly subjects with severe GHD, whereas the effect of GH treatment in healthy elderly subjects is not effective in improving the functional status, even though considerable improvement in body composition has been observed. GHRH and GH secretagogues, which can increase the GH levels physiologically, provide some hope that in the future the hyposomatotropism associated with increasing age can be corrected for a worthwhile purpose. Future studies should focus on frail elderly subjects, and aim to determine if their state of independent living can be prolonged by the induction of such changes in the GH-IGF-1 axis.

References

Arvat E, Gianotti L, Grottoli S et al (1994) Arginine and growth hormone –releasing hormone restore the blunted growth hormone-releasing activity of hexarelin in elderly subjects. J Clin Endocrinol Metab 79: 1440–1443.

Blackman MR, Sorkin JD, Munzer T, Bellantoni MF, Busby-Whitehead J, Stevens TE, Jayme J, O'Connor KG, Christmas C, Tobin JD, Stewart KJ, Cottrell E, St Clair C, Pabst KM, Harman SM(2002) Growth hormone and sex steroid administration in healthy aged women and men. JAMA 288:2282–2292

Cappola AR, Bandeen-Roche K, Wand GS, Volpato S, Fried LP(2001) Association of IGF-1 levels with muscle strength and mobility in older women. J Clin Endocrinol Metab 86(9): 4139–4146

Chan JM, Stampfer MJ, Giovannucci E, Gann PH, Ma J, Wilkinson P, Hennekens CH, Pollak M(1998) Plasma insulin like growth factor-1and prostate cancer risk: a prospective study. Science 279: 563–566

Chapman IM, Bach MA, Van Cauter E, Farmer M, Krupa D, Taylor AM, Schilling LM, Cole KY, Skiles EH, Pezzoli SS, Hartman ML, Veldhuis JD, Gormley GJ, Thorner MO (1996) Stimulation of the GH-IGF-1 axis by daily oral administration of a GH secretagogue (MK-677) in healthy elderly subjects. J Clin Endocrinol Metab 81: 4249–4257

Christmas C, O'Connor KG, Harman SM, Tobin JD, Munzer T, Bellantoni MF, Clair CS, Pabst KM, Sorkin JD, Blackman MR (2002) Growth hormone and sex steroid effects on bone metabolism and bone mineral density in healthy aged women and men. J Gerontol A Biol Sci 57 (1): M12–8

Chu LW, Lam KS, Tam SC, Hu WJ, Hui SL, Chiu A, Chiu KC, Ng P (2001) A randomised controlled trial of low dose recombinant growth hormone in the treatment of malnourished elderly medical patients. J Clin Endocrinol metab 86: 1913–1920

Cohn L, Feller AG, Draper MW, Rudman IW, Rudman D (1993) Carpal tunnel syndrome and gynaecomastia during growth hormone treatment of elderly men with low circulating IGF-1 concentrations. Clin Endocrinol 39: 417–425

Colao A, Cerbone G, Pivonello R, Klain M, Aimaretti G, Faggiano A, Di Somma C, Salvatore M, Lombardi G (1998) Growth hormone deficiency in elderly patients with hypothalamic pituitary tumours. Pituitary 1(1): 59–67

Corpas E, Harman SM, Pineyro MA, Roberson R, Blackman MR (1992) Growth hormone –releasing hormone (1-29) twice daily reverses the decreased GH and insulin like growth factor-1 levels in old men J Clin Endocrinol Metab 75: 530–535.

Corpas E, Harman SM, and Blackman MR (1993) Human growth hormone and human aging Endocrine Rev 14 (1): 20–39

Corpas E, Harman SM, Pineyro MA, Roberson R, Blackman MR (1993) Continuous subcutaneous infusions of growth hormone releasing hormone 1-44 for 14 days increase GH and IGF-1 levels in old men. J Clin Endocrinol Metab 76: 134–138

Elahi D, Muller DC, Tzankoff SP, Andres R, Tobin JD (1982) Effect of age and obesity on fasting levels of glucose, insulin, glucagon, and growth hormone in men. J Gerontol 37:385–391

Fernholm R, Bramnert M, Hagg E, Hilding A, Baylink DJ, Mohan S, Thoren M (2000) Growth hormone replacement therapy improves body composition and increases bone metabolism in elderly patients with pituitary disease. J Clin Endocrinol Metab 85 (11): 4104–12

Finkelstein JW, Roffwarg HP, Boyar RM, Kream J, Hellman L (1972) Age related change in the twenty-four hour spontaneous secretion of growth hormone. J Clin Endocrinol Metab 35: 665–670

Garnero P, Sornay-Rendu E, Chapuy MC, Delmas PD (1996) Increased bone turnover in late postmenopausal women is a major determinant of osteoporosis. J Bone Mineral Res 11: 337–349

Ghigo E, Arvat E, Gianotti L, Lanfranco F, Broglio F, Aimaretti G, Maccario M, Camanni F(2000) Hypothalamic growth hormone-Insulin like growth factor-I axis across the human life Span. J Paed Endocrinol Metab: 13, 1493–1502

Ghiron LJ, Thompson JL, Holloway L, Hintz RL, Butterfield GE, Hoffman AR, Marcus R (1995) Effects of recombinant insulin like growth factor-1 and growth hormone on bone turnover in elderly women. J Bone Miner Res 10(12): 1844–52

Hartman ML, Pezzoli SS, Hellmann PJ, Suratt PM, Thorner MO (1996) Pulsatile growth hormone secretion in older persons is enhanced by fasting without relationship to sleep stages. J Clin Endocrinol Metab 81:2694–2701

Ho KY, Evans WS, Blizzard RM, Veldhuis JD, Merriam GR, Samojlik E, Furlanetto R, Rogol AD, Kaiser DL, Thorner MO (1987) Effects of sex and age on the 24 hour profile of growth hormone secretion in man: importance of endogenous estradiol concentrations. J Clin Endocrinol Metab 64: 51–58

Holmes SJ, Economou G, Whitehouse RW, Adams JE, Shalet SM (1994) Reduced bone mineral density in patients with adult onset growth hormone deficiency. J Clin Endocrinol Metab 78: 669–74.

Iranmanesh A, Lizarralde GB, Veldhuis JD (1991) Age and relative obesity are specific negative determinants of the frequency and amplitude of growth hormone secretory bursts and the half-life of endogenous GH in healthy men. J Clin Endocrinol Metab 73: 1081–1088.

Iranmanesh A, Grisso B, Veldhuis JD (1994) Low basal and persistent pulsatile growth hormone secretion are revealed in normal and hyposomatotropic men studied with a new ultrasensitive chemiluminescence assay. J Clin Endocrinol Metab 78: 526–535.

Janssen JAMJL, Stolk RP, Pols HAP et al (1998) Serum free IGF-I, total IGF-I, IGFBP-I and IGFBP-3 levels in an elderly population: relation to age and sex steroid levels. Clin Endocrinol 48: 471–478

Janssen JA, Burger H, Stolk RP, Grobbee DE, de Jong FH, Lamberts SW, Pols HA (1998) Gender-specific relationship between serum free and total IGF-I and bone mineral density in elderly men and women. Eur J Endocrinol 138: 627–632

Janssen JA, Stolk RP, Pols HA, Grobbee DE, Lamberts SW (1998) Serum free and total insulin like growth factor-1, insulin like growth factor binding protein-1 and insulin like growth factor binding protein-3 levels in healthy elderly individuals. Gerontology. 44: 277–280.

Janssen YJH, Hamdy NAT, Frolich M and Roelfsema F (1998) Skeletal effects of two years of treatment with low physiological doses of recombinant human growth hormone in patients with adult onset GH deficiency. J Clin Endocrinol Metab 83,(6); 2143–48

Juul A, Main K, Blum WF, Lindholm J, Ranke MB, Skakkebaek NE (1994) The ratio between serum levels of insulin-like growth factor (IGF)-I and the IGF binding proteins (IGFBP-1, 2 and 3) decreases with age in healthy adults and is increased in acromegalic patients. Clin Endocrinol 41: 85–93.

Kaiser FE, Silver AJ, and Morley JE (1991) The effect of recombinant human growth hormone on malnourished older individuals. J Am Geriatr Soc 39:235–240

Kalk WJ, Vinik AI, Pimstone BL, Jackson PU (1973) Growth hormone response to insulin hypoglycaemia in the elderly. J Gerontol 28: 431–433

Kalmijn S, Janssen JA, Pols HA, Lamberts SW, Breteler MM (2000) A prospective study on circulating insulin like growth factor-1, IGF-binding proteins, and cognitive function in the elderly. J Clin Endocrinol Metab 85: 4551–4555.

Khorram O, Laughlin GA, Yen SS (1997) Endocrine and metabolic effects of long term administration of (Nle27) growth hormone releasing hormone (1-29)-NH2 in age advanced men and women. J Clin Endocrinol Metab 82(5): 1472–9

Kiel DP, Puhl J, Rosen CJ, Berg K, Murphy JB, MacLean DB (1998) Lack of an association between insulin like growth factor-1 and body composition, muscle strength, physical performance or self reported mobility among older persons with functional limitations. J Am Geriatr Soc 46(7): 822–828

Lange KH, Andersen JL, Beyer N, Isaksson F, Larsson B, Rasmussen MH, Juul A, Bulow J, Kjaer M (2002) GH administration changes myosin heavy chain isoforms in skeletal muscle but does not augment muscle strength or hypertrophy, either alone or combined with resistance exercise training in healthy elderly men. J Clin Endocrinol Metab 87: 513–523

Langlois JA, Rosen CJ, Visser M, Hannan MT, Harris T, Wilson PW, Kiel DP (1998) Association between insulin-like growth factor I and bone mineral density in older women and men: the framingham Heart study. J Clin Endocrinol Metab 83(12): 4257–62

Li Voon Chong JS, Benbow S, Foy P, Wallymahmed ME, Wile D, MacFarlane IA (2000) Elderly people with hypothalamic pituitary disease and growth hormone deficiency: lipid profiles, body composition and quality of life compared with control subjects. Clin Endocrinol 53: 551–559

Li Voon Chong JS, Groves T, Foy P, Wallymahmed ME, MacFarlane IA (2002) Elderly people with hypothalamic pituitary disease and untreated GH deficiency: clinical outcome, body composition, lipid profiles and quality of life after 2 years compared to controls. Clin Endocrinol 56(2): 175–81.

Lissett C and Shalet SM Insulin like growth factor-1 generation test: Peripheral responsiveness to growth hormone is not decreased with ageing Clin Endocrinol (in press)

Ma J, Pollak MN, Giovannucci E, Chan JM, Tao Y, Hennekens CH, Stampfer MJ (1999) Prospective study of colorectal cancer risk in men and plasma levels of insulin-like growth factor (IGF)-I and IGF-binding protein-3. J Natl Cancer Inst 7: 91(7), 620–5.

Maheshwari H, Sharma L, and Baumann G (1996) Decline of plasma growth hormone binding protein in old age. J Clin Endocrinol Metab 81:995–997

Monson JP, Abs R, Bengtsson BA, Bennmarker H, Feldt-Rasmussen U, Hernberg-Stahl E, Thoren M, Westberg B, Wilton P, Wuster C (2000) Growth hormone deficiency and replacement in elderly hypopituitary adults. Clin Endocrinol 53: 281–289

Muggeo M, Fedele D, Tiengo A, Molinari M, Crepaldi G (1975) Human growth hormone and cortisol responses to insulin stimulation in aging. J Gerontol 30: 546–551

Munzer T, Harman SM, Hees P, Shapiro E, Christmas C, Bellantoni MF, Stevens TE, O'Connor KG, Pabst KM, St Clair C, Sorkin JD, Blackman MR (2001) Effects of GH and/ or sex steroid administration on abdominal subcutaneous and visceral fat in healthy aged women and men. J Clin Endocrinol Metab 86: 3604–3610

O'Connor KG, Tobin JD, Harman SM, Plato CC, Roy TA, Sherman SS, Blackman MR (1998) Serum levels of insulin-like growth factor-I are related to age and not to body composition in healthy women and men. J Gerontol A Biol Sci Med Sci: 53(3) M176–82

O'Halloran DJ, Tsatsoulis A, Whitehouse RW, Holmes SJ, Adams JE, Shalet SM (1993) Increased bone density after recombinant growth hormone therapy in adults with isolated GH deficiency. J Clin Endocrinol Metab 76: 1344–1348

Papadakis MA, Grady D, Tierney MJ, Black D, Wells L, Grunfeld C (1995) Insulin-like growth factor-1 and functional status in healthy older men. J Am Geriatr Soc 43(12): 1350–5

Papadakis MA, Grady D, Black D, Tierney MJ, Gooding GA, Schambelan M, Grunfeld C (1996) Growth Hormone replacement in healthy older men improves body composition but not functional ability. Ann Intern Med 124(8):708–16

Pavlov EP, Harman SM, Merriam GR, Gelato MC, Blackman MR (1986) Responses of growth hormone and somatomedin-C to GH releasing hormone in healthy aging men. J Clin Endocrinol Metab 62: 595–600

Pfeilschifter J and Ziegler R (1998) Relationship between IGF-I and skeletal ageing Eur J Endocrinol 138: 617–618

Pyka G, Wiswell RA, and Marcus R (1992) Age-dependent effect of resistance exercise on growth hormone secretion in people. J Clin Endocrinol Metab 75: 404–407

Rosen T, Wiren L, Wilhelmsen L, et al (1994) Decreased psychological wellbeing in adults with growth hormone deficiency. Clin Endocrinol 40: 111–116

Rudman D, Kutner MH, Rogers CM, Lubin MF, Fleming GA, Bain RP (1981) Impaired growth hormone secretion in the adult population: relation to age and adiposity. J Clin Invest 67 (5): 1361–9

Rudman D, Feller AG, Nagraj HS, Gergans GA, Lalitha PY, Goldberg AF, Schlenker RA, Cohn L, Rudman IW, Mattson DE (1990) Effects of human growth hormone in men over 60 years old. N Engl J Med 323: 1–6

Shibasaki T, Shizume K, Nakahara M, Masuda A, Jibiki K, Demura H, Wakabayashi I, Ling N (1984) Age related changes in growth hormone response to growth hormone releasing factor in man. J Clin Endocrinol Metab 58(1): 212–4

Sugimoto T, Nakaoka D, Nasu M, Kanzawa M, Sugishita T, Chihara K (1999) Effect of recombinant human growth hormone in elderly osteoporotic women. Clin Endocrinol 51: 715–724

Taaffe DR, Pruitt L, Reim J, Hintz RL, Butterfield G, Hoffman AR, Marcus R (1994) Effect of recombinant human growth hormone on muscle strength response to resistance exercise in elderly men. J Clin Endocrinol Metab 79: 1361–1366

Taaffe DR, Thompson JL, Butterfield GE, Hoffman AR, Marcus R (2001) Recombinant human growth hormone, but not insulin like growth factor-1, enhances central fat loss in postmenopausal women undergoing a diet and exercise program. Horm Metab Res 33 (3): 156–62

Toogood AA, O'Neill PA, Shalet SM (1996) Beyond the somatopause: growth hormone deficiency in adults over the age of 60 years. J Clin Endocrinol Metab 81: 460–465

Toogood AA, Adams JE, O'Neill PA, Shalet SM (1996) Body composition in growth hormone deficient adults over the age of 60 years. Clin Endocrinol 45: 399–405

Toogood AA, Adams JE, O'Neill PA, Shalet SM (1997) Elderly patients with adult onset growth hormone deficiency are not osteopaenic. J Clin Endocrinol Metab 82: 1462–1466

Toogood AA, Jones J, O'Neill PA, Thorner MO, Shalet SM (1998) The diagnosis of severe growth hormone deficiency in elderly patients with hypothalamic pituitary disease. Clin Endocrinol 48: 569–576

Toogood AA and Shalet SM (1999) growth hormone replacement therapy in the elderly with hypothalamic pituitary disease: A dose finding study J Clin Endocrinol Metab 84: 131–136

Vaessen N, Heutink P, Janssen JA, Witteman JC, Testers L, Hofman A, Lamberts SW, Oostra BA, Pols HA, van Duijn CM (2001) A polymorphism in the gene for IGF-1 functional properties and risk for type 2 diabetes and myocardial infarction. Diabetes 50(3): 637–42

Van Cauter E, Leproult R, and Plat L (2000) Age related changes in slow wave sleep and REM sleep and relationship with growth hormone and cortisol levels in healthy men. JAMA 284 (7); 861–868

Van der Lely AJ, Lamberts SW, Jauch KW, Swierstra BA, Hertlein H, Danielle De Vries D, Birkett MA, Bates PC, Blum WF, Attanasio AF (2000) Use of GH in elderly patients with accidental hip fracture. Eur J Endocrinol 143 (5): 585–592.

Veldhuis JD, Iranmanesh A, Ho KK, Waters MJ, Johnson ML, Lizarralde G (1991) Dual defects in pulsatile growth hormone secretion and clearance subserve the hyposomatotropism of obesity in man. J Clin Endocrinol Metab 72: 51–59

Wallymahmed ME, Foy P, Shaw D, Hutcheon R, Edwards RH, MacFarlane IA (1997) Quality of life, body composition and muscle strength in adult growth hormone deficiency: the influence of GH replacement therapy for up to 3 years. Clin Endocrinol 48: 613–620

Welle S, Thornton C, Statt M, McHenry B (1996) Growth Hormone increases muscle mass and strength but does not rejuvenate myofibrillar protein synthesis in healthy subjects over 60 years old. J Clin Endocrinol Metab 81(9): 3239–43

Estrogen and Cognitive Functioning in Women

Barbara B. Sherwin[1]

During the past two decades, research findings from basic neuroscience have provided a wealth of information concerning the mechanisms of action of estrogen on brain structure and function (discussed in detail in other chapters of this volume). It is now clear that this sex hormone exerts effects on brain morphology and on brain chemistry that provide biological plausibility for the hypothesis that estrogen could enhance and/or preserve aspects of cognitive functioning in women. Before a review of the clinical studies that have provided, or have failed to provide, evidence to support this hypothesis, it will be useful to briefly outline some basic aspects of sex hormone production in women across the life span as well as some key facts regarding cognitive functioning in aging women.

Sex Hormone Production in Women

In females, the hypothalamus produces gonadotropin hormone-releasing hormone (GnRH) as early as 10 weeks of gestation (Speroff et al 1989). This production causes a release of follicle stimulating hormone (FSH) and luteinizing hormone (LH) by the pituitary, which in turn, causes follicular growth and development in the ovaries and secretion of the sex steroids. In childhood, gonadotropin levels are low until the onset of puberty at a mean age of 12.8 years of age. Then, for reasons that are still unclear, episodic LH secretion begins to occur during sleep. In time, the hypothalamic-pituitary-ovarian axis, which had been suppressed during childhood, becomes fully activated during puberty and gives rise to monthly menstrual cycles that are regulated by positive and negative hypothalamic-pituitary-ovarian endocrine feedback mechanisms. During reproductive life (approximately ages 13 to 45 years), the ovary produces over 90% of circulating estrogens in a woman's body (Speroff et al. 1989). Then, at approximately 38-42 years of age, ovulation becomes less frequent and less estrogen is produced until, at a mean age of 51 years, estrogen production is insufficient to provoke menstrual cycles, which then cease. When a woman has missed 12 successive menstrual cycles, she is said to be menopausal. Although estrogen production by

[1] Mc Gill university, Department of Psychology,
1205 Dr. Penfield Ave., Montreal, Quebec, Canada H3X1B1

Chanson et al.
Endocrine Aspects of Successful Aging
© Springer-Verlag Berlin Heidelberg 2004

the ovaries does not continue beyond the menopause, extraglandular conversion of androgen precursors results in some low background of circulating estrogens in postmenopausal women that is variable and modified by a variety of factors (Speroff et al. 1989). During the period of time prior to and during the menopause, the majority of women experience certain symptoms as a result of their diminished estrogen production, most prominently the vasomotor symptoms manifested by hot flashes and cold sweats, atrophic vaginitis, and, sometimes, mood lability and memory disturbances.

Cognitive Functioning in Women

Before reviewing research findings that bear on the relationship between estrogen and cognition in women, it is important to point out that aspects of cognition are differentially mediated by numerous brain areas and neural pathways, so that it is possible, if not likely, that a given chemical compound would have selective and not global effects on cognition. The putative specificity of estrogenic effects on cognition also gains support from the localization of estrogen receptors in certain brain areas, including the hippocampus, although this steroid can also act via nongenomic mechanisms (McEwen 1991). Also, there are sex differences in cognitive functioning; women excel in verbal memory, verbal fluency, and fine motor skills whereas tasks that favor males include visuospatial skills and gross motor coordination (Halpern 1992). These relative sex differences in cognitive functions are thought to occur as a result of prenatal differences in exposure of male and female brains to levels of sex steroids (Sherwin 1994). If it is true that, in adult life, circulating levels of sex hormones upregulate specific neural pathways that had formed under the influence of that same hormone prenatally, then it would be predicted that the administration of estrogen to postmenopausal women would preferentially enhance performance on tasks that favor females. such as verbal memory and verbal fluency.

Age-related changes in cognitive functioning also occur with healthy aging. Recent studies have suggested that the memory system specifically and adversely affected with aging appears to be that which underlies explicit or declarative memory while implicit or nondeclarative memory remains relatively intact (Grady and Craik, 2000). Explicit memory refers to the conscious recollection of facts and events whereas implicit memory involves the performance of nonconscious habits, e.g., tying shoelaces, and repetition priming. A wealth of evidence from rodent, nonhuman primate, and human studies suggests that structures in the medial temporal lobe, including the hippocampus, the dentate gyrus and the entorhinal cortex, are important at the time of learning and for some time thereafter, whereas the neocortical association areas are the permanent repository of memory (Squire and Zola 1996). The ability to retrieve previously learned material (long-term memory) is dependent on the prefrontal cortices (Ungerlieder 1995).

Randomized Controlled Trials

At least eight prospective randomized controlled trials (RCTs) of the efficacy of estrogen on aspects of cognitive functioning in postmenopausal women have been published since 1985. Numerous different estrogen formulations, doses, and routes of administration were used in these RCTs, and serum levels of estradiol ranged from postmenopausal (Paolo-Kantola et al. 1998) to supraphysiological (Sherwin 1988) values at the time of cognitive testing in the groups that received estrogen. Testing was carried out either by computer (Paolo-Kantola et al. 1998; Duka et al. 2000) or conventionally, by a psychologist (Sherwin 1988; Sherwin and Phillips 1990; Ditkoff et al. 1991; Phillips and Sherwin 1992; Wolf et al. 1999) and two studies failed to include any measure of verbal memory (Paolo-Kantola et al. 1998; Ditkoff et al. 1991). Perhaps even more important is the fact that the duration of treatment across studies ranged from 2 weeks to 3 months. Since the latency of onset of the effect of estrogen on the brain is not known for women, the results of studies of very short treatment duration should be regarded with caution. Nonetheless, it is possible to tentatively conclude from these RCTs that short-term estrogen replacement therapy (ERT) acts to selectively maintain verbal memory in healthy, naturally and surgically menopausal women. However, it must be acknowledged that this conclusion is not unanimous among studies, possibly because of the methodological issues cited earlier.

The conclusion that estrogen helps to maintain verbal memory in women was supported by the results of an RCT of young women being treated with a GnRH analog (GnRH-a) for uterine myomas (Sherwin and Tulandi 1996). All experienced a decrease in scores on tests of verbal memory, but not visual memory, following three months of ovarian suppression. In the second phase of the study, those who randomly received add-back estrogen in addition to the GnRH-a had a reversal of their verbal memory deficit that occurred following treatment with the GnRH-a alone, whereas the verbal memory deficit remained in those given add-back placebo in addition to the GnRH-a.

In the Women's Health Initiative Memory Study (WHIMS), there was no difference in the incidence of mild cognitive impairment in women over the age of 65 years who had been randomized to treatment with either 0.625 mg of CEE plus 2.5 mg MPA daily or to a placebo for 4 years (Rapp et al., 2003) However, there was a small increased risk of cognitive decline over time in the combined hormone group compared to placebo.

Cross-sectional Studies

Cross-sectional studies involve the comparison of scores on neuropsychological tests of groups of postmenopausal estrogen users and nonusers from the general population. The subjects are, in the best case, matched for age, level of education, and socioeconomic status, variables that can independently affect cognitive functioning. Except for in one of these longitudinal studies (Hogervorst et al. 1999), women over the age of 50 years who were being treated with estrogen performed significantly better than nonusers on at least one aspect of cognition (Kampen and Sherwin 1994; Robinson et al. 1994; Kimura 1995; Steffens et al. 1999; Carlson and Sherwin 2000; Verghese et al., 2000; Duff and Hampson 2000; Grodstein et al. 2000; Keenan et al. 2001; Maki et al. 2001; Hogervorst et al. 1999). In the majority of studies, the cognitive functions that were most profoundly (but not exclusively) influenced by estrogen were verbal memory and verbal fluency.

Thus, while the data from cross-sectional studies provide substantial support for the idea that estrogen helps to maintain aspects of cognition in postmenopausal women, there is some inconsistency in the findings which may be due to several factors: biases inherent in self-selected populations, the variety of drugs and doses taken by the estrogen users, the failure to confirm that women were being compliant with hormone use by measuring plasma levels of hormones in some studies, the variation in the difficulty, frequency, appropriateness and validity of the neuropsychological tests used in these studies and other confounds, such as the use of psychotropic drugs in some women (Grodstein et al. 2000), the concurrent use of progestins in most groups of estrogen users and the sole use of tests of global cognition that are unable to distinguish between various areas of cognitive function (Steffens et al. 1999).

Longitudinal Studies

Theoretically, longitudinal designs have maximal capacity to test whether ERT protects against cognitive aging because they involve repeated testing of postmenopausal estrogen users and nonusers over a prolonged period of time, when some decrease in aspects of cognitive performance would normally be expected to occur. On the other hand, women were not randomly assigned to ERT in these studies, so a self-selection bias was operative. Nine longitudinal studies of ERT and cognitive functioning were published between 1993 and 2001 (Barrett-Connor and Kritz-Silverstein 1993; Resnick et al. 1997; Jacobs et al. 1998; Matthews et al. 1999; Yaffe et al. 2000; Rice et al. 2000; Carlson et al. 2001; deMoraes et al. 2001; Fillenbaum 2001). The mean age of women tested in these longitudinal studies ranged between 55 and 95 years and the duration between test times varied between 2 years (Rice et al. 2000) and 16.5 years (Barrett-Connor and Kritz-Silverstein 1993). By far, the majority of estrogen users in these longitudinal studies were taking conjugated equine estrogen (CEE) in doses that varied between 0.3 mg and 1.25 mg/day with or without different progestins in different doses. In some studies, the drugs being taken were not reported at all.

Although the findings from these longitudinal studies do not allow causal statements to be made with regard to the influence of estrogen on cognitive aging in women, they nonetheless provide important information. Their findings are quite consistent in showing that the use of estrogen is associated with better cognitive functioning and with less cognitive deterioration in older women over time. Verbal memory and verbal fluency seemed to be preferentially maintained in those longitudinal studies that specifically measured these cognitive functions. However, since the vast majority of these studies were undertaken primarily to measure other endpoints (e.g., osteoporosis, heart disease), they frequently employed only an omnibus test, most often the Mini Mental State Examination (mMMSE), to measure the secondary endpoint of cognition. The mMMSE is generally used as a screening instrument to measure mental status and does not permit the evaluation of specific cognitive functions. If estrogen does preferentially maintain verbal memory and verbal fluency in aging women, as the RCTs suggest, then these effects might not have been apparent in these longitudinal studies due to the use of omnibus tests so that their results may have underestimated the true magnitude of cognitive protection provided by ERT in aging women.

Summary and Conclusions

Findings from basic neuroscience provide considerable biological plausibility for the notion that estrogen could exert beneficial effects on memory in women, although evidence from long-term studies is unavailable. Thus far, results of the available, short-term RCTs suggest that the use of ERT, following either a natural or surgical menopause, maintains verbal memory and verbal fluency in aging postmenopausal women. Findings from the case-control and longitudinal studies are quite consistent in showing that the use of ERT is associated with less cognitive deterioration in older women over time and provide confirmatory support for the results of the RCTs on estrogen and cognition. Verbal memory and verbal fluency seemed to be preferentially maintained in estrogen users in those studies that specifically measured these cognitive domains. That the findings from these studies are not entirely consistent may be due to the fact that there are selection biases in some studies that did not randomly assign participants to ERT, as well as differences in length of estrogen treatment. Others failed to screen for the presence of depression or for the concomitant use of drugs that affect the CNS which might have independently and negatively influenced cognitive performance. Plasma levels of estrogens were not measured in the majority of studies to confirm that ERT users were compliant with medication use. Moreover, since the vast majority of the longitudinal studies were undertaken to measure primary endpoints other than cognition (e.g., osteoporosis, heart disease), they frequently employed only an omnibus test of cognitive functioning, most often the mMMSE, to measure the secondary endpoint of cognition. As mentioned earlier, this test is generally used as a screening instrument to measure cognitive decline and does not allow the evaluation of specific cognitive domains.

Importantly, both human (Zandi, 2002) and animal (Gibbs, 2000) studies have shown that estrogen prevents cognitive decline when it is administered during the peri- or early postmenopause but not when it is given, *de novo*, years following the onset of menopause as occurred in the WHIMS study (Rapp et al., 2003). Therefore, there may be a "window of opportunity" during the early postmenopause when estrogen will protect against cognitive decline. If this is true, then it is not surprising that the WHIMS study did not find a protective effect of hormone therapy on cognitive function since treatment was initiated in women over the age of 65 years. Clearly, the WHIMS findings cannot be generalized to younger, early postmenopausal women, those who are actually treated with hormones in the real world.

Other methodological flaws in the longitudinal studies on estrogen and cognition in aging women may also have confounded their results. Since women with an intact uterus are required to take a progestin in addition to estrogen in order to prevent endometrial hyperplasia, and since progestins can reverse the beneficial effects of estrogen on brain morphology (Gould et al. 1990), the practice, in some studies, of analyzing data from unopposed estrogen users and from estrogen-plus-progestin users together may have also underestimated the beneficial effects of estrogen. Indeed, in the Kame longitudinal study (Rice et al. 2000), whereas scores on a measure of cognitive functioning improved over time in women on unopposed estrogen, the performance of women who took estrogen and a progestin got worse over time. Finally, some inconsistency between these studies can be accounted for by the differing pharmacokinetics and efficacy of the numerous estrogenic drugs administered in different doses via different routes of administration (Ansbacher 2001).

While the substantial evidence that ERT helps to maintain aspects of cognitive function that decline somewhat with normal aging suggests that long-term use of estrogen would protect the quality of life for older women, this treatment decision needs to be balanced against the small, duration-related increase in the risk of invasive breast cancer, coronary heart disease and stroke that occurs with more than four years of estrogen use (Writing Group for the Womens' Health Initiative Investigators 2002), although ERT also reduces all-cause mortality in women (Grodstein et al. 1997).

The fact that female life expectancy has nearly doubled in industrialized countries during the past century means that more and more women are living into old age. In the attempt to preserve the quality of life for elderly women, research efforts have focused on preventing degenerative diseases that may compromise their daily functioning, such as osteoporosis and coronary heart disease. There is increasing recognition that aspects of cognition also decline with normal aging in women and may negatively impact their quality of life. To the extent that ERT may protect women against cognitive decline, this therapy would help to preserve optimal functioning in the elderly. However, there is a possibility that these benefits may be mitigated by the side effects of estrogen treatment, so the decision to treat is highly individual and depends, to some extent, on the woman's current state of health, on her medical history, on her family history and on her lifestyle.

Acknowledgments

The preparation of this manuscript was supported by a grant from the Canadian Institutes of Health Research (# MT-11623).

References

Ansbacher R. (2001) The pharmacokinetics and efficacy of different estrogens are not equivalent. Am J Obstet Gynecol 184: 255–263

Barrett-Connor E, Kritz-Silverstein, D (1993) Estrogen replacement therapy and cognitive function in older women. JAMA 269: 2637–2641

Carlson LE, Sherwin BB (2000) Higher levels of plasma estradiol and testosterone in healthy elderly men compared with age-matched women may protect aspects of explicit memory. Menopause 7: 168–177

Carlson MC, Zandi PP, Plassman BL, Tschanz JT, Welsh-Bohmer KA, Steffens DC, Bastian LA, Mehta KM, Breitner JCS (2001) Hormone replacement therapy and reduced cognitive decline in older women. The Cache County Study. Neurology 57: 2210–2216

de Moraes SA, Szklo M, Knopman D, Park E (2001) Prospective assessment of estrogen replacement therapy and cognitive functioning: Other osclerosis risk in community study. Am J Epidemiol 154: 733–739

Ditkoff EC, Crary WG, Cristo M, Lobo R (1991) Estrogen improves psychological function in asymptomatic postmenopausal women. Obstet Gynecol 78: 991–995

Duff SJ, Hampson E (2000) A beneficial effect of estrogen on working memory in postmenopausal women taking hormone replacement therapy. Horm Behav 38: 262–276

Duka T, Tasker R, McGowan JF (2000) The effects of 3-week estrogen hormone replacement on cognition in elderly healthy females. Psychopharmacol 149: 129–139

Fillenbaum GG, Hanion JT, Landerman LR, Schmader KE (2001) Impact of estrogen use on decline in cognitive function in a representative sample of older community-resident women. Am J Epidemiol, 153: 137–144

Gibbs RB (2000) Long-term treatment with estrogen plus progesterone entrances acquisition of a spatial memory task by ovariectomiged aged rats. Neurobiol of Aging 21: 107–116

Gould E, Woolley CS, Frankfurt M, McEwen BS (1990) Gonadal steroids regulate dendritic spine density in hippocampal pyramidal cells in adulthood. J Neurosci 10: 1286–1291

Grady CL, Craik FIM (2000) Changes in memory processing with age. Curr Opin Neurobiol 10: 224–231

Grodstein F, Stampfer MJ, Colditz GA, Willett WC, Manson JE, Joffe M, Rosner B, Fuchs C, Hankinson SE, Hunter DJ, Hennekens CH, Speizer FE (1997) Postmenopausal hormone therapy and mortality. N Engl J Med. 336:1769–75

Grodstein F, Chen J, Pollen DA, Albert MS, Wilson RS, Folstein, MF, Evans DA, Stampfer MJ (2000) Postmenopausal hormone therapy and cognitive function in healthy older women. J Am Geriatr Soc 48: 746–752

Halpern DF (1992) Sex differences in cognitive abilities. 2nd edition. Hillsdale, NJ: Lawrence Erlbaum Associates

Hogervorst E, Boshuisen M, Riedel W, Willeken C, Jolles J (1999) The effect of hormone replacement therapy on cognitive function in elderly women. Psychoneuroendocrinology 24: 43–68

Jacobs DM, Tang M-X, Stern Y, Sano M, Marder K, Bell KL, Schofield P, Dooneief G, Gurland B, Mayeux R (1998) Cognitive function in nondemented older women who took estrogen after menopause. Neurology 50: 368–373

Janowsky JS, Chavez B, Orwoll E (2000) Sex steroids modify working memory. J Cogn Neurosci 12: 407–414

Kampen DL, Sherwin BB (1994) Estrogen use and verbal memory in healthy postmenopausal women. Obstet Gynecol 83: 979–983

Keenan PA, Ezzat WH, Ginsberg K, Moore GJ (2001) Prefrontal cortex as the site of estrogen's effect on cognition. Psychoneuroendocrinology 26: 577–590

Kimura D (1995) Estrogen replacement therapy may protect against intellectual decline in postmenopausal women. Horm Behav 29: 312–321

Maki PM, Zonderman AB, Resnick SM (2001) Enhanced verbal memory in nondemented elderly women receiving hormone-replacement therapy. Am J Psychiat 158: 227–233

Matthews K, Cauley J, Yaffe K, Zmuda JM (1999) Estrogen replacement therapy and cognitive decline in older community women. J. Am Geriatr Soc 47: 518–523

McEwen BS (1991) Non-genomic and genomic effects of steroids on neural activity. Trends Pharmacol Sci 12: 141–147

Paolo-Kantola P, Portin R, Polo O, Helenius H, Irjala K, Erkkola R (1998) The effect of short-term estrogen replacement therapy on cognition: a randomized, double-blind, cross-over trial in postmenopausal women. Obstet Gynecol 91: 459–466

Phillips S, Sherwin BB (1992) Effects of estrogen on memory function in surgically menopausal women. Psychoneuroendocrinology 17: 485–495

Rapp SR, Espeland MA, Shumaker SA, Henderson VW, Brunner RL, Manson JE, Gass MLS, Stefanick ML, Lane DS, Hays J, Johnson KC, Coker LH, Dailey M, Bowen D (2003) Effect of estrogen plus progestin on global cognitive function in postmenopausal women: The Women's Health Initiative Memory Study. JAMA 289: 2663–2672

Resnick SM, Metter EJ, Zonderman AB (1997) Estrogen replacement therapy and longitudinal decline in visual memory: a possible protective effect? Neurology 49: 1491–1497

Rice MM, Graves AB, McCurry SM, Gibbons LE, Bowen JD, McCormick WC, Larson EB (2000) Postmenopausal estrogen and estrogen-progestin use and 2-year rate of cognitive change in a cohort of older Japanese American women: the Kame project. Arch Intern Med 160: 1641–1649

Robinson D, Friedman L, Marcus R, Tinklenberg J, Yesavage J (1994) Estrogen replacement therapy and memory in older women. J Am Geriatr Soc 42: 919–922

Sherwin BB (1988) Estrogen and/or androgen replacement therapy and cognitive functioning in surgical menopausal women. Psychoneuroendocrinology 13: 345–357

Sherwin BB (1994) Estrogen effects on memory in women. Ann NY Acad Sci 743: 213–239

Sherwin BB, Phillips S (1990) Estrogen and cognitive functioning in surgically menopausal women. Ann NY Acad Sci 592: 474–476

Sherwin BB, Tulandi T (1996) «Add-back» estrogen reverses cognitive deficits induced by a gonadotropin-releasing hormone agonist in women with leiomyomata uteri. J Clin Endocrinol Metab 81: 2545–2549

Squire LR, Zola SM (1996) Structure and function of declarative and nondeclarative memory systems. Proc Natl Acad Sci USA 93: 13515–13522

Speroff L, Glass RH, Kase NG (1989) Clinical gynecologic endocrinology and infertility. Williams & Wilkins, Baltimore, MD.

Steffens DC, Norton MC, Plassman BL, Wyse BW, Welsh-Bohmer KA, Anthony JC, Breitner JC (1999) Enhanced cognitive performance with estrogen use in nondemented community-dwelling older women. J Am Geriat Soc 47: 1171–1176

Ungerlieder LG (1995) Functional brain imaging studies of cortical mechanisms for memory. Science 270: 769–775

Verghese J, Kuslansky G, Sliwinski M, Crystal HA, Bushke H, Lipton RB (2000) Cognitive performance in surgically menopausal women on estrogen. Neurology 55: 872–874

Wolf OT, Kudielka BM, Hellhammer DH, Torber S, McEwen BS, Kirschbaum C (1999) Two weeks of transdermal estradiol treatment in postmenopausal elderly women and its effect on memory and mood: verbal memory changes are associated with the treatment induced estradiol levels. Psychoneuroendocrinology 24: 727–741

Writing Group for the Women's Health Initiative Investigators (2002) Risk and benefits of estrogen plus progestin in healthy postmenopausal women. Principal results from the Women's Health Initiative randomized controlled trial. JAMA 288: 321–333

Yaffe K, Lui L-Y, Grady D, Cauley J, Kramer J, Cummings SR (2000) Estrogen use, APOE, and cognitive decline: evidence of gene-environment interaction. Neurology 54: 1949–195

Zandi PP, Carlson MC, Plassman BL, Welsh-Bohmer KA, Mayer LS, Steffens DC, Breitner JC (2002) Hormone replacement therapy and incidence of Alzheimer's disease in older women: the Cache County study. JAMA 288: 2123–2129

Genetic Polymorphisms and Age-Related Diseases The Example of Osteoporosis

André G. Uitterlinden and *Huibert A.P. Pols*

Summary

Over the past decades epidemiological research of so-called "complex" diseases, such as diabetes, osteoporosis, cancer, and cardiovascular disease, has identified a number of risk factors for these common age-related disorders. Examples include obesity for diabetes, low bone mineral density for osteoporosis, and smoking for cancer and cardiovascular disease. Some of these risk factors are used in clinical practice, for example to identify at-risk subjects, and for monitoring treatment of patients with these diseases.

More recently, a novel class of risk factors, genetic polymorphisms, has gained considerable interest in this respect. This new interest is mostly due to the Human Genome Project, which has identified every human gene and also uncovered a plethora of polymorphic variants of these genes that embody the genetic risk factors. Genetic risk factors are expected to find applications in early identification of at-risk subjects, prediction of response-to-treatment, and development of novel therapeutic options. We will discuss some developments in the field of the genetics of osteoporosis.

Genetics of osteoporosis

Certain aspects of osteoporosis have strong genetic influences. This can be derived, for example, from genetic epidemiological analyses that showed that, in women, a maternal family history of fracture is positively related to fracture risk (Cummings et al. 1995). Most evidence, however, has come from twin studies on bone mineral density (BMD; Smith et al. 1973; Pocock et al. 1987; Flicker et al. 1995). For BMD the heritability has been estimated to be high: 50-80% (Smith et al. 1973; Pocock et al. 1987; Flicker et al. 1995). Thus, although twin studies can overestimate the heritability, a considerable part of the variance in BMD values might be explained by genetic factors while the remaining part could be due to environmental factors. This also implies that there are "bone density" genes, variants of which will result in BMD levels that are different between individuals. These differences can become apparent in different ways, for example, as peak BMD or as differences in the rates of bone loss at advanced age.

The heritablity estimates of osteoporosis indicate a considerable influence of environmental factors that can be modifying the effect of genetic predisposition. Some gene-environment interactions one can think of, in this respect, include

Chanson et al.
Endocrine Aspects of Successful Aging
© Springer-Verlag Berlin Heidelberg 2004

diet, exercise and exposure to sunlight, for example. While genetic predisposition will be constant during life, environmental factors tend to change over the different periods of life, resulting in different "expression levels" of the genetic susceptibility. Ageing is associated with a general functional decline resulting in, for example, less exercise, less time spent outdoors, changes in diet, etc. This can result in particular genetic susceptibilities being revealed only later on in life, after a period when they went unnoticed due to sufficient exposure to an environmental factor.

Taking all this into account, it becomes evident that osteoporosis is, not very surprisingly, considered a "complex" genetic trait. This complex character is shared with other common and often age-related traits with genetic influences such as diabetes, schizophrenia, osteoarthritis, cancer, etc. "Complex" means that a trait is multifactorial as well as multigenic. Thus, genetic risk factors (i.e., certain alleles or gene variants) will be transmitted from one generation to the next but the expression of these factors in the phenotype will be dependent on interaction with other gene variants and with environmental factors.

Genome scans and candidate genes

A first step in the dissection of the genetic factors in osteoporosis is the "genomics" of osteoporosis, i.e., the identification, mapping and characterization of the set of genes responsible for contributing to the genetic susceptibility to aspects of osteoporosis. Finding the responsible gene for monogenic disorders has now become almost a routine exercise for specialized laboratories. However, the complex character of osteoporosis makes it quite resistant to the methods of analysis that, in past decades, have worked so well for the monogenic diseases. Therefore different and often more cumbersome approaches have to be applied (see, e.g., Lander and Schork 1994).

In *top-down* approaches, first large-scale genome searches are performed that indicate which chromosomal areas might contain osteoporosis genes. In an optimal setting such searches are performed in hundreds of relatives (sibs, pedigrees, etc) with hundreds of DNA markers (mostly microsatellites) evenly spread over the genome. Genome searches are based on the assumption that relatives who share a certain phenotype will also share one or more chromosomal areas identical by descent containing one or more gene variants causing (to a certain extent) the phenotype of interest (e.g., low BMD). The gene is then said to be linked with the DNA marker used to "flag" a certain chromosomal region. Upon positive linkage, subsequent research will zoom in on identifying which one of the dozens of genes in the chromosomal area is the one involved in bone metabolism and then identify the particular sequence variant giving rise to (aspects of) osteoporosis. This approach is illustrated in Figure 1.

In contrast, the *bottom-up* approach builds upon the known involvement of a particular gene in aspects of osteoporosis, e.g., bone metabolism. This gene is then referred to as a "candidate gene". The candidacy of such a gene can be established by several lines of evidence:

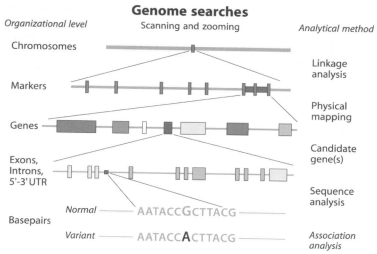

Fig. 1. Schematic flow-diagram depicting the different steps in a '"genome search" or "genome scan." On the left the level of organization of the DNA molecules is presented; on the right the different analytical steps in the process are shown.

1. Cell biological and molecular biological experiments indicating bone-specific expression of the gene.
2. Animal models in which a gene has been mutated (e.g., natural mouse mutants), overexpressed (transgenic mice), or deleted (knock-out mice) and which result in a bone-phenotype.
3. Naturally occurring mutations of the human gene resulting in monogenic Mendelian diseases with a bone phenotype.

Subsequently, in the candidate gene identified by these approaches, frequently occurring sequence variants (polymorphisms) have to be identified which are associated with differences in function of the encoded protein. Such variants will then be tested in association- or linkage -analyses to evaluate its contribution to the phenotype of interest at the population level.

Naturally, top-down and bottom-up approaches will meet each other somewhere down the line, leading to maps of candidate osteoporosis genes and maps of genome areas containing putative osteoporosis genes that will completely or partially overlap. Sequence analysis of a "candidate" osteoporosis gene in a number of different individuals will identify sequence variants, some of which will be just polymorphic (anonymous polymorphisms) while others will have consequences for the activity of the protein encoded (functional polymorphisms). These can include, e.g., sequence variations leading to alterations in the amino acid composition of the protein, changes in the 5' promoter region leading to differences in expression, and/or polymorphisms in the 3' region leading to differences in mRNA degradation. The functional polymorphisms are of prime interest to further test in association analyses to establish if the candidate gene is a true "osteoporosis gene" or not. Because functional polymorphisms lead to meaningful biological differences in function of the encoded "osteoporosis" protein, the interpretation of association analyses using these variants becomes quite straightforward. For functional polymorphisms it is expected that the same allele will be associated with the same phenotype in different populations.

Complicating factors

Several studies have shown that, on average, 1 of every 500 bp is variant in the population. This finding is highlighted, for example, by a comprehensive sequence analysis of 9.7 kb of genomic DNA encoding part of the human lipoprotein lipase gene in 71 different individuals (Nickerson et al. 1998). In this relatively small stretch of genomic sequence, 88 different sites of sequence variation were found, with a mean heterozygosity of 20%. Of these, 79 were single nucleotide polymorphisms (SNPs) and nine involved insertion-deletion types of variations. Thus, candidate gene analyses will have to focus on which of the many variant nucleotides are the ones that actually matter, that is, which sequence variation is functionally relevant by changing expression levels, changing codons, etc. Given the average size of a gene and the relatively young age of human populations, it can be predicted that several sequence variations "that matter" will co-exist in a given sample from a study population. A major challenge of fundamental research will be to unravel the functionality of these variations.

Yet, in spite of such complicating factors, genetic research will contribute to a further understanding of complex diseases. The identification of new genes, or new roles for already known genes, will allow insights into mechanistic pathways that might help in designing therapeutic protocols. Finally, the description of genetic variation underlying phenotypic variation can be used, in concert with existing easy-to-assess risk factors, in prediction of risk for aspects of osteoporosis. In this respect, novel therapeutic protocols but also insights in gene-environment interactions allow for ways to offer treatment to patients.

Osteoporosis candidate genes: Collagen type Iα1 and the vitamin D receptor

The vitamin D receptor (VDR) is the candidate gene that initiated the molecular genetic studies on osteoporosis by Morrison and Eisman (Morrison et al. 1994). They initially reported anonymous 3' polymorphisms, detected as BsmI, ApaI, and TaqI RFLPs, to be associated with differences in BMD and claimed that up to 80% of the population variance in BMD could be explained by this single gene. Although some of their results were later retracted (Morrison et al. 1997), their findings left behind the idea that there could be such a thing as a single osteoporosis gene. For a complex disease such as osteoporosis, this proposal is very unlikely and indeed, by now several large population-based association analyses

(Uitterlinden et al.1996) and metastudies have indicated that – at most – these variants explain only a few percent of the population variance of BMD. Thus, the VDR does not seem to be a powerful marker for predicting BMD. However, in view of their pleiotropic involvement in a number of biological pathways, the vitamin D receptor polymorphisms have also been analysed in relation to a number of other diseases. For example. we have recently shown VDR to be associated with (bony) aspects of osteoarthritis, i.e., osteophytosis (Uitterlinden et al 1997). Yet, a major problem with the vitamin D receptor gene polymorphisms remains the lack of insight into the functional consequences of the polymorphisms used so far. Therefore a major effort, including that of our own laboratory, is focussed on finding additional polymorphic sites, but now in functionally relevant areas of the gene, such as the 3' untranslated region and the 5' promoter area of this gene.

An example of a <u>functional</u> sequence variation in an osteoporosis candidate gene that has quickly shown promising associations is the G to T substitution in the Sp1 binding site in the first intron of the collagen type Iα1 gene. After the discovery and initial association analysis of the T allele by Grant et al. (1996), a large-scale population analysis in the Rotterdam Study showed the T allele to be associated with low BMD and increased fracture risk (Uitterlinden et al. 1998). Interesting observations in our cohort of 1782 elderly women were the increase with age of the genotype-dependent differences and the fact that the genotype-dependent fracture risk was independent of the differences in BMD. Meanwhile, severeal other studies have confirmed these observations (Mann et al 2001; Efstathiadou et al. 2001), making this a promising osteoporosis candidate gene-polymorphism with consistent effects. Also, the molecular way in which this polymorphism is influencing BMD and fracture risk is becoming more and more clear. Work by Ralston and colleagues (Mann et al. 2001) has shown that the T allele has increased affinity for Sp1 binding factor and increased mRNA and protein production, and, in biomechanical experiments on bone biopsies, has been shown to be associated with decreased bone strength. The overrepresentation of collagen type Iα1 homotrimers might explain the decreased bone strength, although this possibility has yet to be proven.

The findings with the COLIA1 Sp1 binding site polymorphism clearly illustrate the accumulation of evidence that is necessary to implicate a gene as an osteoporosis risk gene. The process of finding a functional polymorphism, establishing its molecular mode of action and performing association analysis to see what relevant (disease) endpoints will result from this genotype difference is more useful than analysing a random, anonymous polymorphism and seeing what clinical endpoint is associated with it. Establishing functionality of polymorphisms is therefore a major requirement before genetic polymorphisms will be considered for use in clinical practice.

Clinical Applications

Although still in its infancy with respect to having clinical implications, the field of genetics of osteoporosis is expected to eventually find applications in two main areas:

1. Prediction of response-to-treatment. Polymorphisms in, e.g., drug-metabolizing enzymes will result in different efficiencies with which drugs can exert their effect. Genotype analysis can identify those subjects expected to profit most from a particular treatment or exclude those subjects who will suffer more from side effects (individualised medicine).
2. Identification of at-risk subjects. As was illustrated for COLIA1, subjects carrying risk alleles are more likely to develop osteoporosis. Genotype analysis will allow us to take preventive measures targeted at the individual at an early stage.

So far only one polymorphism is currently being considered as an osteoporosis risk factor (the COLIA1 Sp1 polymorphism), and commercial parties have taken an interest in this genetic marker. Its utility in clinical practice has to be considered with considerable caution, however. For example, analyses in different ethnic populations have shown it to be present mostly in Caucasian subjects (Beavan et al. 1998). Furthermore, interaction of this variant with another polymorphism (the VDR 3' variants) has been demonstrated (Uitterlinden et al. 2001). This latter study also highlights the complex and multigenic nature of osteoporosis. It underlines the need to identify additional osteoporosis risk alleles so as to better understand how particular genetic markers are expressed and result in a phenotype.

Another spin-off of genetic research in osteoporosis is the discovery of new and/or unexpected genes and pathways to be involved in determining, e.g., BMD. A good example is the recent discovery of LRP5 mutations to influence BMD (Gong et al. 2001; Little et al. 2002) and by this the identification of the Wnt-signalling pathway to be involved in bone metabolism. Such discoveries lead to new possibilities of developing drugs to treat osteoporosis. In addition, such genes become osteoporosis risk genes and will be searched for polymorphisms. Risk alleles resulting from such analyses can then be added to the still growing list of osteoporosis genes.

References

Beavan S, Prentice A, Bakary D, Yan L, Cooper C, Ralston SH. (1998)Polymorphism of the collagen type Iα1 gene and ethnic differences in hip fractures rates. N Engl J Med 339: 351–352

Cummings SR, Nevitt MC, Browner WS, Stone K, Fox KM, Ensrud KE, Cauley J, Black D, Vogt TM(1995) Risk factors for hip fracture in white women. New Engl J Med 332:767–773

Efstathiadou Z, Tsatsoulis A, Ioannidis JPA (2001) Association of collagen Iα1 Sp1 polymorphism with the risk of prevalent fractures: a meta-analysis. J Bone Miner Res 16:1586–1592

Flicker L, Hopper JL, Rodgers L, Kaymakci B, Green RM, Wark JD (1995) Bone density determinants in elderly women: a twin study. J Bone Miner Res 10: 1607–1613

Gong Y, Slee RB, Fukai N, Rawadi G, Roman-Roman S, Reginato AM, Wang H, Cundy T, Glorieux FH, Lev D, Zacharin M, Oexle K, Marcelino J, Suwairi W, Heeger S, Sabatakos G, Apte S, Adkins WN, Allgrove J, Arslan-Kirchner M, Batch JA, Beighton P, Black GC, Boles RG, Boon LM, Borrone C, Brunner HG, Carle GF, Dallapiccola B, De Paepe A, Floege B, Halfhide ML, Hall B, Hennekam RC, Hirose T, Jans A, Juppner H, Kim CA, Keppler-Noreuil K, Kohlschuetter A, LaCombe D, Lambert M, Lemyre E, Letteboer T, Peltonen L, Ramesar RS, Romanengo M, Somer H, Steichen-Gersdorf E, Steinmann B, Sullivan B, Superti-Furga A, Swoboda W, van den Boogaard MJ, Van Hul W, Vikkula M, Votruba M, Zabel B, Garcia T, Baron R, Olsen BR, Warman ML, The Osteoporosis-Pseudoglioma Syndrome Collaborative Group (2001) LDL Receptor-related protein 5 (LRP5) affects bone accrual and eye development. Cell 107: 513–523

Grant SFA, Reid DM, Blake G, Herd R, Fogelman I, Ralston SH (1996)Reduced bone density and osteoporotic vertebral fracture associated with a polymorphic Sp1 binding site in the collagen type Iα1 gene. Nature Genet 14: 203–205

Lander ES, Schork NJ (1994) Genetic dissection of complex traits. Science 265: 2037–2048

Little RD, Carulli JP, Del Mastro RG, Dupuis J, Osborne M, Folz C, Manning SP, Swain PM, Zhao SC, Eustace B, Lappe MM, Spitzer L, Zweier S, Braunschweiger K, Benchekroun Y, Hu X, Adair R, Chee L, FitzGerald MG, Tulig C, Caruso A, Tzellas N, Bawa A, Franklin B, McGuire S, Nogues X, Gong G, Allen KM, Anisowicz A, Morales AJ, Lomedico PT, Recker SM, Van Eerdewegh P, Recker RR, Johnson ML (2002) A mutation in the LDL Receptor related protein 5 gene results in the autosomal dominant high bone mass trait. Am J HumanGenet 70: 11–191.

Mann V, Hobson EE, Li B, Stewart TL, Grant SFA, Robins SP, Aspden RM, Ralston SH (2001) A COLIA1 Sp1 binding site polymorphism predisposes to osteoporotic fracture by affecting bone density and quality. J Clin Invest 107: 899–907

Morrison NA, Qi JC, Tokita A, Kelly PJ, Crofts L, Nguyen TV, Sambrook PN, Eisman JA. (1994) Prediction of bone density from vitamin D receptor alleles. Nature 367: 284–287

Morrison NA, Qi JC, Tokita A, Kelly PJ, Crofts L, Nguyen TV, Sambrook PN, Eisman JA (1997) Prediction of bone density from vitamin D receptor alleles (correction). Nature 387: 106

Nickerson DA, Taylor SL, Weiss KM, Clark AG, Hutchinson RG, Stengard J, Salomaa V, Vartiainen E, Boerwinkle E, Sing CF(1998) DNA sequence diversity in a 9.7-kb region of the human lipoprotein lipase gene. Nature Genet 19: 233–240

Pocock NA, Eisman JA, Hopper JL, Yeates GM, Sambrook PN, Ebert S (1987) Genetic determinants of bone mass in adults: a twin study. J.Clin Invest 80: 706–710

Smith DM, Nance WE, Kang KW, Christian JC, Johnston CC (1973) Genetic factors in determining bone mass. J Clin Invest 52: 2800–2808

Uitterlinden AG, Pols HAP, Burger H, Huang Q, van Daele PLA, van Duijn CM, Hofman A, Birkenhäger JC, van Leeuwen JPTM (1996) A large scale population based study of the association of vitamin D receptor gene polymorphisms with bone mineral density. J Bone Miner Res 11: 1242–1248

Uitterlinden AG, Burger H, Huang Q, Odding E, van Duijn CM, Hofman A, Birkenhäger JC, van Leeuwen JPTM, Pols HAP (1997) Vitamin D receptor genotype is associated with osteoarthritis. J Clin Invest 100: 259–63

Uitterlinden AG, Burger H, Huang Q, Yue F, McGuigan FEA, Grant SFA, Hofman A, van Leeuwen JPTM, Pols HAP, Ralston SH (1998) Relation of alleles at the collagen type Iα1 gene to bone density and risk of osteoporotic fractures in postmenopausal women. New Engl J Med 338: 1016–1021

Uitterlinden AG, Weel AEAM, Burger H, Fang Y, van Duijn CM, Hofman A, van Leeuwen JPTM, Pols HAP. (2001)Interaction between the vitamin D receptor gene and collagen type Iα1 gene in susceptibility for fracture. J Bone Miner Res 16: 379–385

Are Estrogens Protective or Risk Factors in the Brain? Insights Derived From Animal Models

Phyllis M. Wise and *Dena B. Dubal*

Summary

We now understand that estrogens are pleiotropic gonadal steroids that influence plasticity and cell survival of the adult brain. Over the past century, the life span of women has increased from approximately 50 to 80 years of age, but the timing of the menopause remains constant and occurs at approximately 50 years of age. This means that women may now live over one-third of their lives in a hypo-estrogenic, postmenopausal state. The impact of prolonged hypoestrogenicity on the the well-being of women and, in particular, on their brains is a critical health concern since it appears that these older women may suffer an increased risk of cognitive dysfunction and neurodegeneration due to a variety of diseases. Accumulating evidence from both clinical and basic science studies indicates that estrogens may exert critical protective actions against neurodegenerative conditions such as Alzheimer's disease (AD) and stroke. However, new evidence purports to suggest that, under some circumstances, hormone replacement may not decrease the risk of neurodegenerative diseases and may, in fact, increase risk of cerebrovascular stroke. Here, we review the discoveries that comprise our current understanding of estrogen action against neurodegeneration. These findings carry far-reaching implications for improving the health and quality of life of aging women.

Introduction

Estrogens are reproductive hormones that act on the reproductive system and on several classical estrogen target organs, including the hypothalamus, anterior pituitary, and organs of the reproductive tract. In addition, we are now beginning to appreciate that they exert trophic and protective actions on multiple tissues including the brain, bone, heart, blood vessels, and immune system. The protective actions of estrogens carry significant repercussions for health and the prevention of disease in postmenopausal women. Since the life span of women has increased from approximately 50 to 80 years, but the age of the menopause remains at about 51 years of age, women may now live 30 years of their lives in a hypoestrogenic, postmenopausal state. The impact of prolonged hypoestrogenicity is an even greater health concern, since we realize that these women may suffer from an increased vulnerability to a variety of diseases. Estrogen replacement therapy (ERT) appears to act in the primary prevention of many disease processes, including neurodegeneration. Estrogens, however, are not always beneficial, since

Chanson et al.
Endocrine Aspects of Successful Aging
© Springer-Verlag Berlin Heidelberg 2004

high doses, particularly in combination with progestins, may increase the risk for certain cancers. It is critical, therefore, to gain a more complete understanding of the spectrum of the targets and mechanisms of estrogens' actions, so that we can design hormone replacement therapies that exert only beneficial effects in the body. To achieve this understanding, we must dissect the mechanisms that underlie the myriad of effects of these steroid hormones.

Neuroprotective actions of estrogens

Included in estrogen's broad spectrum of actions is its apparent ability to protect the brain against injury and to act as a primary preventative against neurodegeneration. Clinical studies demonstrate that ERT in postmenopausal women can 1) improve cognitive function and 2) decrease the risk and delay the onset of degenerative conditions such as AD and stroke. Basic science studies have revealed the cellular and molecular bases that may explain these clinical observations. Recent insights into the molecular events that underlie estrogen-mediated neuroprotection encompass actions that range from its physiological, estrogen receptor-dependent mechanisms to its pharmacological, sometimes receptor-independent antioxidant mechanisms.

However, the conclusions drawn from these studies are not without controversy. During the last year at least three reports have been published that purport to demonstrate lack of protection or increased health risks of hormone replacement therapy (HRT) in the occurrence of cerebrovascular stroke (Viscoli et al. 2001), cardiovascular disease (Hulley et al. 1998), AD (Mulnard et al. 2000) and invasive breast cancer (Writing Group for Women's Health Initiative Investigators 2002). Together, these studies that present seemingly contradictory results make it imperative that we thoroughly understand the circumstances under which estrogens act in the brain to promote enhanced neural function and to exert protective effects against degeneration, and we must compare these to the circumstances under which estrogens may be deleterious to our health. Only then will we be able to design hormones and treatment protocols that exert only beneficial effects in the body.

Estrogen: Effects on cognition and AD

The focus of this review, and the focus of our recent discoveries, is the action of estrogen in the injured and aging brain. Our interest in this area was piqued by the clinical observations that demonstrate that estrogens influence memory and cognition (Kampen and Sherwin 1998; Schmidt et al. 1996; Sherwin 1988, 1994, 1996, 1997; Sherwin and Carlson 1997) and can protect against neurodegenerative diseases such as AD (Asthana et al. 1999; Birge 1997; Fillit 1994; Henderson and Paganini-Hill 1997; Henderson et al. 1996; Kawa et al. 1997; Paganini-Hill and Henderson 1994, 1996; Tang et al. 1996; Waring et al. 1999). As the results of more recent clinical studies have become available, we are beginning to appreciate that the protective actions of estrogens do not apply in all situations (Henderson et al. 2000; Marder and Sano 2000; Wang et al. 2000).

Many studies have examined whether ERT improves cognitive function in normal healthy women. The majority of data show that estrogens enhance cognitive function in both young (Sherwin 1988) and older women (Kampen and Sherwin 1998; Robinson et al. 1994; Schmidt et al. 1996). Furthermore, it appears that, by maintaining normal cognitive function, estrogens may also decrease the risk and delay the onset of AD (Henderson et al. 1994; Kawas et al. 1997; Paganini-Hill and Henderson 1994, 1996; Tang et al. 1996). It is important to emphasize that estrogens do not exert actions on all aspects of memory. Memory is a broad term describing several distinct neural functions; therefore, it is not surprising that estrogens may influence specific subtypes of memory. For example, some (Kampen and Sherwin 1998; Robinson et al. 1994; Sherwin 1997) but not all (Shaywitz et al. 1999) studies show that ERT appears to specifically enhance immediate and delayed recall of verbal information.

Several studies have shown that ERT decreases the risk for AD (Kawas et al. 1997) and/or induces a modest improvement in cognitive function in individuals with the disease (Fillit et al. 1986; Henderson et al. 1994, 1996; Honjo et al. 1995). However, other studies have reported no difference in cognitive function between estrogen- and placebo-treated individuals (Barrett-Connor and Kritz-Silverstein 1993; Brenner et al. 2001; Mulnard et al. 2000). A recent study (Mulnard et al. 2000) of Premarin treatment failed to detect slowing of progression of AD or improvement of cognitive and functional outcomes in women with mild to moderate AD. The results of this study and others (Henderson et al. 2000; Marder and Sano 2000; Wang et al. 2000) strongly suggest that estrogens are not an effective treatment when a disease condition has already initiated. Taken together, the findings of these studies indicate that estrogens may protect the brain through primary prevention and not through repair after a neurodegenerative process is ongoing.

Estrogens and Stroke

Our studies on estrogen action against neurodegeneration have focused attention on whether estradiol plays a role in stroke injury. We, and others, have investigated this question since stroke is a major form of neurodegeneration that grossly impacts our aging population, and experimental models have successfully reproduced a stroke-like injury in several animal models.

To date, most clinical studies have assessed whether ERT alters the risk and mortality of stroke (Paganini-Hill 2001) but have not addressed whether estradiol decreases the degree of brain injury resulting from stroke. In contrast, most studies performed in animal models have examined whether estrogens influence the extent of injury after a stroke-like injury. Experimental methods have been developed to mimic stroke in animal models by blocking blood flow to the cerebral vasculature. The results of these studies have clearly established that estradiol decreases the severity of injury in several in vivo models of permanent or transient cerebral ischemia (Dubal et al. 1998; Rusa et al. 1999; Simpkins et al. 1997; Toung et al. 1998; Wang et al. 1999; Zhang et al. 1998). These studies clearly establish that females uniformly endure less stroke injury than males. Hall and colleagues (1991) showed that female gerbils demonstrate less neuronal pathology than males after ischemia induced by unilateral carotid artery occlusion. Similarly, gonadally intact female rats sustain over 50% less infarction than gonadally intact males and ovariectomized female rats following ischemia induced by transient occlusion of the middle carotid artery (MCA) (Alkayed et al. 1998; Zhang et al. 1998). Further, gonadectomized females (Dubal et al. 1998; Rusa et al. 1999; Simpkins et al. 1997; Toung et al. 1998; Yang et al. 2000) and males (Toung et al. 1998) that are treated with estradiol suffer less MCA occlusion-induced injury than estradiol-depleted controls.

Our work has contributed significantly to the understanding of the neuroprotective actions of physiological levels of estradiol. We have focused our attention on using doses of estradiol that circulate in cycling young rats, since we believe that women will be unwilling to take high concentrations of ERT for three decades of their lives due to the fact that such concentrations have been associated with cancer and deep vein thrombosis. We have found that low, physiological concentrations of estradiol replacement are sufficient to exert dramatic protection in the brains of young female rats (Fig. 1) (Dubal et al. 1998). Further, we found that middle-aged female rats remain equally responsive to the neuroprotective effects of low estradiol levels (Dubal and Wise 2001). Collectively, the results of these studies suggest that, if one can extrapolate from rodents to women, postmenopausal women that have estrogen replacement may suffer a decreased degree of brain injury following a stroke, compared to their hypoestrogenic counterparts.

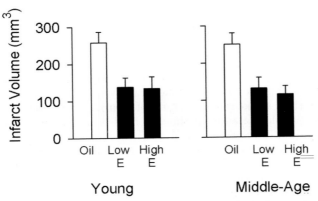

Fig. 1. Estradiol (E) treatment decreases ischemic brain damage in young and middle-aged rats following stroke injury. Pretreatment with low levels of estradiol dramatically decreases the extent of stroke injury, compared with oil-treated controls. Middle-aged rats remain responsive to the protective effects of estradiol (Dubal et al. 1998; Dubal and Wise 2001). Bars represent mean + S.E. of groups of 7-10 rats per experimental group.

We investigated whether estrogen receptor alpha (ERα) and/or ERβ play functional roles in estradiol-mediated protection against stroke injury, and we discovered a novel and unique role for ERα in the brain. Our data revealed that physiological levels of estradiol require this ER subtype to exert protection against cerebral ischemia (Dubal et al. 2001; Wilson et al. 2000). Specifically, we utilized transgenic mice that were knocked out for either ERα or ERβ and found that the classic estrogen receptor, ERα, is the critical mechanistic link in the ability of low levels of estradiol to exert neuroprotection (Fig. 2). We have begun to assess the repertoire of downstream genomic targets of estradiol action through ERs and, to date, have reported that estradiol modulates the expression of several players in ischemic brain injury, including survival factors (Dubal et al. 1999; Fig. 3), immediate early genes (Rau et al. 2001), neuropeptides (Dubal et al. 2000; Fig. 4), and trophic factors (Böttner et al. 2001). We have found that low physiological levels of ERT appear to enhance the expression of several genes that enhance neuronal survival and suppress the expression of those that promote cell death. Furthermore, it appears that ERT may enhance neurogenesis in regions of the brain that give rise to neurons that migrate to the cerebral cortex. ERT may also suppress the proliferation of cells that are involved in the immune response in the peri-infarct region of the brain.

Summary

In summary, clinical and basic science studies have led to a new understanding that estradiol acts far beyond the reproductive axis and exerts multiple actions in the adult and aging brain. We now appreciate that, under some clinical and

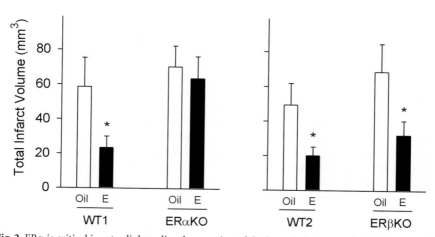

Fig. 2. ERα is critical in estradiol-mediated protection of the brain following stroke injury. Estradiol (E) reduces ischemic infarct in both kinds of wild type (WT) mice, compared to respective oil-treated controls. Estradiol fails to protect in ERαKO mice, compared to oil-treated controls, but continues to protect in ERβKO mice, compared to oil-treated controls (Dubal et al. 2001). Bars represent mean ± S.E. of groups of 6-13 mice per experimental group.

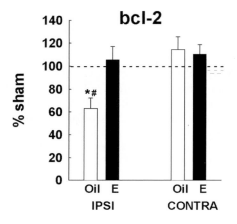

Fig. 3. Estradiol (E) enhances the expression of bcl-2 in rats that underwent middle carotid artery occlusion.
Estradiol treatment prevented the injury-induced down regulation of bcl-2 mRNA levels that occurs close to the site of injury. Data represent mean + S.E.M of groups of between 8 and 12 rats per experimental group. (Modified from Dubal et al. 1999). IPSI, ipsilateral; CONTRA, contralateral.

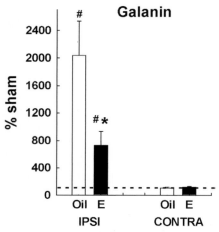

Fig. 4. MCAO injury induces a dramatic increase in galanin gene expression, which is attenuated with pretreatment with estradiol. Stroke-like injury increases galanin mRNA levels over 20-fold. In estradiol-pretreated rats, galanin gene expression increases, but not to the same extent as in ovariectomized, vehicle-treated rats. Bars represent mean ± S.E. of between 8 and 12 rats per experimental group.

experimental conditions, estrogens exert profound protective actions in multiple tissues. Because estrogens may not be protective under some circumstances and may, in fact, lead to increased vulnerability to diseases and injury, it is essential that we understand more thoroughly the cellular and molecular mechanisms of this hormone. A thorough knowledge of estrogen action in the injured brain will ultimately lead to a more complete understanding of the precise mechanisms underlying estradiol-mediated protection. This knowledge is crucial for developing preventative therapies for neurodegenerative conditions and carries great promise in improving the quality of lives in our aging population.

Acknowledgments

This work was supported by the National Institutes of Health: AG02224, AG17164, AG00242, and RR15592.

References

Alkayed NJ, Harukuni I, Kimes AS, London ED, Traystman RJ, Hurn PD (1998) Gender-linked brain injury in experimental stroke. Stroke 29: 159–166

Asthana S, Craft S, Baker LD, Raskind MA, Birnbaum RS, Lofgreen CP, Veith RC, Plymate SR (1999) Cognitive and neuroendocrine response to transdermal estrogen in postmenopausal women with Alzheimer's Disease: results of a placebo-controlled, double-blind, pilot study. Psychoneuroendocrinology 24: 657–677

Barrett-Connor E, Kritz-Silverstein D (1993) Estrogen replacement therapy and cognitive function in older women. JAMA 269: 2637–2641

Birge SJ (1997) The role of estrogen in treatment of Alzheimer's disease. Neurology 48: S36–S41

Böttner M, Dubal DB, Rau SW, Wise PM (2001) Activin gene expression increases after stroke injury: modulation by estradiol. Soc Neurosci 1165 (Abstract)

Brenner DE, Kukull WA, Stergachis A, van Belle G, Bowen JD, McCormick WC, Teri L, Larson EB (1994) Postmenopausal estrogen replacement therapy and the risk of Alzheimer's disease: a population-based case-control study. Am J Epidemiol 140: 262–267

Dubal DB, Wise PM (2001) Neuroprotective effects of estradiol in middle-aged female rats. Endocrinology 142: 43–48

Dubal DB, Kashon ML, Pettigrew LC, Ren JM, Finklestein SP, Rau SW, Wise PM (1998) Estradiol protects against ischemic injury. JCBFM 18: 1253–1258

Dubal DB, Shughrue PJ, Wilson ME, Merchenthaler I, Wise PM (1999) Estradiol modulates Bcl-2 in cerebral ischemia: a potential role for estrogen receptors. J Neurosci 19: 6385–6393

Dubal DB, Wilson ME, Shughrue PJ, Merchenthaler I, Wise PM (2000) Induction of galanin gene expression in estradiol-mediated neuroprotection against cerebral ischemia. Soc Neurosci 1449 (Abstract)

Dubal DB, Zhu B, Yu B, Rau SW, Shughrue PJ, Merchenthaler I, Kindy MS, Wise PM (2001) Estrogen receptor-α, not -β, is a critical link in estradiol-mediated protection against brain injury. Proc Natl Acad Sci USA 98: 1952–1957

Fillit H (1994) Estrogens in the pathogenesis and treatment of Alzheimer's disease in postmenopausal women. Ann NY Acad Sci 743: 233–239

Fillit H, Weinreb H, Cholst I, Luine V, McEwen B, Amador R, Zabriskie J (1986) Observations in a preliminary open trial of estradiol therapy for senile dementia-Alzheimer's type. Psychoneuroendocrinology 11: 337–345

Hall ED, Pazara KE, Linseman KL (1991) Sex differences in postischemic neuronal necrosis in gerbils. JCBFM 11: 292–298

Henderson VW, Paganini-Hill A (1997) Estrogen and Alzheimer's Disease. J Soc Obstet Gynecol Canada 19: 21–28

Henderson VW, Paganini-Hill A, Emanuel CK, Dunn ME, Buckwalter JG (1994) Estrogen replacement therapy in older women. Arch Neurol 51: 896–900

Henderson VW, Watt L, Buckwalter JG (1996) Cognitive skills associated with estrogen replacement in women with Alzheimer's disease. Psychoneuroendocrinology 21: 421–430

Henderson VW, Paganini-Hill A, Miller BL, Elble RJ, Reyes PF, Shoupe D, McCleary CA, Klein RA, Hake AM, Farlow MR (2000) Estrogen for Alzheimer's disease in women.Randomized, double-blind, placebo-controlled trial. Neurology 54: 295–301

Honjo H, Tanaka K, Kashiwagi T, Urabe M, Okada H, Hayashi M, Hayashi K (1995) Senile dementia-Alzheimer's type and estrogen. Horm Metab Res 27: 204–207

Hulley S, Grady D, Bush T, Furberg C, Herrington D, Riggs B, Vittinghoff E (1998) Randomized trial of estrogen plus progestin for secondary prevention of coronary heart disease in postmenopausal women. JAMA 280: 605–613

Kampen DL, Sherwin BB (1998) Estrogen use and verbal memory in healthy postmenopausal women. Obstet Gynecol 83: 979–983

Kawas C, Resnick S, Morrison A, Brookmeyer R, Corrada M, Zonderman A, Bacal C, Lingle D, Metter E (1997) A prospective study of estrogen replacement therapy and the risk of developing Alzheimer's disease: the Baltimore Longitudinal Study of Aging. Neurology 48: 1517–1521

Marder K, Sano M (2000) Estrogen to treat Alzheimer's disease: Too little, too late? So what's a woman to do? Neurology 54: 2035–2037

Mulnard RA, Cotman CW, Kawas C, van Dyck CH, Sano M, Doody R, Koss E, Pfeiffer E, Jin S, Garnst A, Grundman M, Thomas R, Thal LJ (2000) Estrogen replacement therapy for treatment of mild to moderate Alzheimer's disease. JAMA 283:

Paganini-Hill A (2001) Hormone replacement therapy and stroke: risk, protection or no effect? Maturitas 38: 243–261

Paganini-Hill A, Henderson VW (1994) Estrogen deficiency and risk of Alzheimer's disease in women. Amer J Epidemiol 140: 256–261

Paganini-Hill A, Henderson VW (1996) Estrogen replacement therapy and risk of Alzheimer disease. Arch Intern Med 156: 2213–2217

Rau SW, Dubal DB, Wise PM (2001) Immediate early gene regulation by estradiol in ischemic injury. Soc Neurosci p 778 (Abstract)

Robinson D, Friedman L, Marcus R, Tinklenberg J, Yesavage J (1994) Estrogen replacement therapy and memory in older women. J Amer Geriat Soc 42: 919–922

Rusa R, Alkayed NJ, Crain BJ, Traystman RJ, Kimes AS, London ED, Klaus JA, Hurn PD (1999) 17beta-estradiol reduces stroke injury in estrogen-deficient female animals. Stroke 30: 1665–1670

Schmidt R, Fazekas F, Reinhart B, Kapeller P, Fazekas G, Offenbacher H, Eber B, Schumacher M, Freidl W (1996) Estrogen replacement therapy in older women: a neuropsychological and brain MRI study. J Amer Geriat Soc 44: 1307–1313

Shaywitz SE, Shaywitz BA, Pugh KR, Fulbright RK, Skudlarski P, Mencl WE, Canstable RT, Naftolin F, Palter SF, Marchione KE, Katz L, Shankweiler DP, Fletcher JM, Lacadie C, Keltz M, Gore JC (1999) Effect of estrogen on brain activation patterns in postmenopausal women during working memory tasks. JAMA 281: 1197–1202

Sherwin BB (1988) Estrogen and/or androgen replacement therapy and cognitive functioning in surgically menopausal women. Psychoneuroendocrinology 13: 345–357

Sherwin BB (1994) Estrogenic effects on memory in women. Ann NY Acad Sci 743: 213–231

Sherwin BB (1996) Hormones, mood, and cognitive functioning in postmenopausal women. Obstet Gynecol 87: 20S–26S

Sherwin BB (1997) Estrogen effects on cognition in menopausal women. Neurology 48: S21–S26

Sherwin BB, Carlson LE (1997) Estrogen and memory in women. J Soc Obstet Gynecol Canada 19: 7–13

Simpkins JW, Rajakumar G, Zhang Y-Q, Simpkins CE, Greenwald D, Yu CJ, Bodor N, Day AL (1997) Estrogens may reduce mortality and ischemic damage caused by middle cerebral artery occlusion in the female rat. J Neurosurg 87: 724–730

Tang M-X, Jacobs D, Stern Y, Marder K, Schofield P, Gurland B, Andrews H, Mayeux R (1996) Effect of oestrogen during menopause on risk and age at onset of Alzheimer's disease. The Lancet 348: 429–432

Toung TJK, Traystman RJ, Hurn PD (1998) Estrogen-mediated neuroprotection after experimental stroke in male rats. Stroke 29: 1666–1670

Viscoli CM, Brass LM, Kernan WN, Sarrel PM, Suissa S, Horwitz RI (2001) A clinical trial of estrogen-replacement therapy after ischemic stroke. New Engl J Med 345: 1243–1249

Wang PN, Liao SQ, Liu RS, Liu CY, Chao HT, Lu SR, Yu HY, Wang SJ, Liu HC (2000) Effects of estrogen on cognition, mood, and cerebral blood flow in AD. A controlled study. Neurology 54: 2061–2066

Wang Q, Santizo R, Baughman VL, Pelligrino DA, Iadecola C (1999) Estrogen provides neuro-protection in transient forebrain ischemia through perfusion-independent mechanisms in rats. Stroke 30: 630–637

Waring SC, Rocca WA, Petersen RC, O'Brien PC, Tangalos EG, Kokmen E (1999) Postmenopausal estrogen replacement therapy and risk of AD. A population-based study. Neurology 52: 965–970

Wilson ME, Dubal DB, Wise PM (2000) Estradiol protects against injury-induced cell death in cortical explant cultures: a role for estrogen receptors. Brain Res 873: 235–242

Writing Group for the Women's Health Initiative Investigators (2002) Risks and benefits of estrogen plus progestin in healthy postmenopausal women. JAMA 288: 321–333

Yang S-H, Shi J, Day AL, Simpkins JW (2000) Estradiol exerts neuroprotective effects when administered after ischemic insult. Stroke 31: 745–750

Zhang Y-Q, Shi J, Rajakumar G, Day AL, Simpkins JW (1998) Effects of gender and estradiol treatment on focal brain ischemia. Brain Res 784: 321–324

Testosterone Supplementation and Aging-associated Sarcopenia

Shalender Bhasin

Introduction

The use of anabolic agents for the prevention or treatment of sarcopenia associated with aging and chronic illness is based on the premise that these therapies increase muscle mass and that increased muscle mass would be associated with improvements in measures of muscle performance and physical function. We assume that improved physical function in humans with sarcopenia will translate into decreased risk of disability, falls, and fractures and will improve quality of life and other health-related outcomes. The premise that androgen therapy of older men with low testosterone levels can achieve these beneficial effects in health-related outcomes without adverse cardiovascular or prostate effects remains to be critically investigated.

Epidemiology and Health Consequences of Sarcopenia

Sarcopenia, the loss of muscle mass and function, is an important consequence of aging (Baumgartner et al. 1998; Dutta and Hadley 1995; Kohrt et al. 1992; Melton et al. 2000). The prevalence of sarcopenia, defined as appendicular skeletal muscle mass less than two standard deviations below that for healthy young men and women, varies from 10-30% in men over the age of 70 (Baumgartner et al. 1998; Melton et al. 2000) and is as high as 50% in men and women over the age of 80. The principal component of the decrease in fat-free mass is the loss of muscle mass; there is little change in non-muscle lean mass (Borkan et al. 1977, 1983; Cohn et al. 1976; Kohrt et al. 1992; Novak 1972). Between 20 and 80 years of age, the cumulative decline in skeletal muscle mass amounts to 35-40% (Evans 1995; Flegg and Lakatta 1988). The depletion of muscle mass does not result in weight loss because of the corresponding accumulation of body fat (Borkan et al. 1983; Cohn et al. 1976; Kohrt et al. 1992).

The loss of muscle mass results from a decrease in the number as well as cross-sectional area of muscle fibers (Lexell et al. 1983). The number of muscle fibers in the vastus lateralis muscle of older men is 23% lower than in young men (Lexell et al. 1983; Lexell 1995). There is a preferential atrophy of fast-twitch, type II fibers (Lexell 1995), in part because of their reduced reinnervation capacity compared to type I fibers. There is an increase in intramuscular fat and connective tissue (Lexell 1995). These changes reduce the contractile tissue volume available for locomotive and metabolic functions. Aging is associated with decreased synthesis

Chanson et al.
Endocrine Aspects of Successful Aging
© Springer-Verlag Berlin Heidelberg 2004

of skeletal muscle proteins (Proctor et al. 1998), attenuated myosin heavy chain and actin synthesis rates, and decreased generation of the high-energy phosphate (hydrolysis of ATP to ADP) necessary for mechanical energy (Proctor et al. 1998).

The loss of muscle mass that occurs with aging is associated with a reduction in muscle strength (Frontera et al. 1991; Harris 1997; Skelton et al. 1995; Holloszy et al. 1995). There is a substantial decrease in strength and power between 50 and 70 years of age, due primarily to muscle fiber loss and selective atrophy of type II fibers (Frontera et al. 1991; Harris 1997; Skelton et al. 1995). Loss of muscle strength is even greater after the age of 70; in one study, 28% of men over the age of 74 could not lift objects weighing more than 4.5 kg (Skelton et al. 1995). With increasing age, there is a progressive reduction in muscle power (Bassey et al. 1992; Skelton et al. 1995; Metter et al. 1997), the speed of strength generation, and fatigability, i.e., the ability to persist in a task.

Loss of muscle mass and strength leads to impairment of physical function, as indicated by the impaired ability to rise from a chair, climb stairs, generate gait speed, and maintain balance (Bassey et al. 1992; Whipple et al. 1987; Wolfson et al. 1995). Sarcopenia is associated with a 4-fold increased risk of disability, 2-fold increased risk of using a cane or a walker, and 2-3 fold increased likelihood of a balance disorder (Baumgartner et al. 1998; Melton 2000). Decreased muscle mass and muscle strength increase the risk of falls and fractures. Loss of muscle mass and strength is a major cause of frailty, which is associated with increased risk of mortality. Therefore, anabolic interventions such as testosterone that can improve muscle mass physical function would be expected to reduce the risk of disability, falls and fractures.

Changes in Serum Total and Free Testosterone Concentrations in Older Men

There is agreement that serum total, free, and bioavailable testosterone, and DHEA levels are lower in older men than younger men, even after accounting for the potential confounding factors such as time of sampling, concomitant illness and medications, and technical issues related to hormone assays, (Bremner and Prinz 1983; Gray et al. 1991; Harman et al. 1982; Harman and Tsitouras 1980; Harman 2001; Morley et al. 1997; Nankin and Calkins 1986; Nieschlag et al. 1982; Swerdloff and Wang 1993; Tenover et al. 2000; Vermeulen 1991; Zumoff et al. 1982; Zmuda et al. 1997). Several longitudinal studies (Harman 2001; Morley et al. 1997) have confirmed a gradual but progressive decline in serum testosterone concentrations from age 20 to 80. The diurnal rhythm of testosterone secretion is dampened in older men (Bremner and Prinz 1983; Zumoff et al. 1982). Because sex-hormone binding globulin concentrations are higher in older men than younger men (Gray et al. 1991; Pirke and Doerr 1973; Simon et al. 1992), the age-related decline in free and bioavailable testosterone levels is of a greater magnitude than the decline in total testosterone levels. Most of the studies of age-related change in testosterone levels included healthy, older men; it is possible that older men with chronic illness might have an even lower testosterone levels than healthy, older men. The decline in testosterone production in older men is the result of abnormalities at all levels of the hypothalamic-pituitary-testicular axis (Bremner and Prinz 1983; Harman and Tsitouras 1980, 1982; Mulligan et al. 1997; Murono et al. 1982; Tenover et al. 2000): testosterone response to LH is impaired, LH response to GnRH is decreased, and pulsatile GnRH secretion is attenuated. In addition, there are disturbances in the feedback and feed-forward relationships between testosterone and LH secretion (Mulligan et al. 1997; Winters and Atkinson 1997).

Low Testosterone Concentrations are Associated with Decreased Fat-Free Mass and Strength

Healthy, hypogonadal men have lower lean body mass and increased fat mass in comparison to age-matched, eugonadal controls (Katznelson et al. 1996). Induction of androgen deficiency by GnRH agonist treatment in healthy young men is also associated with loss of lean body mass, an increase in fat mass, and a decrease in fractional muscle protein synthesis rates (Mauras et al. 1998). Low bioavailable testosterone concentrations correlate with decreased appendicular skeletal muscle mass and decreased strength of knee extension and flexion in African Americans and Caucasians.

Testosterone Replacement Increases Fat-Free Mass and Maximal Voluntary Strength in Young, Hypogonadal Men

Several studies (Bhasin et al. 1997; Brodsky et al. 1996; Katznelson et al. 1996; Wang et al. 2000; Snyder et al. 2000) have demonstrated that testosterone replacement of young, hypogonadal men increases fat-free mass. Some, but not all, studies have reported a decrease in fat mass during testosterone replacement of androgen-deficient men (Brodsky et al. 1996; Katznelson et al. 1996). Testosterone replacement of hypogonadal men also increases maximal voluntary strength (Bhasin et al. 1997; Wang et al. 2000). In a study by Bhasin et al. (1997), testosterone replacement of young, hypogonadal men was associated with increased muscle strength in the bench press and leg press exercises. Testosterone replacement of young, androgen-deficient men stimulates fractional muscle protein synthesis.

In HIV-infected men with low testosterone levels, testosterone replacement increases fat-free mass (Bhasin et al. 1998), maximal voluntary strength in the leg press, bench press, overhead press, latissimus pull, and leg curls exercises, but the placebo treatment had no significant effect (Bhasin et al. 2000).

Studies of Androgen Supplementation in Older Men

Studies of older men with low normal testosterone levels (Morley et al. 1993; Tenover 1992; Urban et al. 1995; Sih et al. 1997; Snyder et al. 1999; Kenny et al. 2001) have generally shown that testosterone treatment increases fat-free mass and decreases fat mass. However, we do not know whether testosterone treatment improves muscle performance, balance, and physical function. In a recent study by Snyder et al. (1999), testosterone treatment of older men did not increase muscle strength or improve physical performance, but these men were not uniformly hypogonadal and were unusually fit for their age. In addition, their muscle strength was measured by a method (Biodex dynamometer) that did not demonstrate a response even in frankly hypogonadal younger men treated with testosterone (Snyder et al. 2000). Biodex dynamometer measures isometric strength in a range of motion that does not mimic natural movements in activities of daily life. Indeed, more recent studies of androgen supplementation in older men have demonstrated significant improvements in maximal voluntary strength (Schroeder et al. 2003; Ferrando et al. 2002) using the one-repetition maximum method.

It has been hypothesized that testosterone-induced improvements in lean body mass and physical function would improve health-related quality of life; however, this hypothesis has not been tested. Lean body mass is an important determinant of quality of life in HIV-infected individuals (Wilson et al. 1999). Testosterone administration has been shown to improve lean body mass (Bhasin et al. 2000; Grinspoon et al. 1998) and some domains of quality of life in HIV-infected men (Grinspoon et al. 2000). Aging-associated impairment of physical function is a significant contributor to the age-related decrease quality of life (Wilson et al. 2000). A recent study by Bakhshi et al. (2000) demonstrated an improvement in rehabilitation outcomes, including functional independence score and grip strength, in older men treated with testosterone.

Why Have Previous Studies of Testosterone Supplementation in Older Men Failed to Demonstrate Significant Improvements in Physical Function?

Although testosterone replacement of androgen-deficient men increases fat-free mass and maximal voluntary strength, we do not know if testosterone improves physical function. Many previous studies of testosterone replacement in older men did not examine changes in physical function (Bross et al. 1998). The few studies that did examine this issue suffered from methodological problems in the measurements of physical function. We believe a major reason for the failure to demonstrate improvements in physical function is that the measures of physical function used in previous studies were relatively insensitive and "threshold-dependent". The widely used measures, such as 0.625 m stair climb, standing up from a chair, and 20-meter walk, are tasks that require only a small fraction of an individual's maximal voluntary strength. In most healthy older men, the baseline maximal voluntary strength is far higher than the threshold below which these measures would detect impairment. Given the low intensity of the tasks used, these relatively healthy older individuals showed neither impairment in these threshold-dependent measures of physical function at baseline nor an improvement in performance on these tasks during testosterone administration. Because testosterone improves maximal voluntary leg strength, we posit that it would improve measures of physical function that are threshold-independent and require near-maximal strength of critical muscle groups such as the quadriceps. Examples of tests of physical function that allow the subject to make near-maximal effort include the Margaria power test and load carry test. Another confounder of the effects of anabolic interventions on muscle function is the learning effect. For instance, subjects who are unfamiliar with weight-lifting exercises often demonstrate improvements in measures of muscle performance simply because of increased familiarity with the exercise equipment and technique. Therefore, in efficacy trials of anabolic interventions, it is important to incorporate strategies to minimize the confounding influence of the learning effect. Because of the considerable test-to-test variability in tests of physical function, it is possible that previous studies (Snyder et al. 1999; Tenover 2000) did not have adequate power to detect meaningful differences in measures of physical function between the placebo and testosterone-treated groups. Furthermore, previous studies of testosterone replacement included men who had low normal testosterone levels at baseline and used relatively low doses of testosterone; consequently, the increments in serum testosterone concentrations during treatment were modest, resulting in relatively small changes in muscle mass.

In a recent proof-of-concept study (Schroeder et al. 2003), we determined the effects of oxymetholone on body composition and muscle strength in older men, 65-80 years old, who were randomized to placebo (Group 1), 50 mg (Group 2) or 100 mg (Group 3) daily for 12 weeks. Total LBM increased by 3.3 ± 1.2 and 4.2 ± 2.4 kg and upper extremity LBM increased by 0.7 ± 0.4 and 0.7 ± 0.2 kg in Groups 2 and 3, respectively, compared to placebo ($p<0.02$). Total (-2.6 ± 1.2 and -2.5 ± 1.6 kg) and trunk (-1.7 ± 1.0 and -2.2 ± 0.9 kg) fat decreased in Groups 2 and 3, respectively ($p<0.02$). Relative increases in 1-repetition maximum (1-RM) strength for seated biaxial chest press of $8.2 \pm 9.2\%$ and $13.9 \pm 8.1\%$ in Groups 2 and 3 were both significantly greater than those in placebo group ($p<0.03$). For lat pull-down, 1-RM changed by $-0.6 \pm 8.3\%$, $8.8 \pm 15.1\%$ and 18.4 ± 21.0 ($p=0.049$). Repeated measures ANOVA of LBM and upper body strength suggested that changes were related to dose. ALT increased by 72 ± 67 U/dL in Group 3 ($p<0.001$) and HDL cholesterol decreased by -19 ± 9 and -23 ± 18 mg/dL in Groups 2 and 3, respectively ($p=0.04$ and $p=0.008$). Thus, when proper androgen-responsive measures of muscle performance are used, and confounding variable are controlled, androgens can be shown to improve maximal voluntary muscle strength in older men.

Testosterone Dose-Response Relationships

Testosterone supplementation increases muscle mass and strength (Bhasin et al. 1996; Bhasin et al. 1997; Griggs et al. 1999a and 1999b; Young et al. 1993) and regulates other physiologic processes, but we do not know whether testosterone effects are dose-dependent and whether dose requirements for maintaining various androgen-dependent processes are similar (Bhasin et al. 2000; Bhasin et al. 2001a). Androgen receptors in most tissues are either saturated or down-regulated at physiologic testosterone concentrations (Antonio et al. 1999;

Dahlberg 1981; Rance and Max 1984); Wilson 1988), leading to speculation that there might be two separate dose-response curves: one in hypogonadal range, with maximal response at low normal testosterone concentrations, and a second in supraphysiologic range, representing a separate mechanism of action (Wilson 1988; Bhasin et al. 2000). However, testosterone dose-response relationships for a range of androgen-dependent functions in humans have not been studied.

To determine the effects of graded doses of testosterone on body composition, muscle size, strength, power, sexual and cognitive functions, PSA, plasma lipids, hemoglobin, and IGF-1 levels, 61 eugonadal men, 18-35 years of age, were randomized to one of five groups to receive monthly injections of a long-acting GnRH agonist to suppress endogenous testosterone secretion and weekly injections of 25, 50, 125, 300 or 600 mg testosterone enanthate for 20 weeks (Bhasin et al. 2001a; Singh et al. 2002; Storer et al. 2003). Energy and protein intake were standardized. The administration of gonadotropin-releasing hormone (GnRH) agonist plus graded doses of testosterone resulted in mean nadir testosterone concentrations of 253, 306, 542, 1345, and 2370 ng/dL at 25, 50, 125, 300, and 600 mg doses, respectively. Fat-free mass increased dose-dependently in men receiving 125, 300 or 600 mg of testosterone weekly (change +3.4, 5.2, and 7.9 kg, respectively). The changes in fat-free mass were highly dependent on testosterone dose (Fig. 1, P = 0.0001) and correlated with log testosterone concentrations (R=0.73, P=0.0001). Changes in leg press strength, leg power, thigh and quadriceps muscle volumes, hemoglobin, and IGF-1 were positively correlated with testosterone concentrations, whereas changes in fat mass and plasma HDL cholesterol were correlated negatively. Sexual function, visual-spatial cognition, mood, and PSA levels did not change significantly at any dose. These data demonstrate that changes in circulating testosterone concentrations, induced by GnRH agonist and testosterone administration, are associated with testosterone dose- and concentration-dependent changes in fat-free mass, muscle size, strength and power, fat mass, hemoglobin, HDL cholesterol, and IGF-1 levels, in conformity with a single linear dose-response relationship. However, different androgen-dependent processes have different testosterone dose-response relationships.

Mechanisms of Testosterone's Anabolic Effects on the Muscle

The prevalent view that testosterone produces muscle hypertrophy by increasing fractional muscle protein synthesis (Urban et al. 1995; Brodsky et al. 1996) is supported by a number of studies. However, as discussed below, recent observations suggest that the increase in muscle protein synthesis probably occurs as a secondary event and may not be the sole or the primary mechanism by which testosterone induces muscle hypertrophy (Sinha-Hikim et al. 2002).

To determine whether testosterone-induced increase in muscle size is due to muscle fiber hypertrophy or hyperplasia, muscle biopsies were obtained from *vastus lateralis* in 39 men before and after 20 weeks of combined treatment with GnRH agonist and weekly injections of 25, 50, 125, 300 or 600 mg of testosterone enanthate (Sinha-Hikim et al. 2002). Graded doses of testosterone administration

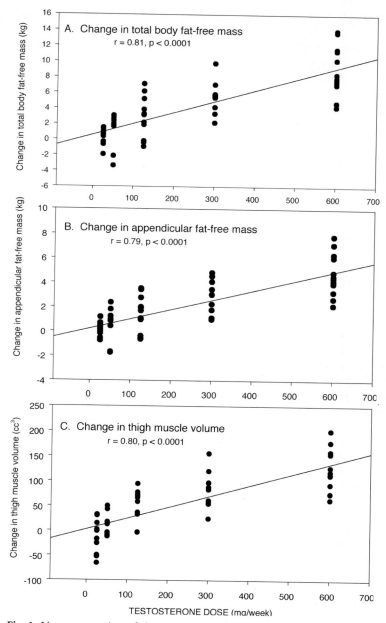

Fig. 1. Linear regression of the testosterone enanthate (TE) dose and change in: total body fatfree mass (panel A), appendicular fat-free mass (panel B) and thigh muscle volume (panel C) demonstrate the heterogeneity of individual responses, within each TE dose, despite strong and significant correlations overall (Pearson product-moment correlation coefficients of r = 0.79 to 0.81, p<0.0001 for each model).

were associated with testosterone dose and concentration-dependent increase in muscle fiber cross-sectional area (Sinha-Hikim et al. 2002). Changes in cross-sectional areas of both type I and II fibers were dependent on testosterone dose and significantly correlated with total (r = 0.35, and 0.44, P <0.0001 for type I and II fibers, respectively) and free (r=0.34 and 0.35, P <0.005) testosterone concentrations during treatment. The men receiving 300 and 600 mg of testosterone enanthate weekly experienced significant increases from baseline in areas of type I (baseline vs. 20 weeks, 3176 ± 163 vs. 4201 ± 163 μm^2, P<0.05 at the 300-mg dose, and 3347 ± 253 vs. 4984 ± 374 μm 2, P = 0.006 at the 600-mg dose) muscle fibers; the men in the 600-mg group also had significant increments in cross-sectional area of type II (4060 ± 401 vs. 5526 ± 544 μm^2, P = 0.03) fibers. The relative proportions of type I and type II fibers did not change significantly after treatment in any group. The myonuclear number per fiber increased significantly in men receiving the 300- and 600-mg doses of testosterone enanthate and was significantly correlated with testosterone concentration and muscle fiber cross-sectional area (Sinha-Hikim et al. 2002). These data demonstrate that increases in muscle volume in healthy eugonadal men treated with graded doses of testosterone are associated with concentration-dependent increases in muscle fiber cross-sectional area and myonulcear number, but not muscle fiber number. We conclude that the testosterone-induced increase in muscle volume is due to muscle fiber hypertrophy. In our study, the myonuclear number increased in direct relation to the increase in muscle fiber diameter. Therefore, it is possible that muscle fiber hypertrophy and increase in myonuclear number were preceded by a testosterone-induced increase in satellite cell number and their fusion with muscle fibers. The mechanisms by which testosterone might increase satellite cell number are not known. An increase in satellite cell number could occur by an increase in satellite cell replication, inhibition of satellite cell apoptosis, and/or increased differentiation of stem cells into the myogenic lineage. We do not know which of these processes is the site of regulation by testosterone. The hypothesis that testosterone promotes muscle fiber hypertrophy by increasing the number of satellite cells should be further tested. Because of the constraints inherent in obtaining multiple biopsy specimens in humans, the effects of testosterone on satellite cell replication and stem cell recruitment would be more conveniently studied in an animal model.

The molecular mechanisms, which mediate androgen-induced muscle hypertrophy, are not well understood. Urban et al. (1995) have proposed that testosterone stimulates the expression of insulin-like growth factor-I (IGF-I) and down-regulates insulin-like growth factor binding protein-4 (IGFBP-4) in the muscle. Reciprocal changes in IGF-1 and its binding protein thus provide a potential mechanism for amplifying the anabolic signal.

It is not clear whether the anabolic effects of supraphysiologic doses of testosterone are mediated through an androgen receptor-mediated mechanism. In vitro binding studies (Saartok et al. 1984) suggest that the maximum effects of testosterone should be manifest at about 300 ng/dL, i.e., serum testosterone levels that are at the lower end of the normal male range. Therefore, it is possible that the supraphysiologic doses of androgen produce muscle hypertrophy through androgen – receptor-independent mechanisms, such as through an anti-glucocorticoid effect (Konagaya and Max 1986). We cannot exclude the possibility that some androgen effects may be mediated through non-classical binding sites. Testosterone effects on the muscle are modulated by a number of other factors, such as the genetic background, growth hormone secretory status (Fryburg et al. 1997), nutrition, exercise, cytokines, thyroid hormones, and glucocorticoids. Testosterone may also affect muscle function by its effects on neuromuscular transmission (Leslie et al. 1991; Blanco et al. 1997).

The Role of 5-alpha Reduction and Aromatization of Testosterone in the Muscle

Although the enzyme 5-alpha-reductase is expressed at low concentrations within the muscle (Bartsch et al. 1980), we do not know whether conversion of testosterone to dihydrotestosterone is required for mediating the androgen effects on the muscle. Men with benign prostatic hypertrophy who are treated with the 5-alpha reductase inhibitor do not experience muscle loss. Similarly, individuals with congenital 5-alpha-reductase deficiency have normal muscle development at puberty. These data suggest that 5-alpha reduction of testosterone is not obligatory for mediating its effects on the muscle.

Studies of aromatase knockout mice have revealed higher fat mass and lower muscle mass in mice that are null for the P450-linked CYP aromatase gene. Data from these gene-targeting experiments suggest that aromatization of testosterone might also be important in mediating androgen effects on the muscle.

Testosterone Effects on Fat Metabolism

Percent body fat is higher in hypogonadal men in comparison to eugonadal controls (Katznelson et al. 1998). Induction of androgen deficiency in healthy men by administration of a GnRH agonist leads to an increase in fat mass (Mauras et al. 1998). Some studies of young, hypogonadal men have reported a decrease in fat mass with testosterone replacement therapy (Katznelson et al. 1996; Brodsky et al. 1996) whereas others (Bhasin et al. 1997; Wang et al. 1996; Snyder et al. 2000) found no change. In contrast, long-term studies of testosterone supplementation of older men have consistently demonstrated a decrease in fat mass (Snyder et al. 1999). Epidemiologic studies (Seidell et al. 1990; Barrett-Connor and Khaw 1988) have shown that serum testosterone levels are lower in middle-aged men with visceral obesity. Serum testosterone levels correlate inversely with visceral fat area and directly with plasma HDL levels. Testosterone replacement of middle-aged men with visceral obesity improves insulin sensitivity and decreases blood glucose and blood pressure (Marin et al. 1992, 1995). In our dose-response studies, administration of graded doses of testosterone to men was associated with a dose-dependent decrease in fat mass (Bhasin et al. 2001a). Loss of fat mass at higher doses was evenly distributed in the trunk and appendices and in the superficial and deep compartments. Thus, there was a decrease in intra-abdominal fat as well as intermuscular fat in association with the high doses of testosterone. Testosterone is an important determinant of regional fat distribution and metabolism in men (Marin et al. 1995).

Potential Concerns About Testosterone Supplementation in Older Men

While short-term testosterone administration is relatively safe in young, androgen-deficient men, the risks of long-term testosterone supplementation in older men remain largely unknown. The risks of testosterone administration include erythrocytosis, induction or exacerbation of sleep apnea, and breast tenderness or enlargement (Rolf and Nieschlag 1998). However, the two major areas of concern are the effects of long-term testosterone administration on prostate cancer and on progression of atherosclerotic heart disease. There is agreement that testosterone does not cause prostate cancer. Also, there is no consistent relationship between endogenous serum testosterone levels and the risk of prostate cancer. However, there are a number of areas of concern. Prostate cancer is a common, androgen–dependent tumor, and androgen administration may promote tumor growth. Testosterone administration is absolutely contraindicated in men with a history of prostate cancer. Many older men have microscopic foci of cancer in their prostates. We do not know whether testosterone administration will make these subclinical foci of cancer grow and become clinically overt. In addition, older men with prostate cancer may have low testosterone levels. Morgentaler and colleagues (Hoffman et al. 2000; Morgentaler et al. 1996) reported a high prevalence of biopsy-detectable prostate cancer in men with low total or free testosterone levels despite normal PSA levels and results of digital rectal examination. However, this study did not have a control group, and we do not know whether sextant biopsies of age-matched controls with normal testosterone levels would yield a similarly high incidence of biopsy-detectable cancer. Serum PSA levels are lower in testosterone–deficient men and are restored to normal following testosterone replacement (Behre et al. 1994; Cooper et al.1998; Meikle et al. 1997; Sasagawa et al. 1989; Svetec et al. 1997). However, serum PSA levels do not increase progressively in healthy hypogonadal men with replacement doses of testosterone. In two placebo-controlled trials of testosterone administration in older men, the change in serum PSA levels over three years was not significantly different between placebo – and testosterone – treated men (Snyder et al. 1999; Tenover 2000). The increase in PSA levels during testosterone replacement might trigger evaluation and biopsy in some patients. More intensive PSA screening and follow-up of men receiving testosterone replacement might lead to an increased number of prostate biopsies and detection of subclinical prostate cancers that would have otherwise remained undetected. Serum PSA levels tend to fluctuate when measured repeatedly in the same individual over time. Therefore, when serum PSA levels in androgen-deficient men on testosterone replacement therapy show a change from a previously measured value, the clinician has to decide whether the change warrants detailed evaluation of the patient for prostate cancer, or whether it is simply due to test–to–test variability in PSA measurement. Adequately powered, long-term, placebo-controlled studies are needed to determine the risks and clinical benefits of testosterone replacement in older men with low testosterone levels.

References

Bakhshi V, Elliott M, Gentili A, Godschalk M, Mulligan T (2000) Testosterone improves rehabilitation outcomes in ill older men. J Am Geriatr Soc 48: 550–553

Bardin CW (1996) The anabolic action of testosterone. New Engl J Med 335: 52–53

Barrett-Connors E, Khaw K-T (1988) Endogenous sex hormones and cardiovascular disease in men. A prospective population-based study. Circulation 78: 539–545

Bartsch W, Krieg M, Voigt KD (1980) Quantitation of endogenous testosterone, 5-alpha-dihydrotestosterone and 5-alpha-androstane-3-alpha, 17-beta-diol in subcellular fractions of the prostate, bulbocavernosus/levator ani muscle, skeletal muscle, and heart muscle of the rat. J Steroid Biochem 13: 259–267

Bassey EJ, Fiatarone MA, O'Neill EF, Kelly M, Evans WJ (1992) Leg extensor power and functional performance in very old men and women. Clin Sci 82: 321–327

Baumgartner RN, Koehler KM, Gallagher D, Romero L, Heymsfield SB, Ross RR, Garry PJ, Lindeman RD (1998) Epidemiology of sarcopenia among the elderly in New Mexico [published erratum appears in Am J Epidemiol (1999) 149:1161]. Am J Epidemiol 147: 755–763

Behre HM, Bohmeyer J, Nieschlag E (1994) Prostate volume in testosterone-treated and untreated hypogonadal men in comparison to age-matched normal controls. Clin Endocrinol 40:341–349

Bhasin S, Storer TW, Berman N, Callegari C, Clevenger BA, Phillips J, Bunnell T, Tricker R, Shirazi A, Casaburi R (1996) The effects of supraphysiologic doses of testosterone on muscle size and strength in men. New Eng J Med 335: 1–7

Bhasin S, Storer TW, Berman N, Yarasheski K, Phillips J, Clevenger B, Lee WP, Casaburi R (1997) A replacement dose of testosterone increases fat-free mass and muscle size in hypogonadal men. J Clin Endocrinol Metab 82: 407–413

Bhasin S, Storer TW, Asbel-Sethi N, Kilbourne A, Hays R, Sinha-Hikim I, Shen R, Arver S, Beall G (1998) Effects of testosterone replacement with a non-genital, transdermal system, Androderm, in human immunodeficiency virus-infected men with low testosterone levels. J Clin Endocrinol Metab 83: 3155–3162

Bhasin S, Storer TW, Javanbakht M, Berman N, Yarasheski KE, Phillips J, Dike M, Sinha-Hikim I, Shen R, Hays RD, Beall G (2000) Effects of testosterone replacement and resistance exercise on muscle strength, and body composition in human immunodeficiency virus-infected men with weight loss and low testosterone levels. JAMA 283: 763–770

Bhasin S, Woodhouse L, Casaburi R, Singh AB, Bhasin D, Berman N, Chen X, Yarasheski KE, Magliano L, Dzekov C, Dzekov J, Bross R, Phillips J, Sinha-Hikim I, Shen R, Storer TW (2001a) Testosterone dose-response relationships in healthy young men. Am J Physiol Endocrinol Metab. 281: 1172–1181

Bhasin S, Woodhouse L, Storer TW (2001b) Proof of the effect of testosterone on skeletal muscle. J Endocrinol. 170: 27–38

Blanco CE, Popper P, Micevych P (1997) Anabolic-androgenic steroid induced alterations in choline acetyltransferase messenger RNA levels of spinal cord motoneurons in the male rat. Neuroscience 78: 973–982

Borkan GA, Norris AH (1977) Fat redistribution and the changing body dimensions of the adult male. Hum Biol 49: 495–513

Morley JE, Perry HMd, Kaiser FE, Kraenzle D, Jensen J, Houston K, Mattammal M, Perry HM Jr (1993) Effects of testosterone replacement therapy in old hypogonadal males: a preliminary study. J Am Geriatr Soc 41: 149–152

Morley JE, Kaiser F, Raum WJ, Perry HM 3rd, Flood JF, Jensen J, Silver AJ, Roberts E (1997) Potentially predictive and manipulable blood serum correlates of aging in the healthy human male: progressive decreases in bioavailable testosterone, dehydroepiandrosterone sulfate, and the ratio of insulin-like growth factor 1 to growth hormone. Proc Natl Acad Sci 94: 7537–7542

Mulligan T, Iranmanesh A, Johnson ML, Straume M, Veldhuis JD (1997)Aging alters feed-forward and feedback linkages between LH and testosterone in healthy men. Am J Physiol 273: 1407–1413

Murono EP, Nankin HR, Lin T, Osterman J (1982) The aging Leydig cell: VI. Response of testosterone precursors to gonadotropin in men. Acta Endocrinol 100:455–461

Nankin HR, Calkins JH (1986) Decreased bioavailable testosterone in aging normal and impotent men. J Clin Endocrinol Metab 63: 1418–1420

Nieschlag E, Lammer U, Freischem CW, Langer K, Wickings EJ (1982) Reproductive function in young fathers and grandfathers. J Clin Endocrinol Metab 51: 675–681

Novak LP (1972) Aging, total body potassium, fat free-mass, and cell mass in males and females between ages 18–85 years. J Gerontol 27: 438–443

Pirke KM, Doerr P (1973) Age related changes and interrelationships between plasma testosterone, oestradiol and testosterone-binding globulin in normal adult males. Acta Endocrinol 74: 792–800

Proctor DN, Balagopal P, Nair KS (1998) Age-related sarcopenia in humans is associated with reduced synthetic rates of specific muscle proteins. J Nutrit 128: 351S–355S

Rance NE, Max SR (1984) Modulation of the cytosolic androgen receptor in striated muscle by sex steroids. Endocrinology. 115: 862–866

Rolf C, Nieschlag E(1998) Potential adverse effects of long-term testosterone therapy. Baillieres Clin Endocrinol Metab. 12: 521–534

Saartok T, Dahlberg E, Gustaffsson JA (1984) Relative binding affinity of anabolic-androgenic steroids, comparison of the binding to the androgen receptors in skeletal muscle and in prostate as well as sex hormone binding globulin. Endocrinology 114: 2100–2107

Sasagawa I, Nakada T, Kazama T, Terada T, Katayama T (1989) Testosterone replacement therapy and prostate/seminal vesicle volume in Klinefelter's syndrome. Arch Androl. 22: 245–249

Schroeder ET, Singh A, Bhasin S, Storer TW, Azen C, Davidson T, Martinez C, Sinha-Hikim I, Jaque SV, Terk M, Sattler FR (2003) Effects of an oral androgen on muscle and metabolism in older, community-dwelling men. Am J Physiol Endocrinol Metab. 284: 120–128

Seidell J, Bjorntorp P, Sjostrom L, Kvist H, Sannerstedt R (1990) Visceral fat accumulation in men is positively associated with insulin, glucose and C-peptide levels, but negatively with testosterone levels. Metabolism 39: 897–901

Sheffield-Moore M, Urban RJ, Wolf SE, Ferrando AA (1999) Short-term oxandrolone administration stimulates net muscle protein synthesis in young men. J Clin Endocrinol Metab 84: 2705–2711

Sih R, Morley JE, Kaiser FE, Perry HM 3rd, Patrick P, Ross C (1997) Testosterone replacement in older hypogonadal men: a 12-month randomized controlled trial (see comments). J ClinEndocrino Metab 82: 1661–1667

Simon D, Preziosi P, Barrett-Connor E, Roger M, Saint-Paul M, Nahoul K, Papoz L (1992) The influence of aging on plasma sex hormones in men: the Telecom Study. Am J Epidemiol 135: 783–791

Singh AB, Hsia S, Alaupovic P, Sinha-Hikim I, Woodhouse L, Buchanan TA, Shen R, Bross R, Berman N, Bhasin S (2002) The effects of varying doses of T on insulin sensitivity, plasma lipids, apolipoproteins, and C-reactive protein in healthy young men. J Clin Endocrinol Metab 87:136–143

Sinha-HiKim I, Artaza J, Woodhouse L, Gonzalez-Cadavid N, Singh AB, Storer TW, Bhasin S (2002). Testosterone-induced increase in muscle size in healthy young men is associated with muscle fiber hypertrophy. Am J Physiol (Endocrinol Metab) 283: 154–164

Skelton DA, Greig CA, Davies JM, Young A (1995) Strength, power, and related functional ability of healthy people aged 65–89 years. Age Aging 23: 371–377

Snyder PJ, Peachey H, Hannoush P, Berlin JA, Loh L, Lenrow DA, Holmes JH, Dlewati A, Santanna J, Rosen CJ, Strom BL (1999) Effect of testosterone treatment on body composition and muscle strength in men over 65. J Clin Endocrinol Metab 84: 2647

Snyder PJ, Peachey H, Berlin JA, Hannoush P, Haddad G, Dlewati A, Santanna J, Loh, L, Lenrow DA, Holmes JH, Kapoor SC, Atkinson LE, Strom BL (2000) Effects of testosterone replacement in hypogonadal men. J Clin Endocrinol Metab 85: 2670–2677

Storer TW, Magliano L, Woodhouse L, Casaburi R, Bhasin S (2003) Testosterone dose-dependently increases muscle strength and leg power, but not specific tension in healthy, young men. J Clin Endocrinol Metab, 88: 1478–1485

Svetec DA, Canby ED, Thompson IM, Sabanegh ES Jr (1997) The effect of parenteral testosterone replacement on prostate specific antigen in hypogonadal men with erectile dysfunction. J Urol. 158: 1775–1777

Swerdloff RS, Wang C (1993) Androgen deficiency and aging in men [see comments]. West J Med 159: 579–585

Tenover JS (1992) Effects of testosterone supplementation in the aging male. J Clin Endocrinol Metab 75: 1092–1098

Tenover JL (2000) Experience with testosterone replacement in the elderly. Mayo Clin Proc 75 Suppl: S77–81; discussion S82

Urban RJ, Bodenburg YH, Gilkison C, Foxworth J, Coggan AR, Wolfe RR, Ferrando A (1995) Testosterone administration to elderly men increases skeletal muscle strength and protein synthesis. Am J Physiol: E820–E826

Vermeulen A (1991) Clinical review 24: Androgens in the aging male. J Clin Endocrinol Metab 73: 221–224

Wang C, Eyre DR, Clark R, Kleinberg D, Newman C, Iranmanesh A, Veldhuis J, Dudley RE, Berman N, Davidson T, Barstow TJ, Sinow R, Alexander G, Swerdloff RS (1996) Sublingual testosterone replacement improves muscle mass and strength, decreases bone resorption, and increases bone resorption markers in hypogonadal men – a Clinical Research Center Study. J Clin Endocrinol Metab 81: 3654–3662

Wang C, Swerdloff RS, Iranmanesh A., Dobs A, Snyder PJ, Cunningham G, Matsumoto AM, Weber T, Berman N (2000) Transdermal testosterone gel improves sexual function, mood, muscle strength, and body composition parameters in hypogonadal men. Testosterone Gel Study Group. J Clin Endocrinol Metab 85: 2839–2853

Wilson JD (1988) Androgen abuse by athletes. Endocrinol Rev 9: 181–199

Wilson IB, Roubenoff R, Knox TA, Spiegleman D, Gorbach SL (2000) Relation of lean body mass to health-related quality of life in persons with HIV. J Acquir Immune Defic Syndrome 24: 137–146

Winters SJ, Atkinson L (1997) Serum LH concentrations in hypogonadal men during transdermal testosterone replacement through scrotal skin: further evidence that ageing enhances testosterone negative feedback. The Testoderm Study Group. Clin Endocrinol 47: 317–322

Wolfson L, Judge J, Whipple R, King M (1995) Strength is a major factor in balance, gait, and the occurrence of falls. J Gerontol 50: 64–67

Young NR, Baker HWG, Liu G, Seeman E (1993) Body composition and muscle strength in healthy men receiving testosterone enanthate for contraception. J Clin Endocrinol Metab 77: 1028–1032

Zmuda JM, Cauley JA, Kriska A, Glynn NW, Gutai JP, Kuller LH (1997) Longitudinal relation between endogenous testosterone and cardiovascular disease risk factors in middle-aged men. A 13-year follow-up of former Multiple Risk Factor Intervention Trial participants. Am J Epidemiol. 146: 609–617

Zumoff B, Strain GW, Kream J, O'Connor J, Rosenfeld RS, Levin J, Fukushima DK (1982) Age variation of the 24-hour mean plasma concentrations of androgens, estrogens, and gonadotropins in normal adult men. J Clin Endocrinol Metab. 54: 534–538

The Long Thread of GFAP in Aging, Steroids, and Synaptic Plasticity

Caleb E. Finch, Todd E. Morgan, Irina Rozovsky, and *Min Wei*

Summary

Glial fibrillary acidic protein (GFAP), an intermediate filament of astrocytes, shows progressive increases per cell during normal aging in the absence of neurodegenerative diseases. Increased transcription mediates the increase of GFAP expression. We hypothesize that increased GFAP expression is a factor in age-related impairments of synaptic plasticity, and we are developing an in vitro model to test this hypothesis.

Introduction

In the 1998 IPSEN Foundation Symposium, «Neuro-Immune Interactions in Neurologic and Psychiatric Disorders,» we developed the concept that glial hyperactivity in Alzheimer's disease is an intensification of a general neuroinflammatory process of aging (Finch et al. 2000). Here, we examine the basis for glial hyperactivity during aging, with a focus on astrocytes and their increased expression of GFAP. The emerging evidence suggests that increased GFAP expression during normal aging is a consequence of oxidative stress and is an upstream factor in impaired synaptogenesis. GFAP expression may be linked to neuronal growth through the secretion of extracellular trophic and matrix factors.

The age-related increases of glial activities present major puzzles. In general, brain glial activation is associated with damage, such as primary neurodegeneration, blood-brain barrier disruption, or autoreactive lymphocytes (see reviews in Patterson et al. 2000; de Vellis 2002; Streit 2002). However, much evidence shows that the activation of astrocytes (astrocytic fibrosis) occurs spontaneously during aging.

Astrocytic Fibrosis during Normal Aging

This story may be traced 25 years ago to the discovery of astrocytic changes during normal aging in the rodent hippocampus and hypothalamus. Astrocytic hypertrophy (fibrous astrocytosis) was found in the rat hippocampus (by Landfield, Lynch et al., at UC Irvine, and by Geinisman, Bondareff et al., at Northwestern University), and in the hypothalamus (by Brawer, Naftolin, Schipper

Chanson et al.
Endocrine Aspects of Successful Aging
© Springer-Verlag Berlin Heidelberg 2004

et al., at McGill University). In the rat hippocampus, several-fold increases in astrocytic fibrosis were detected by metal stains for cytoskeletal elements (Geinisman et al. 1978; Landfield et al. 1977, 1981a,b; Landfield 1978). These major astrocytic changes appeared to be cell hypertrophy rather than hyperplasia, because no age changes were detected in astrocyte cell density (Lindsey et al. 1979). Using a histochemical indicator of phagocytic activity (astrocyte inclusion bodies), Brawer et al. (1978) noted that astrocytes in the hypothalamic arcuate nucleus of middle-aged rodents showed modest activation.

The outer molecular layer of the dentate gyrus shows prominent astrocytic changes that are germane to Alzheimer's disease (AD) as an age-related disease. In AD, the outer molecular layer shows extensive synaptic loss because of the death of projecting perforant path neurons from the entorhinal cortex. Although there is no evidence for neuron loss during normal aging in the perforant path neurons or in their hippocampal targets (Rasmussen et al.1996), there is modest loss of hippocampal synapses during aging (Geinisman et al. 1977, 1995).

These findings were extended as specific immunoreagents became available to identify the particular cytoskeletal elements involved. The fibrous characteristic of activated astrocytes was attributed to the intermediate filament, glial fibrillary acidic protein (GFAP; Eng et al. 2000; Bjorklund et al. 1985), the «long-thread» in this article's title. GFAP-positive astrocytes in rats showed major increases in cell size during postnatal maturation followed by slower increases in cell size continuing through old age (Bjorklund et al.1985). Similarly, in normal human cerebral cortex, the numbers of GFAP-immunopositive fibrous astrocytes increased linearly with age up to 100 years in brains without clinical or pathological evidence of dementia (Hansen et al.1987). Figure 1 also shows the increased size of GFAP-immunostained astrocytes from cerebral cortex in vivo and after primary culture (Rozovsky, Morgan, and Finch, unpublished). The hypothalamic astrocyte inclusion bodies contain peroxidase activity and redox-active iron and may be derived from degenerating mitochondria (Schipper 1996). GFAP expression also increases during aging in the arcuate nucleus (Anderson et al. 2002), but its relationship to the inclusion bodies is not known.

Steroidal Regulation of Astrocytic Aging

A remarkable aspect of these astrocytic aging changes is their modulation by steroid hormones. In the hippocampus of aging rats, individual brain differences in astrocytic hypertrophy were correlated with blood corticosterone. The importance of corticosterone as a primary variable was further demonstrated by two physiological manipulations of the astrocytic changes: long-term adrenalectomy (adrenalectomy of young adults allowed to age with low corticosteroid) attenuated the astrocytic hypertrophy in aging rats, whereas chronic corticosterone accelerated astrocytic hypertrophy (Landfield et al. 1978; reviewed in Finch and Landfield 1985).

In the hypothalamus of female mice and rats, age-like astrocytic changes were induced by intense exposure of young male or female rats to estradiol (Brawer

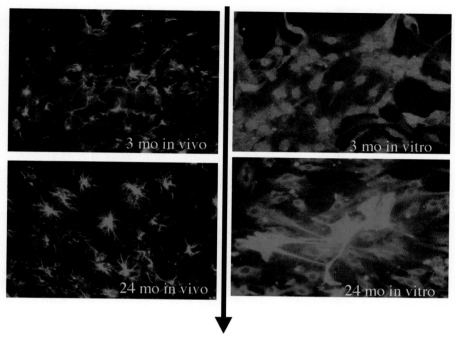

Fig. 1. Glial fibrillar acidic protein (GFAP) immunocytochemistry showing cerebral cortex from young adult and old adult rat (left) and primary cultures of astrocytes derived from cerebral cortex of these ages. (From I. Rozovsky and C. Finch, unpublished; culture methods in Rozovsky et al. 1998)

and Sonnenschein 1975; Brawer et al. 1978, 1980), whereas collaborations with our lab found that the hypothalamic astrocytic activation of aging was attenuated by long-term ovariectomy (Schipper et al. 1981). These manipulations of estrogen exposure caused changes in hypothalamic function in parallel with changes in hypothalamic glia. On the one hand, age-related impairments in the preovulatory surge of gonadatropins was attenuated by long-term ovariectomy, whereas aging changes were accelerated by sustained physiological elevations of estradiol (Finch et al. 1984; Kohama et al. 1989). The primary cell targets of estradiol in the hypothalamus are not known.

GFAP and Aging

Our lab re-entered the astrocyte field as an outcome of screening for changes in gene expression during AD from 1987-1995. Because AD increases strikingly during aging, we searched for genes that are activated during normal aging and show further increases during AD. In view of evidence for the role of sex and adrenal steroids in rodent glial aging, we also screened these genes for steroidal influences. GFAP emerged in all screens.

The search was based on the first cDNA libraries from AD and normal aging human and rat brains and on two-day gels of in vitro translation products (May et al. 1990; Poirier et al. 1991b; Day et al. 1992; Nichols et al. 1994). Another cDNA library used brains given perforant path lesions as models of AD (Day et al. 1992). The increases of GFAP were validated by Northern blot hybridization (Goss et al. 1990, 1991; Nichols et al. 1993, 1995). In situ hybridization showed that the GFAP mRNAs was increased per astrocyte in the outer molecular layer of the dentate gyrus (Yoshida et al. 1996; Morgan et al. 1999). GFAP increases during normal aging were also recently confirmed by microarray technology (Lee et al. 2000). These approaches showed relatively few major mRNA age changes, about 1-2% of the prevalent mRNA species detected. This number is consistent with our early analysis of mRNA inventory using solution hybridization to single copy DNA (Colman et al. 1980). Rats showed no age changes in the yield of polysomal poly(A)mRNA or in its sequence complexity. The statistics set upper limits to the number of different mRNA changes, which approximate the microarrray finding of 1-2% of brain mRNAs change with age. At that time, some believed that aging was caused by gross impairments of gene expression (Cutler 1975). However, this dire view of aging has not been supported by several lines of evidence. The total RNA content of most brain regions of aging mice does not change with aging (Chaconas and Finch 1973). Brain RNA sequence diversity changes very little during normal aging (Colman et al. 1980). Lastly, brain histology shows normal cell phenotypes of neurons and glia in aging rodents which depend on precisely maintained, cell-specific patterns of gene expression.

GFAP shows progressive, age-related increases of expression in most brain regions in all mammals examined: lab mice, rats, dogs, and monkeys (Goss et al. 1990, 1991; Morgan et al. 1999). This and other laboratories have found increases of GFAP mRNA and protein in mice and rats (12-18 months) in hippocampus, striatum, and other brain regions that reach greater than two-fold increases above those of young adults. The similar age-related increases in brains of neurologically normal humans (Nichols et al. 1993) render the increased expression of GFAP as one of the most generalizable molecular, age-related changes in the mammalian brain (Johnson et al. 1996). In general, the age-related increases are progressive and can be detected by mid-life in rodents and humans. GFAP can thus be considered to be a marker for aging in mammals, along with other markers of microglial hyperactivity. It is remarkable that, at the same ages when glial activity is increasing, there are also small progressive losses of neurotransmitter receptors (Fig. 2). Together, there changes may be considered as a canonical pattern of aging in mammals that begins soon after maturity in the absence of definable neurodegeneration or neuropathology (Finch 1993; Laping et al. 1994a) and decreases by 50% after glucocorticoid treatment (Laping et al. 1994b; Rozovsky et al. 1995). Although these run-on assays did not reach statistical significance in overall trends for increased GFAP transcription rates in cerebral cortex of old rats (Laping 1994a; Laping et al.1994c), another lab observed statistically significant increases in GFAP transcription by run-on (Krekowki et al. 1996).

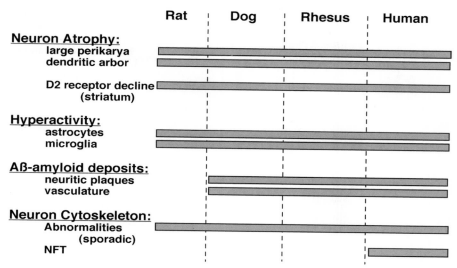

Fig. 2. Canonical patterns of brain aging, showing age changes in species of increasing life span: rat (2 y), dog (15 y), rhesus monkey (25 y) human 70 y). For details, see Finch 1993. NFT, neurofibrillary tangles.

In situ hybridization with an intron-probe was used to detect astrocyte subpopulations that might show greater effects of aging. The subcellular grain distribution obtained by in situ hybridization with the intron 1-containing probe is localized to the region of the cell nucleus, whereas that of an exon 1-containing probe is more widely distributed throughout the cytoplasm, as expected (Fig. 3). Three subregions display marked age changes: the outer molecular layer of the dentate gyrus, the internal capsule, and the corpus callosum (Fig. 4). Age-related increases of > 50% in the mean intron signal were significant in each region (Morgan et al. 1997, 1999).

GFAP is the first example of a gene to show progressive increases in expression across the life span. Age changes in GFAP expression diverge strikingly from the decreased expression of certain other genes during aging in non-neural tissues. For example, the expression of hepatic α_{2u}-globulin and androgen receptor genes decrease >90% during aging in male rats, as measured by run-on transcription rates and by mRNA and protein per cell (Van Remmen et al. 1994).

Why do astrocytes become activated during aging? We discuss three possibilities: neuron death; changes in neuron activity and in response to other glia; and response to oxidation.

First, innumerable histopathological observations show increased expression of GFAP in association with dying neurons. Thus, it seems plausible a priori that glial changes are secondary to neuron degeneration. However, glial activation is too general and arises too early during aging to be secondary to neuron death in all examples, e.g., in genotypes that do not show neuron loss with age (Rasmussen in the outer sheaths of myelin that are remote from cytoplasmic repair processes. Oxidized lipids can activate microglia and peripheral macrophages and are recognized by scavenger receptors. Alternatively, glycated adducts (AGE) form in association with hyperglycemia of diabetes in many tissues with long-lived proteins and lipids.

To test the possibility that GFAP transcription was sensitive to oxidative stress, we examined the effects of hydrogen peroxide on transcription. Two assays in primary astrocyte cultures gave similar induction in response to hydrogen peroxide: GFAP mRNA levels and activity of a transfected, full length GFAP promoter construct (Rozovsky et al. 1998). The upstream GFAP promoter contains a rich inventory of physiologically sensitive response elements in domains that show extensive conservation between human and rodents (Laping et al. 1994a; Fig. 5). A candidate for mediating the responses of GFAP transcription to hydrogen peroxide is an overlapping NF-1/NF6B response element (TGGGGGTGCTGCCAGGAA) that also mediates responses to TGF-β1 and IL-1 (Krohn et al. 1999). The responses to hydrogen peroxide are abolished by selective mutagenesis (Wei et al., in preparation).

Caloric restriction slows GFAP induction during aging

In view of the potential role of oxidized proteins on glial activation, it is of great interest that many age changes in mRNA can be attenuated by caloric restriction (CR). Restricting the ad libitum food intake by 10-40% robustly increases rodent life spans and slows many aging processes. Whether begun early or at middle-age, CR increases the life span and reduces and delays spontaneous abnormal growths, kidney degeneration, and many other age-related diseases (Weindruch and Walford 1988; Finch 1990). We also showed that CR attenuated the age increases in GFAP transcription (Morgan et al. 1997, 1999; Fig. 4).

The mechanisms involved in CR are poorly understood despite intensive study. In the brain, CR decreases the accumulation of AGE and other oxidized products, possibly by lowering blood glucose, which is one substrate for the formation of AGE (Dubey et al. 1996; Forster et al. 2000). CR reduces not only oxygen consumption on a whole-animal basis but also thyroid hormones and body temperature, which suggests that CR lowers the metabolic rate (Weindruch and Walford 1988; Sohal and Weindruch 1996). These findings on GFAP were verified by microarray analysis of cerebellum and cerebral cortex (Lee et al. 2000). More generally, of the brain mRNAs that changed by more than 70%, about 30% were either completely or partially prevented by CR. We are examining the possibility that a limited set of transcription factors may in coordination regulate the activities of many genes during aging and responses to CR.

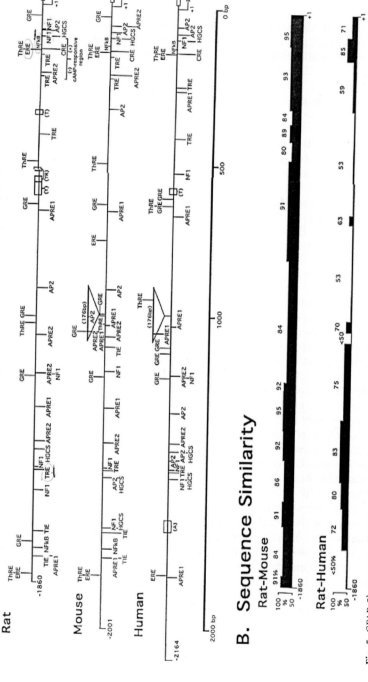

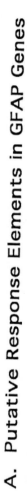

Fig. 5. GFAP 5'-upstream promoter organization. A. putative response elements identified by canonic sequences from rat, mouse, and human. B. Sequence similarity. Redrawn from Laping et al. 1994b

Estrogen regulation of GFAP

GFAP expression is also sensitive to estradiol, which we hypothesize is a factor in the support of synaptic sprouting after lesions. As shown in rodent models for the hippocampal deafferentation of AD (see Introduction), neuronal outgrowth is enhanced by estradiol in ovariectomized female rodents (Stone et al. 1998a, 2000). Astrocytes are among the targets of estradiol in complex interactions with neurons that may support, or alternatively inhibit, neuronal remodeling. On one hand, neurite outgrowth is supported by astrocytic secretions, which include laminin and other adhesion substrates (e.g., Garcia-Abreu et al. 2000; Weissmuller et al. 2000; Costa et al. 2002). However, reactive astrocytes can inhibit neurite outgrowth through the formation of glial scars, which contain fibrous astrocytes with high expression of GFAP (e.g., Alonso and Privat 1993). Deficits of estradiol after ovariectomy enhance astrocytic fibrosis after several types of brain lesions, as well as in unlesioned brains (e.g., Day et al. 1993). In confluent primary cultures of astrocytes, estradiol modulates GFAP transcription through the estrogen receptor ER-alpha, which we showed by site directed mutagenesis to bind a functional estrogen response element in the upstream promoter (Stone et al.1998b).

To approach the complex processes of astrocyte-neuron interactions after deafferenting lesions, we are analyzing these effects of estradiol on astrocyte responses to «wounding-in-a-dish» in cell culture models at two levels of complexity, which allows examination of effects of estradiol on astrocytes alone or on cocultures of astrocyte and neurons (McMillian et al. 1994; Lefrancois et al. 1997). In astrocyte-neuron cocultures, antisense GFAP cRNA enhanced neurite outgrowth in association with the reorganization of astrocytic laminin, as well as the diminution of GFAP protein (Lefrançois et al. 1997). Laminins are secreted by astrocytes and, as constituents of the basement membrane that interact with the cytoskeleton, can guide neurite sprouting and other cell movements. Because estradiol inhibits GFAP expression in vivo and in vitro, we hypothesized that estradiol treatment would be physiologically equivalent to antisense GFAP treatment. In fact, physiological levels of estradiol suppress GFAP responses to wounding and enhance neurite outgrowth in association with reorganization of astrocytic laminin (Rozovsky et al. 2002; Fig. 6).

The importance of transcriptional controls to these processes was shown above, in which the attenuation of GFAP protein increase after wounding by estradiol was paralleled by decreased GFAP transcription. It is therefore likely that the attenuation of GFAP expression by estradiol after wounding in vivo is transcriptionally mediated. The upstream region necessary for wounding responses is highly conserved, with 84-95% similarity between mouse and rat (-642 to 1867 bp) and >70% similarity of the rat, mouse, and human promoter for -1000 to -1800 bp (Fig. 5). This unusually extensive response implies a conserved set of regulatory responses to integrate steroidal and inflammatory mechanisms (Laping et al. 1994b).

Mechanisms appear to include a near 5'-upstream estrogen response element (ERE-1). Mutations of ERE-1, which blocked transcritional regulation of GFAP by

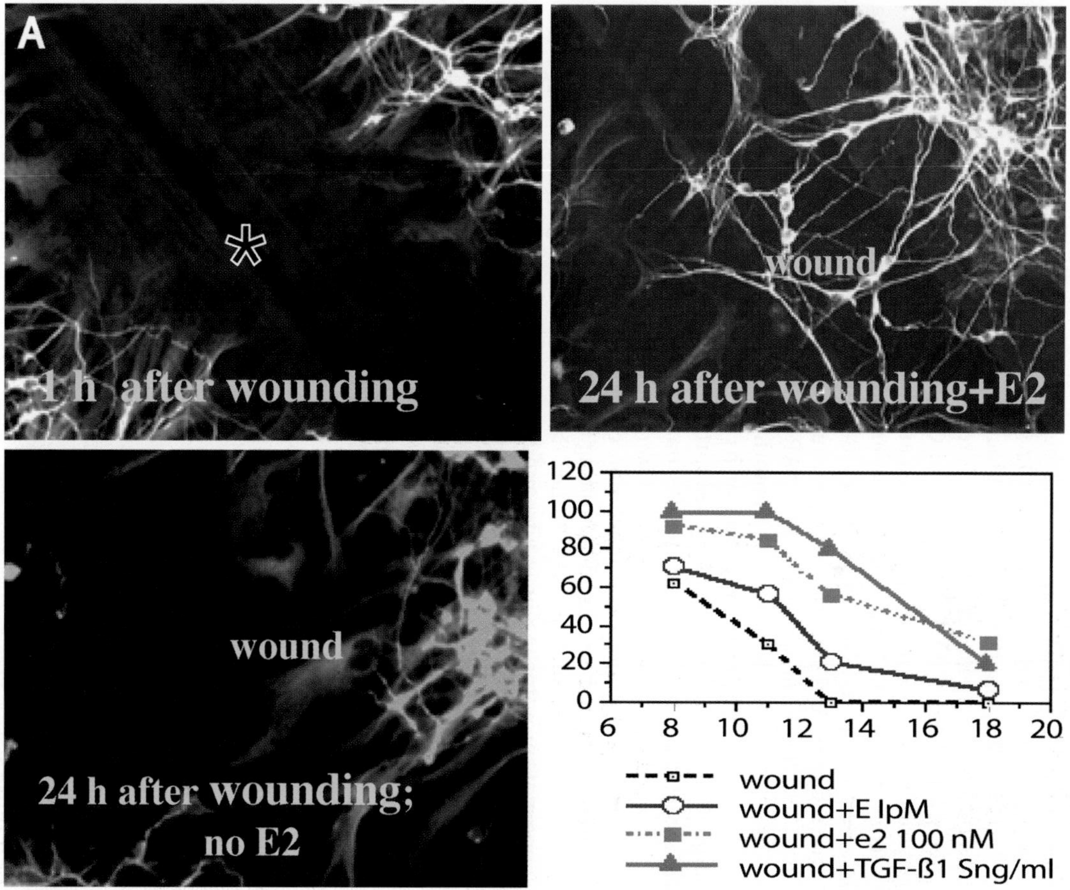

Fig. 6. In the wounding-in-a-dish model, primary cultures of astrocytes from cerebral cortex are overlaid with embryo E18 cortical neurons (McMillian et al. 1994). Scratch wounding induces neurite outgrowth (MAP-5 immunohistochemistry) if GFAP is down- regulated by anti-sense (Lefrancois et al. 1997; Costa et al. 2002) or by estradiol (Rozovsky et al. 2002)

estradiol alone, also partially blocked the effects of estradiol on GFAP induction by wounding, but did not impair the GFAP induction by wounding in the absence of estradiol. This mutation in ERE-1 blocks binding of the transcriptional factor ERα (Stone et al. 1998b). Because ERα is required for neuroprotection by estradiol after stroke (Dubal et al. 2001), ERα in GFAP regulation by estradiol may have general significance in neuroprotection and neuronal sprouting.

The inhibition of GFAP expression by estradiol in response to scratch wounding in either astrocytes alone or in astrocyte-neuron cocultures is consistent with in vivo responses of female rats. In stab wounds to the cerebral cortex, ovariectomy increased the local induction of GFAP immunoreactivity (Garcia-Estrada et al. 1993). Similarly, lesions of the entorhinal cortex distal to the hippocampus, causing downstream degeneration of its terminals and astrocyte hyperactivity, responded to estradiol with increased sprouting and diminished GFAP expression (Stone et al. 2000). Because neurite outgrowth is enhanced by treatment of astrocyte-neuron cocultures with antisense GFAP before wounding (Lefrancois et al. 1997), we propose that repression of GFAP expression is important in the estradiol mechated increase of sprouting by neurons.

Lastly, we mention ongoing studies that indicate that aging alters astrocytic support of sprouting in this in vitro model. We have shown that primary cultures of astrocytes from aging brains retain the activated phenotype with higher GFAP expression (Rozovsky et al. 1998; Fig. 1). Moreover, astrocytes derived from aging adults support neuron outgrowth much less well than astrocytes from young adults. GFAP is a major candidate in this effect of aging, because treatment with RNAi, which lowered GFAP in old-derived cultures, also restored neuron sprouting and outgrowth to young levels (Rozovsky et al., in preparation). In view of the inverse association of GFAP expression and neurite-promoting organizations of laminin, the expression of GFAP may have a broader role than usually considered in the context of glial scaring.

Acknowledgments

CEF is grateful for support from the N.I.A. and the John Douglas French Alzheimer's Foundation.

References

Alonso G, Privat A (1993) Reactive astrocytes involved in the formation of lesional scars differ in the mediobasal hypothalamus and in other forebrain regions. J Neurosci Res 34: 523–538
Anderson CP, Rozovsky I, Stone DJ, Song Y, Lopez LM, Finch CE (2002) Aging and increased hypothalamic glial fibrillary acid protein (GFAP) mRNA in F344 female rats.
Dissociation of GFAP inducibility from the luteinizing hormone surge. Neuroendocrinology 76: 121–130
Bjorklund H, Eriksdotter-Nilsson M, Dahl D, Rose G, Hoffer B, Olson L (1985) Image analysis of GFA-positive astrocytes from adolescence to senescence. Exp Brain Res 58: 163–170
Brawer JR, Sonnenschein C (1975) Cytopathological effects of estradiol on the arcuate nucleus of the female rat. A possible mechanism for pituitary tumorigenesis. Am J Anat 144: 57–88

Brawer JR, Naftolin F, Martin J, Sonnenschein C (1978) Effects of a single injection of estradiol valerate on the hypothalamic arcuate nucleus and on reproductive function in the female rat. Endocrinology 103: 501–512

Brawer JR, Schipper H, Naftolin F (1980) Ovary-dependent degeneration in the hypothalamic arcuate nucleus. Endocrinology 107: 274–279

Butterfield DA, Kanski J (2001) Brain protein oxidation in age-related neurodegenerative disorders that are associated with aggregated proteins. Mech Ageing Dev 122: 945–962

Canady KS, Hyson RL, Rubel EW (1994) The astrocytic response to afferent activity blockade in chick nucleus magnocellularis is independent of synaptic activation, age, and neuronal survival. J Neurosci 14: 5973–5985

Chaconas G, Finch CE (1973) The effect of ageing on RNA-DNA ratios in brain regions of the C57BL-6J male mouse. J Neurochem 21: 1469–1473

Colman PD, Kaplan BB, Osterburg HH, Finch CE (1980) Brain poly(A)RNA during aging: stability of yield and sequence complexity in two rat strains. J Neurochem 34: 335–345

Costa S, Planchenault T, Charriere-Bertrand C, Mouchel Y, Fages C, Juliano S, Lefrancois T, Barlovatz-Meimon G, Tardy M (2002) Astroglial permissivity for neuritic outgrowth in neuron-astrocyte cocultures depends on regulation of laminin bioavailability. Glia 37: 105–113

Cutler RG (1975) Transcription of unique and reiterated DNA sequences in mouse liver and brain tissues as a function of age. Exp Gerontol 10: 10–37

Day JR, Min BH, Laping NJ, Martin G, 3rd, Osterburg HH, Finch CE (1992) New mRNA probes for hippocampal responses to entorhinal cortex lesions in the adult male rat: a preliminary report. Exp Neurol 117: 97–99

Day JR, Laping NJ, Lampert-Etchells M, Brown SA, O'Callaghan JP, McNeill TH, Finch CE (1993) Gonadal steroids regulate the expression of glial fibrillary acidic protein in the adult male rat hippocampus. Neuroscience 55: 435–443

de Vellis J (2002) The MRRC at the University of California (UCLA), Los Angeles, CA. Int J Dev Neurosci. 20: 287–288. Review. No abstract available.

Dubal DB, Zhu H, Yu J, Rau SW, Shughrue PJ, Merchenthaler I, Kindy MS, Wise PM (2001) Estrogen receptor alpha, not beta, is a critical link in estradiol-mediated protection against brain injury. Proc Natl Acad Sci USA 98: 1952–1957

Dubey A, Forster MJ, Lal H, Sohal RS (1996) Effect of age and caloric intake on protein oxidation in different brain regions and on behavioral functions of the mouse. Arch Biochem Biophys 333: 189–197

Eng LF, Ghirnikar RS, Lee YL (2000) Glial fibrillary acidic protein: GFAP-thirty-one years (1969-2000). Neurochem Res 25: 1439–1451

Finch CE (1990) Longevity, senescence, and the genome. Chicago: University of Chicago

Finch CE (1993) Neuron atrophy during aging: programmed or sporadic? Trends Neurosci 16: 104–110

Finch CE, Landfield PW (1985) Neuroendocrine and autonomic function in aging mammals. In: Finch CE, Schneider EL (eds) Handbook of the biology of aging. 2nd edition. New York: Van Nostrand, pp 79–90

Finch CE, Felicio LS, Mobbs CV, Nelson JF (1984) Ovarian and steroidal influences on neuroendocrine aging processes in female rodents. Endocrinol Rev 5: 467–497

Finch CE, Morgan TE,Xie Z, Stone D, Lanzrein AS, Rosovsky I. (2000) Glial hyperactivity during aging as a neuroinflammatory process.In Patterson P, Kordon C, Christen Y(eds)°Neuro-immune interactions in neurologic and psychiatric disorders. Heidelberg: Springer-Verlag 47–56

Forster MJ, Sohal BH, Sohal RS (2000) Reversible effects of long-term caloric restriction on protein oxidative damage. J Gerontol A Biol Sci Med Sci 55: B522–529

Garcia-Abreu J, Mendes FA, Onofre GR, De Freitas MS, Silva LC, Moura Neto V, Cavalcante LA (2000) Contribution of heparan sulfate to the non-permissive role of the midline glia to the growth of midbrain neurites. Glia 29: 260–272

Garcia-Estrada J, Del Rio JA, Luquin S, Soriano E, Garcia-Segura LM (1993) Gonadal hormones down-regulate reactive gliosis and astrocyte proliferation after a penetrating brain injury. Brain Res 628: 271–278

Geinisman Y, Bondareff W, Dodge JT (1977) Partial deafferentation of neurons in the dentate gyrus of the senescent rat. Brain Res 134: 541–545

Geinisman Y, Bondareff W, Dodge JT (1978) Hypertrophy of astroglial processes in the dentate gyrus of the senescent rat. Am J Anat 153: 537–543

Geinisman Y, Detoledo-Morrell L, Morrell F, Heller RE (1995) Hippocampal markers of age-related memory dysfunction: behavioral, electrophysiological and morphological perspectives. Prog Neurobiol 45: 223–252.

Goss JR, Finch CE, Morgan DG (1990) GFAP RNA increases during a wasting state in old mice. Exp Neurol 108: 266–268

Goss JR, Finch CE, Morgan DG (1991) Age-related changes in glial fibrillary acidic protein mRNA in the mouse brain. Neurobiol Aging 12: 165–170

Hansen LA, Armstrong DM, Terry RD (1987) An immunohistochemical quantification of fibrous astrocytes in the aging human cerebral cortex. Neurobiol Aging 8: 1–6

Johnson S, Young-Chan CS, Laping NJ, Finch CE. (1996) Perforant path transection induces complement C9 deposition in hippocampus. Exp Neurol 138: 198–205

Kohama SG, Anderson CP, Osterburg HH, May PC, Finch CE (1989) Oral administration of estradiol to young C57BL/6J mice induces age-like neuroendocrine dysfunctions in the regulation of estrous cycles. Biol Reprod 41: 227–232

Krekoski CA, Parhad IM, Fung TS, Clark AW (1996) Aging is associated with divergent effects on Nf-L and GFAP transcription in rat brain. Neurobiol Aging 17: 833–841

Krohn K, Rozovsky I, Wals P, Teter B, Anderson CP, Finch CE (1999) Glial fibrillary acidic protein transcription responses to transforming growth factor-beta1 and interleukin-1beta are mediated by a nuclear factor-1-like site in the near-upstream promoter. J Neurochem 72: 1353–1361

Landfield PW, Rose G, Sandles L, Wohlstadter TC, Lynch G (1977) Patterns of astroglial hypertrophy and neuronal degeneration in the hippocampus of ages, memory-deficient rats. J Gerontol 32: 3–12

Landfield PW (1978) An endocrine hypothesis of brain aging and studies on brain-endocrine correlations and monosynaptic neurophysiology during aging. Adv Exp Med Biol 113: 179–199

Landfield PW, Waymire JC, Lynch G (1978) Hippocampal aging and adrenocorticoids: quantitative correlations. Science 202: 1098–1102

Landfield PW, Baskin RK, Pitler TA (1981a) Brain aging correlates: retardation by hormonal-pharmacological treatments. Science 214: 581–584

Landfield PW, Braun LD, Pitler TA, Lindsey JD, Lynch G (1981b) Hippocampal aging in rats: a morphometric study of multiple variables in semithin sections. Neurobiol Aging 2: 265–275

Laping NJ, Teter B, Nichols NR, Rozovsky I, Finch CE (1994a) Glial fibrillary acidic protein: regulation by hormones, cytokines, and growth factors. Brain Pathol 4: 259–275

Laping NJ, Morgan TE, Nichols NR, Rozovsky I, Young-Chan CS, Zarow C, Finch CE (1994b) Transforming growth factor-beta 1 induces neuronal and astrocyte genes: tubulin alpha 1, glial fibrillary acidic protein and clusterin. Neuroscience 58: 563–572

Laping NJ, Teter B, Anderson CP, Osterburg HH, O'Callaghan JP, Johnson SA, Finch CE (1994c) Age-related increases in glial fibrillary acidic protein do not show proportionate changes in transcription rates or DNA methylation in the cerebral cortex and hippocampus of male rats. J Neurosci Res. 39: 710–717

Lee CK, Weindruch R, Prolla TA (2000) Gene-expression profile of the ageing brain in mice. Nature Genet 25: 294–297

Lefrancois T, Fages C, Peschanski M, Tardy M (1997) Neuritic outgrowth associated with astroglial phenotypic changes induced by antisense glial fibrillary acidic protein (GFAP) mRNA in injured neuron-astrocyte cocultures. J Neurosci 17: 4121–4128

Lindsey JD, Landfield PW, Lynch G (1979) Early onset and topographical distribution of hypertrophied astrocytes in hippocampus of aging rats: a quantitative study. J Gerontol 34: 661–671

May PC, Lampert-Etchells M, Johnson SA, Poirier J, Masters JN, Finch CE (1990) Dynamics of gene expression for a hippocampal glycoprotein elevated in Alzheimer's disease and in response to experimental lesions in rat. Neuron 5: 831–839

McMillian MK, Thai L, Hong JS, O'Callaghan JP, Pennypacker KR (1994) Brain injury in a dish: a model for reactive gliosis. Trends Neurosci 17: 138–142

Morgan TE, Rozovsky I, Goldsmith SK, Stone DJ, Yoshida T, Finch CE (1997) Increased transcription of the astrocyte gene GFAP during middle-age is attenuated by food restriction: implications for the role of oxidative stress. Free Rad Biol Med 23: 524–548

Morgan TE, Xie Z, Goldsmith S, Yoshida T, Lanzrein AS, Stone D, Rozovsky I, Perry G, Smith MA, Finch CE (1999) The mosaic of brain glial hyperactivity during normal ageing and its attenuation by food restriction. Neuroscience 89: 687–699

Nichols NR, Masters JN, May PC, de Vellis J, Finch CE (1989) Corticosterone-induced responses in rat brain RNA are also evoked in hippocampus by acute vibratory stress. Neuroendocrinology 49: 40–46

Nichols NR, Day JR, Laping NJ, Johnson SA, Finch CE (1993) GFAP mRNA increases with age in rat and human brain. Neurobiol Aging 14: 421–429

Nichols NR, Finch CE (1994) Gene products of corticosteroid action in hippocampus. Ann N Y Acad Sci. 30: 145–154

Nichols NR, Finch CE, Nelson JF (1995) Food restriction delays the age-related increase in GFAP mRNA in rat hypothalamus. Neurobiol Aging 16: 105–110

Patterson P, Kordon C, Christen Y, (eds) (2000) Neuro-immune interactions in neurologic and psychiatric disorders. Heidelberg: Springer-Verlag

Poirier J, Hess M, May PC, Finch CE (1991a) Astrocytic apolipoprotein E mRNA and GFAP mRNA in hippocampus after entorhinal cortex lesioning. Brain Res Mol Brain Res 11: 97–106

Poirier J, Hess M, May PC, Finch CE (1991b) Cloning of hippocampal poly(A) RNA sequences that increase after entorhinal cortex lesion in adult rat. Brain Res Mol Brain Res 9: 191–195

Rasmussen T, Schliemann T, Sorensen JC, Zimmer J, West MJ (1996) Memory impaired aged rats: no loss of principal hippocampal and subicular neurons. Neurobiol Aging 17: 143–147

Rozovsky I, Laping NJ, Krohn K, Teter B, O'Callaghan JP, Finch CE (1995) Transcriptional regulation of glial fibrillary acidic protein by corticosterone in rat astrocytes in vitro is influenced by the duration of time in culture and by astrocyte-neuron interactions. Endocrinology 136: 2066–2073

Rozovsky I, Finch CE, Morgan TE (1998) Age-related activation of microglia and astrocytes: in vitro studies show persistent phenotypes of aging, increased proliferation, and resistance to down-regulation. Neurobiol Aging 19: 97–103

Rozovsky I, Wei M, Stone DJ, Zanjani H, Anderson CP, Morgan TE, Finch CE (2002) Estradiol (E2) enhances neurite outgrowth by repressing glial fibrillary acidic protein expression and reorganizing laminin. Endocrinology 143: 636–646

Schipper HM (1996) Astrocytes, brain aging, and neurodegeneration. Neurobiol Aging 17: 467–480

Schipper H, Brawer JR, Nelson JF, Felicio LS, Finch CE (1981) Role of the gonads in the histologic aging of the hypothalamic arcuate nucleus. Biol Reprod 25: 413–419

Sohal RS, Weindruch R (1996) Oxidative stress, caloric restriction, and aging. Science 273: 59–63

Stone DJ, Rozovsky I, Morgan TE, Anderson CP, Finch CE (1998a) Increased synaptic sprouting in response to estrogen via an apolipoprotein E-dependent mechanism: implications for Alzheimer's disease. J Neurosci 18: 3180–3185

Stone DJ, Song Y, Anderson CP, Krohn KK, Finch CE, Rozovsky I (1998b) Bidirectional transcription regulation of glial fibrillary acidic protein by estradiol in vivo and in vitro. Endocrinology 139: 3202–3209

Stone DJ, Rozovsky I, Morgan TE, Anderson CP, Lopez LM, Shick J, Finch CE (2000) Effects of age on gene expression during estrogen-induced synaptic sprouting in the female rat. Exp Neurol 165: 46–57

Streit WJ (2002) Microglia as neuroprotective, immunocompetent cells of the CNS. Glia 40: 133–139

Van Remmen H, Ward WF, Sabia RV, Richardson A (1994) Effect of age on gene expression and protein degradation. In: Masoro E (ed) Handbook of physiology. Volume on Aging. New York: Oxford University Press, pp 171–234

Weindruch RH, Walford R (1988) The retardation of aging and disease by dietary restriction. Springfield IL, Thomas

Weissmuller G, Garcia-Abreu J, Mascarello Bisch P, Moura Neto V, Cavalcante LA (2000) Glial cells with differential neurite growth-modulating properties probed by atomic force microscopy. Neurosci Res 38: 217–220

Yoshida T, Goldsmith SK, Morgan TE, Stone DJ, Finch CE (1996) Transcription supports age-related increases of GFAP gene expression in the male rat brain. Neurosci Lett 215: 107–110

Circadian Rhythmicity and Aging: the Molecular Basis of Oscillatory Gene Expression

Paolo Sassone-Corsi

Summary

Circadian rhythmicity in hormone synthesis and secretion is a characteristic feature of a large number of biological systems. These rhythms are essential in the regulation of most physiological functions, and studies over the past several years have started to elucidate the molecular mechanisms governing them. Importantly, there is evidence that fundamental changes occur in the quality of circadian rhythmicity during the aging process. These changes occur via differential adaptation to the environment. The day-night rhythm is translated into hormonal oscillations governing the metabolism of all living organisms. In mammals, circadian synthesis of the hormone melatonin occurs in the pineal gland in response to signals originating from the endogenous clock located in the hypothalamic suprachiasmatic nucleus (SCN). The molecular mechanisms involved in rhythmic synthesis of melatonin involve the CREM (cAMP-responsive element modulator) gene, which encodes transcription factors responsive to activation of the cAMP signalling pathway. ICER (inducible cAMP early repressor) is a product of the CREM gene that is rhythmically expressed and participates in a transcriptional autoregulatory loop. ICER also controls the amplitude of oscillations of serotonin N-acetyl transferase, the rate-limiting enzyme of melatonin synthesis. Thus, processes of transcriptional regulation are central to the physiological mechanisms of oscillatory hormonal production that are known to change during aging.

Introduction

Day-night and seasonal changes in the environment dominate the lives of plants and animals; thus many facets of physiology are adapted to anticipate these changes. In vertebrates, the endocrine system plays a key role in synchronizing physiology with the environment. Circadian and seasonal rhythmicity characterize the action of many hormones that ultimately direct long-term changes in gene expression (Felig et al. 1987; Krieger 1979). Thus, the properties of transcription factors and the signaling pathways that regulate them constitute an essential link in the relay of temporal information. Fundamental to temporal adaptations made by animals is the presence of an internal circadian clock (Aschoff 1981; Fig. 1). Daily inputs of light and other stimuli continually reset this clock and synchronize it with the environment. Clock output pathways subsequently modulate various aspects of

Chanson et al.
Endocrine Aspects of Successful Aging
© Springer-Verlag Berlin Heidelberg 2004

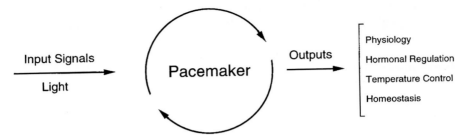

Fig. 1. The classical view of the circadian clock includes three components: a pacemaker or oscillator, which generates and sustains rhythms, even in constant conditions; input pathways, regulating oscillator response to various stimuli (for example, light-dark cycles); and output pathways, which convey rhythmic information from the pacemaker to other physiological systems. During the aging process, signals from the central pacemaker decrease in intensity, causing changes in the amplitude of hormonal synthesis.

physiology. One key hormonal output from the clock is the nighttime production of melatonin. In vertebrates, this is synthesized by the retina and pineal gland.

Linking the Circadian clock and the pineal gland

A small anatomical structure located in the center of the skull between the two cerebral hemispheres is identified as the pineal gland in mammals. This structure is directly light-sensitive in birds, reptiles, amphibia and fish, justifying its popular name as "the third eye" (Collin 1971; Dodt 1973; Okshe 1984). The pineal gland possesses an independent circadian clock in these animals (Takahashi et al. 1980; Menaker and Wisner 1983). In mammals, however, pinealocytes are not light-sensitive and do not possess a clock. The central pacemaker is instead located in the hypothalamic suprachiasmatic nucleus (SCN), from where it directs a number of peripheral clocks (Pando et al. 2002; Schibler and Sassone-Corsi, 2002). Light stimuli are conveyed to the SCN via the retino-hypothalamic pathway.

Production of the hormone melatonin occurs principally in the pineal gland. Primary roles of melatonin in mammals are 1) the regulation of seasonal changes in reproductive activity in response to changes in day length, 2) entrainment of the SCN clock to ensure synchronicity with the environment, and 3) in the retina, where melatonin is also synthesized, the regulation of photopigment disc shedding, phagocytosis and the inhibition of retinal dopamine release (Cahill 1996; Tosini and Menaker 1996). Melatonin mediates its biological effects by binding to high affinity receptors belonging to the seven transmembrane G-protein coupled receptor superfamily. The synthesis of melatonin begins with the N-acetylation of serotonin followed by addition of a methyl group at the 5-hydroxy position via the enzyme, hydroxyindole-O-methyltransferase (HIOMT; Axelrod and Weissbach 1960). The pathway connecting light signals to melatonin synthesis is shown in Figure 2.

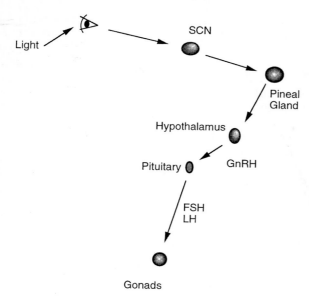

Fig. 2. A neuronal pathway regulating pineal melatonin synthesis in the rodent. Photic information is received by the retina and transmitted via the retino-hypothamic tract to the suprachiasmatic nucleus (SCN), the central circadian pacemaker. Oscillating signals from the SCN are transmitted to the pineal gland through the superior cervical ganglion (SCG) and induce circadian synthesis of the hormone melatonin. The pineal gland communicates with the hypothalamus and the pituitary gland to regulate gonadotropic hormonal synthesis and seasonal variations in gonadal function.

Melatonin synthesis in the pineal gland follows a powerful circadian rhythm. Whereas serotonin levels are much lower at night than in the day, melatonin concentrations display a reversed rhythm, with highest concentration at night associated with elevated circulating levels of melatonin. The link between these two reciprocal rhythms is the rate-limiting enzyme for melatonin synthesis, serotonin N-acetyltransferase (AANAT). This enzyme displays a diurnal rhythm of activity, with levels at nighttime peaking up to 100 times higher than in daytime (Klein and Weller 1970). The AANAT and melatonin rhythms derive from nighttime activation of the pineal's sympathetic innervation in mammals. Norepinephrine binds to β-adrenoceptors and thus stimulates adenylate cyclase activity. The resulting increase in cAMP levels has been shown to stimulate AANAT transcription and translation and also to maintain the enzyme in an active form (Takahashi 1994). α1-Adrenergic receptors also participate in AANAT stimulation (Klein et al. 1983), apparently by activating the phosphoinositide (PI) cycle and protein kinase C (PKC), which potentiates β-receptor-induced cAMP production.

Cloning of the gene encoding the AANAT enzyme was achieved from sheep by screening a cDNA expression library using an enzymatic assay for acetylation of arylalkylamine substrates (Coon et al. 1995). The rat cDNA was subsequently isolated using a PCR-based subtractive hybridization technique using day and night pineal gland RNA (Borjigin et al. 1995). The night-enriched AANAT cDNA displayed a diurnal rhythm of expression in the pineal gland that was identical to that of AANAT activity. Interestingly AANAT expression in the rat contrasts with the ovine pineal, where levels of the AANAT transcript change only slightly between day and night while AANAT activity oscillates strongly (Coon et al. 1995;

Borjigin et al. 1995; Roseboom et al. 1996). The rapid rise and fall in rat AANAT mRNA levels indicate that transcriptional regulation is a primary determinant of AANAT function in this species.

Introducing essential molecular players: cAMP-responsive transcription factors

The nocturnal release of norepinephrine in the mammalian pineal gland activates β adrenoreceptors, resulting in the stimulation of adenylate cyclase activity. The associated intracellular rise in cAMP is a key step in the subsequent upregulation of AANAT and melatonin synthesis (Klein 1985; Sugden et al. 1985; Vanecek et al. 1985). In the avian pineal gland these changes in cAMP occur under endogenous circadian clock control. Increases in intracellular cAMP levels lead to activation of cAMP-dependent protein kinase A (PKA) and the transport of active catalytic subunits to the nucleus (Krebs and Beavo 1979). Nuclear phosphorylation targets include a group of transcription factors that modulate the expression of cAMP-responsive genes (Sassone-Corsi 1995). These factors constitute a family of both activators and repressors that bind as homo- and heterodimers to cAMP-responsive elements (CREs). They belong to the basic leucine zipper (bZip) class of transcription factors, and their function is tightly regulated by phosphorylation (Sassone-Corsi 1995). Constitutively expressed factors such as CREB (CRE-binding protein) are phosphorylated by PKA and thereby converted into transcriptional activators. Their transcriptional activation domain contains a phosphorylation box (P-box) with consensus phosphorylation sites for several protein kinases, including PKA (Sassone-Corsi 1995). This is flanked by glutamine-rich regions, termed Q1 and Q2, which are believed to make contacts with the basal transcriptional machinery.

The gene encoding CREM (CRE-modulator) is closely related to CREB and, in common with other cAMP-responsive factors, generates a family of alternatively spliced isoforms (Foulkes et al. 1991; Laoide et al. 1993). A unique feature of CREM, however, is the presence of two alternative DNA binding domains, interchanged by the alternate use of splicing acceptor sites (Foulkes et al. 1991). CREM isoforms function as both activators and repressors of cAMP-directed transcription and have a characteristic cell- and tissue-specific pattern of expression, with high levels of CREM activators notably in the testis (Foulkes et al. 1992). In addition, the use of an alternative cAMP-inducible promoter (P2) at the 3' end of the CREM gene generates the factor ICER (Inducible cAMP Early Repressor; Stehle et al. 1993; Molina et al. 1993). This small factor contains only the DNA binding domain consisting of the leucine zipper and basic region and functions as a dominant repressor of cAMP-induced transcription. It acts by binding to CRE elements either as a homodimer or as heterodimeric complexes with other CRE activators. Since it lacks the activation domains, ICER repression function is primarily regulated by its intracellular concentration (Stehle et al. 1993; Molina et al. 1993). Stimuli that increase CREB phosphorylation have thus been associated with increased levels of ICER. ICER subsequently represses the same genes that are activated by phospho-

CREB. Furthermore, ICER participates in a negative autoregulatory loop (Molina et al. 1993) since ICER protein binds to the CRE elements in its own promoter and represses its own transcription.

The control of rhythmic melatonin synthesis

The transcripts of both AANAT and ICER display diurnal rhythmicity in the pineal gland (Stehle et al. 1993). The peak of ICER mRNA occurs during the second part of the night, just preceding the decline of melatonin synthesis. Interestingly, this pattern is developmentally regulated, being absent at birth and maturing only between the first and second week of postnatal development (Stehle et al. 1995). This coincides with the maturation of a functional sympathetic innervation linking the SCN and pineal as well as maturation of cAMP inducibility of gene expression within the pineal and the appearance of elevated nighttime melatonin synthesis (Stehle et al. 1995). Together these observations suggest that ICER might function as a downregulator of melatonin production by repressing cAMP-induced AANAT transcription at the end of the night (Stehle et al. 1995). A direct evaluation of the relationship between ICER and AANAT has been made possible by the generation of mice that carry a null mutation at the CREM locus (Nantel et al. 1996).

The study of AANAT regulation in the mouse posed potential problems, since the majority of inbred strains used for transgenic and homologous recombination experiments have genetic defects in melatonin synthesis (Goto et al. 1989). Biochemical and genetic analyses have implicated defects in AANAT or AANAT regulators and HIOMT in this deficiency (Ebihara et al. 1986). Thus the first step was to test whether AANAT mRNA is expressed in the 129/sv strain used for the CREM knockout studies. By using RNAse protection assay to analyze mouse pineal RNA, it was demonstrated that this mouse strain does indeed show a nighttime induction in AANAT expression, the timing of which is identical to that in the rat. The same AANAT expression pattern was encountered in C3H/He mice, an outbred mouse strain that does produce melatonin (Foulkes et al. 1996a). This finding indicates that the genetic defect in melatonin biosynthesis cannot be accounted for at the level of AANAT transcription. The two mouse strains also display equivalent profiles of elevated ICER nighttime expression, again with the timing being the same as that in the rat (Foulkes et al. 1996a). Expression of the transcription factor Fra-2 (Fos-related antigen) was also tested in the mouse pineal. Fra-2 mRNA and protein have been documented to vary diurnally in the rat pineal gland, with an elevation in the early part of the night that appears to be directed by adrenergic signals (Baler and Klein 1995). Furthermore, Fra-2 has been implicated as a negative regulator of AANAT expression (Baler and Klein 1995). The kinetics of Fra-2 expression in the mouse are the same as those in the rat. Thus, the patterns of ICER, AANAT and Fra-2 expression indicate that rat and mouse pineal glands can be considered equivalent in terms of adrenergically regulated gene expression (Foulkes et al. 1996a).

With the exception of time points during the day when mutant and wild-type control animals display an equivalent low basal level of expression, the mutant animals have significantly higher levels of nighttime AANAT mRNA than do their wild-type counterparts (Foulkes et al. 1996a). Specifically, a rise in AANAT transcript is detected earlier at the beginning of the night in the CREM-null mutants. AANAT expression reaches a higher peak and then persists longer than in wild-type siblings. Thus the consequence of removal of ICER protein seems to be the relief of a general dampening effect upon nighttime AA-NAT expression. In contrast, the timing and magnitude of Fra-2 expression is equivalent in wild-type and mutant animals. Normal Fra-2 expression in the mutant animals demonstrates that the deregulation of AANAT expression does not extend to all adrenergically regulated genes. Furthermore the Fra-2 result indicates that clock-derived adrenergic signals are not grossly altered in the knockout animals.

We have also analyzed the molecular mechanisms by which ICER down-regulates AANAT expression by cloning and characterizing the AANAT promoter. A CRE element (TGACGCCA), divergent from the consensus (TGACGTCA; Sassone-Corsi 1995) by only one mismatch, was identified at position -108. A 378 bp promoter fragment including this region is sufficient to direct cAMP-inducible transcription of a reporter gene and also the down-regulation of cAMP-activated transcription by coexpressed ICER. ICER protein generated in bacteria binds to the AANAT CRE. Moreover a high mobility complex binds to this CRE element in nuclear extracts prepared from mouse and rat pineal glands which is absent in extracts prepared from the CREM knockout mice. Thus, ICER protein binds to the AANAT promoter at the CRE element in vivo.

In CREM-null mice the AANAT transcript is upregulated at all stages of its nighttime induction, as compared to wild-type controls. This finding indicates that ICER dampens AANAT transcription throughout the night and not, as originally predicted, at the end of the night, when melatonin synthesis falls. Consistent with this function, the ICER protein persists throughout the day-night cycle, in contrast to the strong diurnal variations in its mRNA (Foulkes et al. 1996b).

Our findings indicate that ICER elicits a central function in the rat pineal gland (Fig. 3). Adrenergic stimulation at the onset of the night induces CREB phosphorylation whereas the termination of adrenergic stimulation towards morning is associated with CREB dephosphorylation (Foulkes et al. 1996a). Abundant evidence indicates that CREB phosphorylation involves PKA (Sassone-Corsi 1995) whereas a phosphatase that dephosphorylates CREB in the pineal has yet to be identified. Phosphorylated CREB binds to the CREM P2 promoter and thereby activates nighttime transcription of ICER. Dephosphorylation of CREB and the instability of the ICER transcript cause ICER mRNA levels to fall to low basal levels by the beginning of the day. In contrast, the ICER protein is more stable and persists at elevated levels throughout the day and night. Via binding to the CRE element in the AANAT promoter, ICER modulates the rate and magnitude of melatonin induction in response to adrenergic signals by exerting a dampening effect (Fig. 3). Thus the negative regulatory role of ICER operates throughout the 24-hour cycle and not exclusively during the down-regulation of melatonin synthesis that occurs at the end of the night. Normal Fra-2 expression in the

CREM mutant mice indicates that negative regulation by ICER in the pineal gland does not extend equally to all adrenergically regulated genes. Differential binding affinities of activators and repressors to the respective CRE elements may explain this observation. An additional, important conclusion from our studies concerns the oscillations of hormonal synthesis. Indeed, regulation of AANAT by the CREM feedback loop may constitute a paradigm for how transcriptional autoregulatory loops control oscillatory responses (Fig. 3; Sassone-Corsi 1994).

Perspectives

A number of questions concerning circadian physiology might be resolved by our findings. In particular, the dampening of melatonin oscillatory synthesis during aging could be directly linked to intrinsic changes in the molecular mechanism of AANAT transcriptional regulation by ICER. Indeed, the cloning of the AANAT gene and the demonstration that it is regulated by ICER have provided important insights. For example, in some species, such as the sheep, AANAT transcripts oscillate only weakly compared with the rat. Also in the mouse, overall levels of AANAT transcript are substantially lower than in rat. This finding implies an inherent variability in the mode of AANAT regulation between different mammalian species. These differences might reflect different relative contributions of ICER and other transcriptional regulators to AANAT transcriptional regulation.

The transcriptional mechanisms within mammalian pinealocytes documented here are potentially of much wider importance. However, the functioning of the mammalian pineal gland is regulated only indirectly by the SCN clock. It will thus be of great interest to assess the relative contribution of ICER and other transcriptional regulators to rhythmic melatonin production in lower vertebrates where the cAMP fluxes that drive melatonin synthesis are generated by an endogenous pinealocyte clock. The diurnal oscillation of AANAT mRNA in chick pinealocyte cultures combined with the pattern of cAMP inducibility of AANAT expression has lead to the speculation that cAMP regulation of AANAT activity is primarily post- transcriptional in the chick pineal (Bernard et al. 1997). Furthermore, it has been proposed that transcriptional regulation in the chick pinealocyte is clock driven via a mechanism independent of cAMP (Bernard et al. 1997). Additional studies are needed to uncover the molecular pathways involved in the aging process of circadian rhythmicity. These are likely to provide us with some exciting discoveries that will be relevant to our general knowledge of clock biology, but also to the implication that it has in the procees of aging.

Acknowledgments

Our studies are funded by CNRS, INSERM, CHUR, Human Frontiers Scientific Program (RG-240), Fondation pour la Recherche Médicale and Association pour Recherche sur le Cancer.

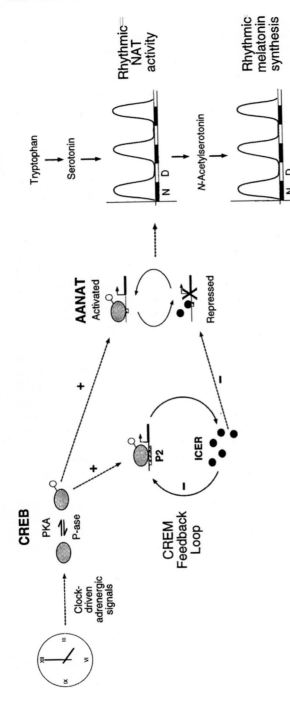

Fig. 3. Circadian oscillation of melatonin synthesis in the mouse is determined by the CREM feedback loop, which transduces rhythmic clock-derived signals at the transcriptional level. Serotonin is acetylated by serotonin N-acetyltransferase (AANAT) to produce N-acetylserotonin. N-acetylserotonin is in turn methylated by the enzyme hydroxyindole-o-methyltransferase (HIOMT). The rate-limiting step in the synthesis of melatonin is the AANAT enzyme. A schematic representation of the regulatory pathway responsible for generating rhythmic melatonin synthesis. Nighttime adrenergic signals originating from the clock activate PKA and thus phosphorylate CREB. During the day, dephosphorylation is achieved by phosphatase (P-ase) action. Thus clock-directed signals determine the equilibrium position. Phosphorylated CREB activates the P2 promoter of the CREM gene and thus induces the expression of ICER. ICER down-regulates its own expression constituting the CREM feedback loop. The balance between the proportion of phosphorylated CREB (positive effect) and ICER protein levels (negative effect) determines the transcriptional activity of the AANAT promoter. Thus the promoter cycles between activated and repressed states as a function of time. In this way, AANAT mRNA oscillates between high nighttime and low basal daytime levels and determines the characteristic day-night oscillation of AANAT activity. This directly determines rhythmic melatonin synthesis.

References

Aschoff J (1981) Biological rhythms. In: Handbook of behavioral neurobiology (Aschoff J. Ed.) Plenum Press, New York, pp 3–10

Axelrod J, Weissbach H (1960) Enzymatic O-methylation of N-acetylserotonin to melatonin. Science 131: 1312

Baler R, Klein DC (1995) Circadian expression of transcription factor Fra-2 in the rat pineal gland. J Biol Chem 270: 27319–27325

Bernard M, Klein DC, Zatz M (1997) Chick pineal clock regulates serotonin N-acetyltransferase mRNA rhythm in culture. Proc NatlAcad Sci USA 94: 304–309

Borjigin J, Wang MM, Snyder SH (1995) Diurnal variation in mRNA encoding serotonin N-acetyltransferase in pineal gland. Nature 378: 783–785

Cahill GM (1996) Circadian regulation of melatonin production in cultured zebrafish pineal and retina. Brain Res 708: 177–181

Collin JP (1971) Differentiation and regression of the cells of the sensory line in the epiphysis cerebri, in The pineal gland. (eds G.E.W. Wolstenhome and J. Knight), Churchill Livingstone, Edinburgh, pp.79–125

Coon SL, Roseboom PH, Baler R, Weller JL, Namboodiri MAA, Koonin EV, Klein DC (1995) Pineal serotonin N-acetyltransferase: expression cloning and molecular analysis. Science 270: 1681–1683

Dodt E (1973) Handbook of sensory physiology. Elsevier, New York pp113–140

Ebihara S, Marks T, Hudson DJ, Menaker M (1986) Genetic control of melatonin synthesis in the pineal gland of the mouse. Science 231: 491–493.

Felig P, Baxter JD, Broadus AE, Frohman LA (1987) Endocrinology and metabolism. McGraw-Hill, New York.

Foulkes NS, Borrelli E, Sassone-Corsi P (1991) CREM gene: Use of alternative DNA-binding domains generates multiple antagonists of cAMP-induced transcription. Cell 64: 739–749

Foulkes NS, Mellström B, Benusiglio E, Sassone-Corsi P (1992) Developmental switch of CREM function during spermatogenesis: from antagonist to transcriptional activator. Nature 355: 80–84.

Foulkes NS, Borjigin J, Snyder SH, Sassone-Corsi P (1996a) Transcriptional control of Circadian Hormone Synthesis by the CREM Feedback Loop. Proc Natl Acad Sci USA 93: 14140–14145

Foulkes NS, Duval G, Sassone-Corsi P (1996b) Adaptive inducibility of CREM as transcriptional memory of circadian rhythms. Nature 381: 83–85

Goto M, Oshima I, Tomita T, Ebihara S (1989) Melatonin content of the pineal gland in different mouse strains. J Pineal Res 7: 195–204

Klein DC, Weller JL (1970) Indole metabolism in the pineal gland: a circadian rhythm in N-acetyltransferase. Science 169: 1093–1095

Klein DC, Sugden D, Weller JL (1983) Postsynaptic α-adrenergic receptors potentiate the β-adrenergic stimulation of pineal serotonin N-acetyltrasferase. Proc Natl Acad Sci USA 80: 599–603

Klein DC (1985) Photoneural regulation of the mammalian pineal gland. Ciba Found. Symp. 117: 38–56

Krebs EG, Beavo JA (1979) Phosphorylation-dephosphorylation of enzymes. Ann Rev Biochem 48: 923–959

Krieger DT (1979) Endocrine rhythms. Raven Press, New York.

Laoide BM, Foulkes NS, Schlotter F, Sassone-Corsi P (1993) The functional versatility of CREM is determined by its modular structure. EMBO J 12: 1179–1191

Menaker M, Wisner S (1983) Temperature-compensated circadian clock in the pineal of Anolis. Proc Natl Acad Sci USA 80: 6119–6121

Molina CA, Foulkes NS, Lalli E, Sassone-Corsi P (1993) Inducibility and negative autoregulation of CREM: an alternative promoter directs the expression of ICER, an early response repressor. Cell 75: 875–886

Nantel F, Monaco L, Foulkes NS, Masquilier D, LeMeur M, Henriksén K, Dierich A, Parvinen M, Sassone-Corsi P (1996) Spermiogenesis deficiency and germ cell apoptosis in CREM-mutant mice. Nature 380: 159–162

Okshe A (1984) Evolution of the pineal complex: correlation of structure and function. Opthalmic Res 16: 88–95

Pando MP, Morse D, Cermakian N, Sassone-Corsi P (2002) Phenotypic rescue of a peripheral clock genetic defect via SCN hierarchical dominance. Cell 110: 107–117

Roseboom PH, Coon SL, Baler R, McCune SK, Weller JL, Klein DC (1996) Melatonin synthesis: analysis of the more than 150-fold nocturnal increase in serotonin N-acetyltransferase messenger ribonucleic acid in the rat pineal gland. Endocrinology 137: 3033–3044

Sassone-Corsi P (1994) Rhythmic transcription and autoregulatory loops: winding up the biological clock. Cell 78: 361–364

Sassone-Corsi P (1995) Transcription factors responsive to cAMP. Annu Rev Cell Dev Biol 11: 355–377

Schibler, U, Sassone-Corsi, P (2002) A web of circadian pacemakers. Cell 111: 919–922

Stehle JH, Foulkes NS, Molina CA, Simonneaux V, Pévet P, Sassone-Corsi P (1993) Adrenergic signals direct rhythmic expression of transcriptional repressor CREM in the pineal gland. Nature 365: 314–320

Stehle JH, Foulkes NS, Pévet P, Sassone-Corsi P (1995) Developmental maturation of pineal gland function: synchronised CREM inducibility and adrenergic stimulation. Mol Endocrinol 9: 706–716

Sugden D, Vanecek J, Klein DC, Thomas TP, Anderson WB (1985) Activation of protein kinase C potentiates isoprenaline-induced cyclic AMP accumulation in rat pinealocytes. Nature 314: 359–361

Takahashi JS (1994) Circadian rhythms. ICER is nicer at night (sir!). Curr Biol 4: 165–168

Takahashi JS, Hamm H, Menaker M (1980) Circadian rhythms of melatonin release from individual superfused chicken pineal glands in vitro. Proc Natl Acad SciUSA 77: 2319–2322

Tosini G, Menaker M (1996) Circadian rhythms in cultured mammalian retina. Science 272: 419–421

Vanecek J, Sugden D, Weller JL, Klein DC (1985)(Atypical synergistic alpha 1- and beta-adrenergic regulation of adenosine 3',5'-monophosphate and guanosine 3',5'-monophosphate in rat pinealocytes. Endocrinology 116: 2167–2173

Prediction of Death in Elderly Men: Endocrine Factors

Annewieke W. van den Beld and *Steven W. J. Lamberts*

Summary

There are numerous definitions of successful aging. Rowe and Kahn (1987, 1997) defined it as including three main components: low probability of disease and disease-related disability, high cognitive and physical functional capacity, and active engagement with life. This definition was taken as a starting point in a study among 403 independently living elderly men. Since low muscle strength and functional ability were highly predictive of four-year mortality in this population, muscle strength and functional ability might be considered as the key characteristics of the physical functional status of independently living elderly men. Growth hormone and testosterone seem to play a role in the physical decline that occurs during aging. In addition, both serum IGF-I and testosterone concentrations are related to the presence of atherosclerosis. However, serum concentrations of both hormones are not predictive of death. Further, the effect of growth hormone and testosterone replacement on quality of life has hardly been examined in the elderly population.

Aging can be approached in two different ways: one can direct attention to the ensuing deficits or to the factors that play a protective role in the decline in function. These different approaches, which are reflected in the concepts of "frailty" and "successful aging," need to be explained. Frailty is defined as a syndrome of multi-system reduction in physiological capacity as a result of which an older person's function may be severely compromised by minor environmental challenges, giving rise to the condition "unstable disability" (Campbell and Buchner 1997). The variable presence of co-morbidity makes research findings more difficult to generalize. Therefore, the alternative of focussing research on the least frail and "non-diseased," which implies the successfully aged, might be easier. Older persons with minimal physiologic loss, or none at all, when compared to the average of their younger counterparts, can be regarded as having aged more broadly successful in physiologic terms (Rowe and Kahn 1987). The concept of frailty focuses mainly on the physical aspects of aging, whereas the concept of successful aging includes a broader range of aspects, such as physical, psychological and social aspects. Neither concept is easy to define in a single measure, and there are no generally accepted criteria to categorize a certain individual.

Chanson et al.
Endocrine Aspects of Successful Aging
© Springer-Verlag Berlin Heidelberg 2004

Although definitions of successful aging in gerontology are numerous, there is still no consensus on the definition of successful aging. Rowe and Kahn (1997) defined it as including three main components: low probability of disease and disease-related disability, high cognitive and physical functional capacity, and active engagement with life (Fig. 1). A definition proposed by Day et al. (2002) focused on psychological well-being, capacity for self care and social support. Fries (1988)   defined successful aging as optimizing life expectancy while simultaneously minimizing physical, psychological and social morbidity. Vaillant and Vaillant (1990) argued that, in addition to physical health, there are three further dimensions, or outcomes, of successful aging: mental health, psychosocial efficiency and life satisfaction.

In our study population we focused on the least frail, which implies the successfully aged. To decrease the number of subjects with severe diseases to a minimum, we invited subjects who lived independently, had no severe mobility problems and did not have signs or symptoms of dementia. Finally, 403 men, aged between 73 and 94 years, participated in this study. The definition of successful aging as illustrated in the model by Rowe and Kahn (1987) was taken as a starting point in order to gain insight into the role and the interactions of the different physical and endocrine factors, aspects that are assumed to be important to age

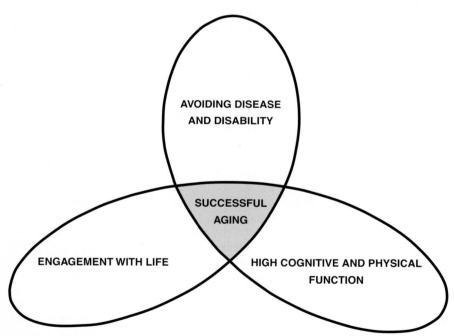

Fig. 1. The concept of "successful aging" as illustrated by the model Rowe and Kahn (1987, 1997) with "maintaining high cognitive and physical functional capacity," "avoiding disease and disability," and "maintaining active engagement with life" as main determinants.

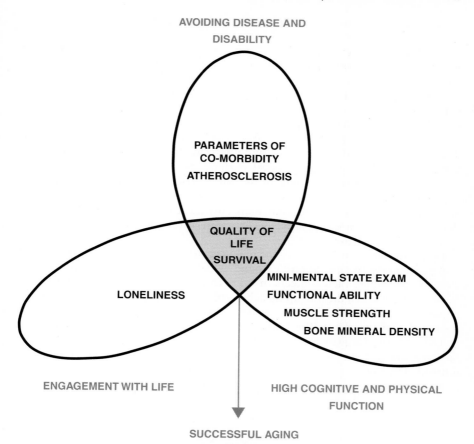

Fig. 2. Parameters measured in our study of 403 elderly men implemented in the model of "successful aging" by Rowe Rowe and Kahn (1987, 1997).

successfully. However, for an individual assessment of successful aging, adequate, reproducible, and if possible predictive measures are needed. Consequently one of the aims of our study was to find parameters that reliably reflect the three different parts of the model. To measure overall successful aging we used two parameters; quality of life and survival. We acknowledge that we were not able to determine all aspects that compromise or influence successful aging, as described by Rowe and Kahn (1987) and illustrated in Figure 2.

How to define chronological and successful aging?

Chronological aging. Many of the predictors of physical functional status appear to be potentially modifiable, and research must be done to refine diagnostic criteria and develop practical methods of measurement of key physiological capacities. This in order to identify proper targets for interventions with disabled elderly or of preventive interventions in 'normal' elderly individuals, with the ultimate goal to enhance the proportion of the older population that ages successfully. Among the physical characteristics measured in this study, several relationships were observed. It is hypothesized that good muscle strength is necessary to maintain high physical performance. A person needs a certain amount of leg extensor strength to be able to rise from a chair. Although the opposite direction is also possible: a good physical performance might lead to a high activity level, which in turn might improve muscle strength. It is hypothesized that muscle strength is a positive determinant of functional ability, whereas fat mass is a negative determinant.

Isometric leg extensor strength was measured as described by Hsieh and Philips using the Hoggan MicroFET hand held dynamometer (Hsieh and Phillips 1990). In our study, a few subjects (n = 12) with isometric grip strength between 30 and 50 kg reached the maximum achievable value of the microFET, as shown in Figure 2. The marked associations between isometric grip strength (IGS) and all the measurements of LES (Fig. 3) indicate that measuring knee extensor strength at 120 with the Hoggan microFET dynamometer provides an easy method to measure strength in elderly men, especially in a home-based setting. This is also illustrated by the normal distribution in our population (Fig. 4).

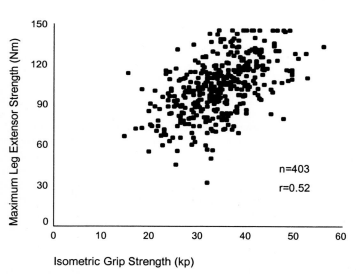

Fig. 3. Association between isometric grip strength and leg extensor strength.

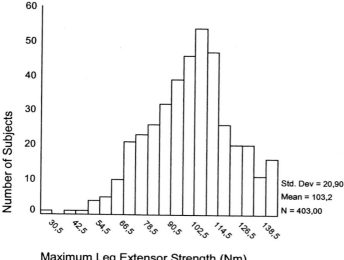

Maximum Leg Extensor Strength (Nm)

Fig. 4. Distribution of leg extensor strength in 403 elderly men.

To define proper targets for intervention and to establish a prognosis, it is necessary to define what the physical capacity of an individual is in relation to his or her chronological age. So far this capacity is not known. As there are probably large inter-individual differences, and these capacities are probably dependent on multiple individual and environmental conditions, it is hypothesized that this capacity should at least be that of an older individual free of disease. This capacity can then serve as a reference for subjects with disease.

The most attractive way, however, to define the key physical characteristic of aging in this study seems to be its predictive value of death. Since low muscle strength and functional ability were highly predictive of four-year mortality in our population (Table 1), we suggest that muscle strength and functional ability (objectively measured with the physical performance test) can be considered the key characteristics of the physical functional status of independently living elderly men. With regard to physical functional capacity, it is suggested that measuring physical performance according to the method described by Guralnik et al. (1994) and muscle strength might be sufficient to be informed about this aspect. However, physical performance may not be modified directly by interventions; it is more likely modified by changes in muscle strength, balance, bone mineral density and perhaps body composition. To select those who might benefit from intervention therapy and to monitor therapy, it may be useful to measure muscle strength and bone mineral density rather than, or in combination with, physical performance.

Table 1. Predictors of 4-year mortality. General characteristics: Relative Risk (95% CI) P-value; Age (yr) 1.39 (1.14 – 1.70) 0.001; Number of diseases (0 – 5) 1.50 (1.03 – 2.17) 0.04. Physical characteristics: Physical Performance (points) 0.71 (0.57 – 0.89) 0.004; Activities of daily living (points) 1.19 (1.00 – 1.43) 0.06; Maximum Leg Extensor Strength (Nm) 0.75 (0.60 – 0.95) 0.02. Somatotropic hormones: Insulin-like Growth Factor-I (ng/l) 0.95 (0.75 – 1.21) 0.68; Insulin (mU/l) 1.09 (0.89 – 1.35) 0.40; Glucose (mmol/l) 0.82 (0.52 – 1.30) 0.40. Gonadal hormones: Total Testosterone (nmol/l) 0.92 (0.74 – 1.14) 0.45. Adrenal hormones: DHEA (nmol/l) 1.07 (0.87 – 1.31) 0.51; DHEAS (µmol/l) 0.84 (0.64 – 1.10) 0.20. Activities of Daily Living (ADL) denotes the number of problems in ADL.

General characteristics	Relative Risk (95% CI)	P-value
Age (yr)	1.39 (1.14 – 1.70)	0.001
Number of diseases (0 - ≥5)	1.50 (1.03 – 2.17)	0.04
Physical characteristics		
Physical Performance (points)	0.71 (0.57 – 0.89)	0.004
Activities of daily living (points)	1.19 (1.00 – 1.43)	0.06
Maximum Leg Extensor Strength (Nm)	0.75 (0.60 – 0.95)	0.02
Somatotropic hormones		
Insulin-like Growth Factor-I (ng/l)	0.95 (0.75 – 1.21)	0.68
Insulin (mU/l)	1.09 (0.89 – 1.35)	0.40
Glucose (mmol/l)	0.82 (0.52 – 1.30)	0.40
Gonadal hormones		
Total Testosterone (nmol/l)	0.92 (0.74 – 1.14)	0.45
Adrenal hormones		
DHEA (nmol/l)	1.07 (0.87 – 1.31)	0.51
DHEAS (µmol/l)	0.84 (0.64 – 1.10)	0.20

Activities of Daily Living (ADL) denotes the number of problems in ADL.

Successful aging. We cannot fully define and assess successful aging, and it is certainly not possible to assess it in one single measurement. Quality of life (QoL), however, is often used in the context of terms like successful aging, and it might be used as a relatively good indicator. We therefore decided to use it as an end-point in this study. In this study we used a QoL questionnaire (QLS) that was recently developed by Herschbach et al. (2001). In the development of this questionnaire, an attempt was made to deal adequately with the problem of the relative importance of individual aspects of QoL. Recent studies with QLS have shown that weighing of the individual items for their importance to the respondent is an effective way to incorporate the concept of subjectivity of QoL in the QoL instrument (8).

As expected, physical functional ability was strongly related with QLS. Although this finding was expected, it has never been demonstrated as clearly that muscle strength was also strongly positively related with QLS and it emphasizes the importance of maintaining muscle strength in old age. Whether a good QoL is a consequence of an overall good physical functional status or whether a good QoL leads to a good physical functional status cannot be established from the results of this study.

In conclusion, the measurement of a combination of both physical performance and muscle strength in older men seems to give optimal information about a subject's chronological age and his life satisfaction. To emphasize the importance of the relationships between physical characteristics and QoL, it was demonstrated that subjects with the lowest QoL had a higher risk of mortality compared to subjects with higher QoL. It is important to know, however, whether these relationships might at least in part be explained by lower hormone concentrations as well.

Endocrine aspects of aging

Several significant relationships exist between serum hormone concentrations of the different axes and physiological determinants of functional capacity, such as physical performance, muscle strength, body composition, and QoL.

Somatotropic axis. Remarkably, but in agreement with other studies, serum IGF-I (total nor the free fraction) was not related to measures of physical functional status (Boonen et al. 1996; Johansson et al. 1994; Erfurth et al. 1996; Rudman et al. 1994; Goodman-Gruen and Barrett-Connor 1997; Papadakis et al. 1995). IGF-I might not be a good marker of the activity of the somatotropic axis during aging. In agreement with this, normal serum IGF-I levels are frequently found in elderly individuals with growth hormone (GH) deficiency (Ghigo et al. 1996). It is known that GH itself exerts anabolic effects (Ho et al. 1996). In addition, serum IGF-I concentrations might not reflect the bio-activity of IGF-I in the different target organs or tissues in a proper manner.

The effect of growth hormone on QoL has hardly been examined in the elderly population. Therefore intervention programs using growth hormone to increase QoL might be an option to investigate the effect of GH on QoL. However, it has to be taken into account that GH is likely to induce many side-effects as well.

Gonadal axis. With regard to the gonadal axis, we demonstrated before that luteinizing hormone (LH), independent of testosterone, reflects serum androgen activity in a different way than testosterone, possibly reflecting more closely the combined feedback effect of estrogen and androgen (van den Beld et al. 1999). Testosterone was positively related to muscle strength and bone mineral density and inversely related to fat mass (van den Beld et al. 2000). Remarkably, no significant association was present with physical performance measured objectively, or with lean body mass.

It might therefore be that the measurement of both testosterone and LH will define elderly men who might benefit better from testosterone replacement therapy. It remains to be established whether LH, perhaps in combination with testosterone, might serve as a parameter of the optimal dose and the effect of androgen replacement therapy.

Although it has been demonstrated in elderly men that bioavailable testosterone levels are lower in men with defined depression compared to other men (Barrett-Connor et al. 1999), the benefits of testosterone replacement therapy on mood and QoL have not been well investigated. In post-menopausal women, estrogen replacement therapy is known to improve subjective well-being (Karlberg et al. 1995), and testosterone replacement in hypogonadal men has been reported to improve well-being (Howell and Shalet 2001). Future research should focus on the conversion of testosterone to estradiol, and its serum concentrations, during testosterone replacement studies, with QoL as an outcome measure.

Although serum testosterone levels were not directly associated with an increased or decreased risk of mortality four years after the initial investigation (Table 1), taking the results of the literature as well as the results of this study into account, it seems beneficial to replace testosterone in some elderly men. In most studies on testosterone replacement therapy, the beneficial effects seem to be greater than the potential risks. However, only a few studies have investigated properly the effects of testosterone replacement therapy on QoL and the mechanism of such a potential effect on QoL. In addition, it is still unclear which elderly men should be treated with testosterone therapy. Are these men defined by lowered serum testosterone levels or subjects with clinical symptoms of androgen deficiency? How should we interpret serum levels and symptoms in the presence of other diseases? Androgen deficiency is very difficult to define, since many symptoms overlap with those of disease and of aging. In conclusion, testosterone replacement should be administered only to very well-defined groups of otherwise "healthy" elderly men with clear clinical symptoms of androgen deficiency, in the presence of lowered serum testosterone and/or high LH levels. Also the use of androgen and estrogen receptor modulators might further elucidate the role of estrogens in men.

Adrenal axis. In agreement with previous findings, serum dehydro-epiandrosterone (DHEA) and its sulfate (DHEAS) both decreased with age in our population (van den Beld et al. 2003). DHEA is sold in the United States in large amounts and has been called the "fountain of youth." Most knowledge concerning the potential function of DHEA, however, was derived from animal studies, mainly from rodents, which do not produce DHEA themselves. Looking at the results of these studies, DHEA (S) is supposed to have a variety of functions, like preventing obesity, cancer, and cardiovascular disease, and it might improve physical as well as psychological well being. However, several studies on DHEA replacement in humans yielded inconsistent and controversial results (Flynn et al. 1999; Morales et al. 1998; Arlt et al. 1999, 2001; Yen et al. 1995; Baulieu et al. 2000). It has well been demonstrated that women with adrenal insufficiency, and therefore very low DHEA levels, benefit from DHEA therapy (Arlt et al. 1999).

In conclusion, data recently published on the potential beneficial effects of DHEA administration in men, which induced a slight improvement on mood scores (Arlt et al. 2001), suggest that this steroid itself only plays a minor role in the aging process. It remains intriguing, however, that DHEAS circulates in the human serum in such high concentrations, probably being a reservoir which is at the tissue level transformed to biologically active sex steroids. The dream of DHEA as a "fountain of youth" remains far away, however.

Atherosclerosis

Avoiding disease and disability is the second component of the model by Rowe and Kahn (1987). In this population, men with certain diseases had a lower functional ability, measured subjectively as well as objectively. This finding indicates the correctness of the model. It is suggested that (subclinical) atherosclerosis is also an aspect of this part of the model. Reducing the atherosclerotic process might lead to a decrease in cerebro- and cardiovascular events, which in turn helps people to age successfully.

We have described recently that serum-free IGF-I concentrations, as well as testosterone and estrone concentrations, are inversely related to the intima-media thickness of the carotid artery (van den Beld et al. 2003). In a previous study, high fasting serum-free IGF-I levels were associated with a reduced number of atherosclerotic plaques, symptomatic cardiovascular disease and lower serum triglyceride levels (Janssen et al. 1998). In our population, free IGF-I, rather than total IGF-I, was independently related to the mean intima-media thickness of the carotid bifurcation, suggesting that it is the easily dissociable IGF-I fraction that may be able to act directly on the vascular wall. On the other hand, a potential effect of free IGF-I on the vascular wall may also be indirect via changes in cholesterol levels or insulin sensitivity. However, in this cross-sectional study the relation between free IGF-I and intima-media thickness was not dependent on cholesterol, glucose or insulin levels.

Testosterone concentrations have never previously been described as being related to the intima-media thickness of the carotid artery. The first question is whether testosterone influences the vascular wall directly or indirectly, via for example changes in the lipid profile or the physical functional ability? The relationship between testosterone and intima-media thickness is independent of serum cholesterol concentrations. However, a definitive answer to this question may only be obtained by performing a placebo-controlled trial with testosterone administration and monitoring the effect on intima-media thickness. Secondly, it can be asked whether, as with IGF-I, serum-free or non-SHBG-bound testosterone levels are more strongly related to the intima-media thickness. This was not the case in our study (data not shown).

References

Arlt W, Callies F, van Vlijmen JC, Koehler I, Reincke M, Bidlingmaier M, Huebler D, Oettel M, Ernst M, Schulte HM, Allolio B (1999) Dehydroepiandrosterone replacement in women with adrenal insufficiency. N Engl J Med 341: 1013–1020

Arlt W, Callies F, Koehler I, van Vlijmen JC, Fassnacht M, Strasburger CJ, Seibel MJ, Huebler D, Ernst M, Oettel M, Reincke M, Schulte HM, Allolio B (2001) Dehydroepiandrosterone supplementation in healthy men with an age- related decline of dehydroepiandrosterone secretion. J Clin Endocrinol Metab 86: 4686–4692

Barrett-Connor E, Von Muhlen DG, Kritz-Silverstein D (1999) Bioavailable testosterone and depressed mood in older men: the Rancho Bernardo Study. J Clin Endocrinol Metab 84: 573–577

Baulieu EE, Thomas G, Legrain S, Lahlou N, Roger M, Debuire B, Faucounau V, Girard L, Hervy MP, Latour F, Leaud MC, Mokrane A, Pitti-Ferrandi H, Trivalle C, de Lacharriere O, Nouveau S, Rakoto-Arison B, Souberbielle JC, Raison J, Le Bouc Y, Raynaud A, Girerd X, Forette F (2000) Dehydroepiandrosterone (DHEA), DHEA sulfate, and aging: contribution of the DHEAge Study to a sociobiomedical issue. Proc Natl Acad Sci USA 97: 4279–4284

Boonen S, Lesaffre E, Dequeker J, Aerssens J, Nijs J, Pelemans W, Bouillon R (1996) Relationship between baseline insulin-like growth factor-I (IGF-I) and femoral bone density in women aged over 70 years: potential implications for the prevention of age-related bone loss. J Am Geriatr Soc 44: 1301–1306

Campbell AJ, Buchner DM (1997) Unstable disability and the fluctuations of frailty [see comments]. Age Ageing 26: 315–318

Day R, Salzet M (2002) The neuroendocrine phenotype, cellular plasticity, and the search for genetic switches: redefining the diffuse neuroendocrine system. Neur Lett 23: 447–451

Erfurth EM, Hagmar LE, Saaf M, Hall K (1996) Serum levels of insulin-like growth factor I and insulin-like growth factor-binding protein 1 correlate with serum free testosterone and sex hormone binding globulin levels in healthy young and middle-aged men. Clin Endocrinol (Oxf) 44: 659–664

Flynn MA, Weaver-Osterholtz D, Sharpe-Timms KL, Allen S, Krause G (1999) Dehydro-epiandrosterone replacement in aging humans. J Clin Endocrinol Metab 84: 1527–1533

Fries JF (1988) Aging, illness, and health policy: implications of the compression of morbidity. Perspect Biol Med 31: 407–428

Ghigo E, Aimaretti G, Gianotti L, Bellone J, Arvat E, Camanni F (1996) New approach to the diagnosis of growth hormone deficiency in adults. Eur J Endocrinol 13: 352–356

Goodman-Gruen D, Barrett-Connor E (1997) Epidemiology of insulin-like growth factor-I in elderly men and women. The Rancho Bernardo Study [published erratum appears in Am J Epidemiol 1997 Aug 15;146(4):357]. Am J Epidemiol 145: 970–976

Guralnik JM, Seeman TE, Tinetti ME, Nevitt MC, Berkman LF (1994) Validation and use of performance measures of functioning in a non- disabled older population: MacArthur studies of successful aging. Aging (Milano) 6: 410–419

Herschbach P, Heinrich G, Strasburger CJ, Feldmeier H, Marin F, Attanasio AM, Blum WF Development and psychometric properties of a disease-specific quality of life questionnaire for adult patients with growth hormone deficiency. Eur J Endocrinol 145: 255–265

Ho KK, O'Sullivan AJ, Hoffman DM (1996) Metabolic actions of growth hormone in man. Endocr J 43 Suppl: S57–63

Howell S, Shalet S (2001) Testosterone deficiency and replacement. Horm Res 56(Suppl 1): 86–92

Hsieh CY, Phillips RB (1990) Reliability of manual muscle testing with a computerized dynamometer. J Manip Physiol Ther 13: 72–82

Janssen JA, Stolk RP, Pols HA, Grobbee DE, Lamberts SW (1998) Serum total IGF-I, free IGF-I, and IGFB-1 levels in an elderly population: relation to cardiovascular risk factors and disease. Arterioscler Thromb Vasc Biol 18: 277–282

Johansson AG, Forslund A, Hambraeus L, Blum WF, Ljunghall S (1994) Growth hormone-dependent insulin-like growth factor binding protein is a major determinant of bone mineral density in healthy men. J Bone Miner Res 9: 915–921

Karlberg J, Mattsson LA, Wiklund I (1995) A quality of life perspective on who benefits from estradiol replacement therapy. Acta Obstet Gynecol Scand 74(5): 367–372.

Morales AJ, Haubrich RH, Hwang JY, Asakura H, Yen SS (1998) The effect of six months treatment with a 100 mg daily dose of dehydroepiandrosterone (DHEA) on circulating sex steroids, body composition and muscle strength in age-advanced men and women. Clin Endocrinol (Oxf) 49: 421–432

Papadakis MA, Grady D, Tierney MJ, Black D, Wells L, Grunfeld C (1995) Insulin-like growth factor 1 and functional status in healthy older men. J Am Geriatr Soc 43: 1350–1355

Rowe JW, Kahn RL (1987) Human aging: usual and successful. Science 237: 143–149

Rowe JW, Kahn RL (1997) Successful aging [see comments]. Gerontologist 37: 433–440

Rudman D, Drinka PJ, Wilson CR, Mattson DE, Scherman F, Cuisinier MC, Schultz S (1994) Relations of endogenous anabolic hormones and physical activity to bone mineral density and lean body mass in elderly men. Clin Endocrinol (Oxf) 40: 653–661

Vaillant GE, Vaillant CO (1990) Natural history of male psychological health, XII: a 45-year study of predictors of successful aging at age 65. Am J Psychiat 147: 31–37

van den Beld A, Huhtaniemi IT, Pettersson KS, Pols HA, Grobbee DE, de Jong FH, Lamberts SW (1999) Luteinizing hormone and different genetic variants, as indicators of frailty in healthy elderly men. J Clin Endocrinol Metab 84: 1334–1339

van den Beld AW, de Jong FH, Grobbee DE, Pols HA, Lamberts SW (2000) Measures of bioavailable serum testosterone and estradiol and their relationships with muscle strength, bone density, and body composition in elderly men. J Clin Endocrinol Metab 85: 3276–3282

Van Den Beld AW, Bots ML, Janssen JA, Pols HA, Lamberts SW, Grobbee DE (2003) Endogenous hormones and carotid atherosclerosis in elderly men. Am J Epidemiol 157: 25–31

Yen SS, Morales AJ, Khorram O (1995) Replacement of DHEA in aging men and women. Potential remedial effects. Ann NY Acad Sci 774: 128–142

Subject Index

Printing: Saladruck Berlin
Binding: Stürtz AG, Würzburg

DATE DUE

FEB 1 8 2010

The Wonder of Food

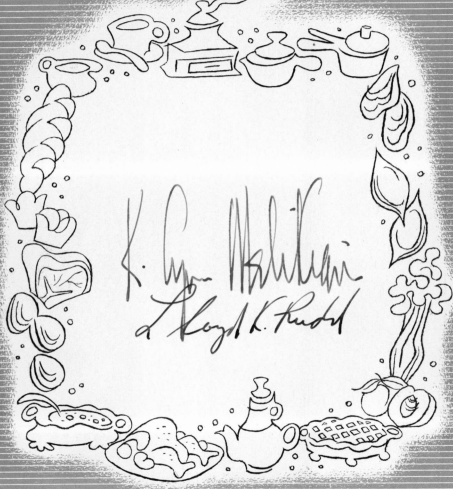

THE WONDER OF FOOD

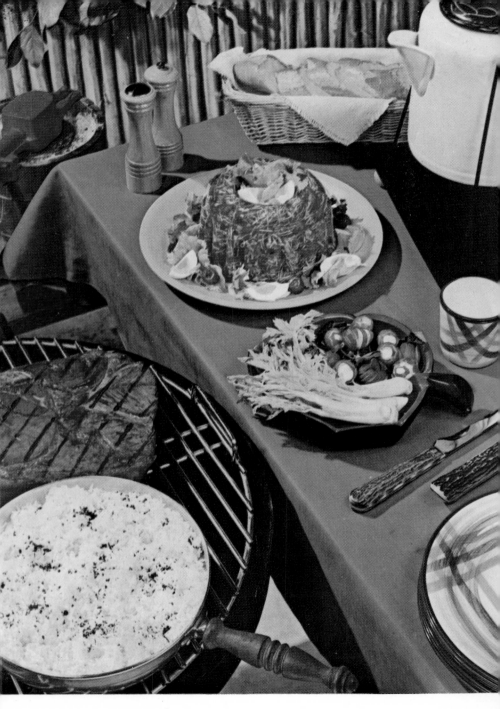

Culinary Magic For Outdoor Enjoyment.

The Wonder of Food

By K. Cyrus Melikian
and Lloyd K. Rudd

Appleton-Century-Crofts, Inc.
New York

FOREWORD

The subject of food holds boundless fascination for us. As executives of a successful concern which manufactures equipment for dispensing food and beverages automatically, and as enthusiastic food hobbyists, it is a subject we discuss, and learn something new about, almost constantly. The special knowledge and appreciation of food thus acquired gave us the idea for this book.

We discarded immediately the notion of compiling a cookbook. What we wanted to do was to try to create a work that would stir in the reader the same excitement and fascination for food, in all its forms, that we have. This called, we felt, not merely for a collection of recipes interspersed with information on food preparation and menu planning, but rather for a penetrating yet informal look at some of the historical aspects of food and food processing, using recipes we had collected to supplement and illustrate our story.

From what, for example, does our word "supper" derive? Why do we call potatoes "spuds?" Did they originally come from Ireland? How is coffee harvested and processed? What are the ancient origins of bread? It is the answers to this type of question that make up the greater part of THE WONDER OF FOOD.

The intent of this book, then, is to incite the reader to

a greater interest in and enjoyment of food by increasing his knowledge of it. It includes recipes—some old stand-bys with a new twist, others that are special favorites of ours that may or may not have been previously found in print. We have also added some personal pointers on the preparing and serving of meals both indoors and out.

Whether his dish be old-fashioned beef stew or *moules a l'escargot,* if some of the romance and the true wonder of food come through to the reader—if, after a perusal of these pages, the meals he eats at home or away from home become a bit more meaningful and pleasurable to him— then we have accomplished our purpose.

K. C. M.

L. K. R.

November 1961

CONTENTS

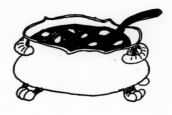

1

"Soup, Beautiful Soup..."

by K. Cyrus Melikian

Soup has a history almost as old as humanity itself. As soon as primitive man had fire to cook with he hollowed out a stone, set it in the center of his fire outside his cave, and soup was born. Maybe his dish was something between soup and stew, yet it is still the great-grand-daddy of all meat-stock soups today. And now, as then, it can be either the first course of a dinner or a whole nourishing meal in itself.

Soup. Where did the word come from? Its origin dates back to before the Middle Ages. The ancient ancestor, so the dictionaries say, was Teutonic, but its descendants became citizens of all the countries of Europe and later, America. It is a distant relative of our words "supper" and "sup" and probably of "sop," as in the sense of sopping-up good-tasting soups and gravies with bread. It comes to us from those days when dinner, whether for hard-working folk or the landed aristocracy who gorged themselves in the banquet hall of the castle, took place at midday and supper was—you guessed it—soup.

1

In Old French we find the word *soupe,* although today the French use the word *potage,* which is related to the pot in which the soup is made. To this day, everywhere in the world, soups are made in pots, whether they be of iron, copper, stainless steel, aluminum, or glassware.

But let's get down to components. Soup is essentially an extract of the various soluble solid ingredients that go into a pot along with water. Soups, except for the strictly vegetable purees, such as bean, pea and potato, start with a stock—beef, mutton, fowl, fish or shellfish. That's the beginning and from that point on there's no end to the variety of soups—clear or cream, thick or thin, crystalline bouillon or rich, square-meal gumbo. A thousand soups are yours for the mere inventing—and the care and ingenuity you put into them. All human nourishment, health and strength, come from Mother Earth, either directly or in roundabout ways. The heartier soups convey, in one spoonful, the most variegated nourishment of any dish you can put on the table. First, a brief classification of soups:

Protein Soups

These might be called the "essence soups"—clear distillations of meat stock with only, perhaps, the addition of rice or noodles. They are refinements of old-time beef tea, a domestic standby of other years. They are quick energizers, pickups with special values for fast-growing children and convalescents. In the form of consommé and bouillon they are nonfilling and quickly absorbed, leaving the appetite stimulated rather than dulled as heavy soups would do. As soup stock, they form the very foundation of all meat-stock soups, simple or elaborate.

Cream Soups

Cream soups are more than merely dairy-rich. Besides their ingredients of milk or cream and butter they also contain the vegetable values of other basic ingredients, as in cream of spinach, cream of cauliflower, cream of celery, and cream of tomato. Many cream soups start with a cream of chicken stock and are built up from there. Yet such a base is not at all necessary. Cream-of-corn soup, for instance, calls for no assistance from meat or fish or fowl. The sugar element in corn, beets, and peas might conflict with these stocks.

Chilled Soups

These are not necessarily hot weather soups, although they are undoubtedly most appreciated in summer. Cold soup has a refreshing quality as a first course of a dinner at any time of year. If a full meal is to follow, cold soup should be served in cups, since too much chill will retard the flow of digestive juices. The imaginative hostess can add piquancy to her party dinner by serving a chilled soup to begin a hot meal. Cold soups can be clear bouillons or cream soups, and nothing is lost in the chilling. Among the non-stock soups are such gastronomical treats as iced cream of avocado, cream of cucumber, cream of tomato, cream of asparagus, cream of watercress, and that popular importation, borsch, a beet and cabbage combination.

Sea Food Soups

The sea is rich in the minerals that go into the physical composition of man. There's a theory—I can't vouch for it—that food from the sea is brain food. That should make seashore dwellers, fishermen and their families and lobster-potters the world's leading intellectuals. But in nutritional value there's no doubt about the value of as well as the deliciousness of sea food soups. Perhaps they do take a little more "doing" than what might be called land-based soups, but in tastiness they are well worth it.

Sea food soups chiefly fall somewhere between soups

and stews. For the housewife they involve more preparation than other soups, but, being originally bland in flavor,
they invite—indeed demand—the use of herbs and spices
which often would be out of place in other soups. Oyster
bisque, clam bisque, turtle soup, snapper soup (actually
made from turtle base) and cream of crab all call for a
well-stocked herb shelf. Sea food soups largely fall in the
category of full-meal soups, since they usually include
such vegetables as potatoes, beans, and carrots. They call
for such flavorings as bay leaf, thyme, and nutmeg. But,
sir or madam, don't attempt a real all-out bouillabaisse
unless you are ready for it. It involves some really devoted
kitchen work.

That defines briefly the major categories of soups. Now
for some of what I might call soup stories, experiences,
comments and conclusions of famous cooks who, with
their art, have given the world the great soups we enjoy
today.

It has been said that Monsieur Grimod d'la Regnier,
one of the illustrious gastronomes of all time, proclaimed
that soup was to a dinner what a porch or gateway was to
a building; that not only must it be the foremost portion
thereof but also it must be so devised as to convey a fore-
taste of the whole to which it belongs. Indeed, lifting
soup into the field of art, it should be what an orchestral
overture is to an operetta, comprising some of the main
phrases of the melodies to come.

In contrast, hear this: Famous restaurateurs of Paris
know that there has been a current of thought among
epicures during the past thirty years toward eliminating
soup entirely from the *haute cuisine* because soup is so
very filling that the delicate flavors and gustatory pleasures
of the meal to come may be grossly impaired. And of

course, nothing must impair the ecstasy of an epicure or a gourmet when he sits down to table.

Perhaps there may be, someday, eating spots in Paris that will omit soups, but in the provinces—never! The provincial housewife will continue to maintain the soup pot on the back of the range and will add good things to it from day to day, enriching it with nutritious meat and bones left over from the family servings. Her children will grow strong and healthy on the tempting, steamy contents of that perennial *pot-au-feu*. More power to her.

It is quite possible that the people of France—both the housewives and the professional chefs—have done more for the artistic (yes, that's the word) development of soups than the cooks of any other country. Or perhaps that belief arises because French cuisine got such a head start internationally that the great cooks of other countries have never been able to catch up in renown.

The great restaurants of the world have sought out and publicized their French chefs to the extent that these men have become known by name to millions of fastidious diners and famed restaurants bear their names. Such a person is M. Careme, a fabulous chef, for whom the Sheraton Hotel in Philadelphia has recently completed the Café Careme. And how did M. Careme achieve his fame? Largely by initiating many improvements in the methods of preparing soups.

Who would have supposed that a famous French soup was actually born in America? Or, anyway, it has a famous French name. It is Vichyssoise, and here's the story. Louis Diat, a Frenchman, was head chef at the Ritz Hotel in New York and, experimenting in his art, he devised a potato soup and named it Vichyssoise. It was accepted with gusto by his patrons, who assumed it was a native of France. But, it seems, the Parisians had never heard of it.

Presenting it as a French soup was a mischievous and engaging hoax but Vichyssoise was so delicious and immediately popular that no one could resent the misrepresentation. Actually, today Vichyssoise is making some of the menus in the fine restaurants of Paris. It is a magnificent soup, a gastronomic delight, especially when served over a bowl of cracked ice and garnished with finely chopped chives. Yet to enjoy it at its best, one must be in America.

Here is a labor-saving way to prepare it. Chop finely together four well-washed leeks and one medium-size onion and sauté them in a pan with a tablespoonful of butter, letting them get tender but not brown. Remove to soup pot and add three cups of chicken stock—canned chicken bouillion or consommé will do nicely. Cook for about fifteen minutes, then strain the mixture through a coarse sieve. Add one-quarter cup of dehydrated mashed potato powder, stirring it in thoroughly until smooth and blended. Season with salt and freshly ground pepper to taste. Add a tablespoon of butter and a cup of light cream. Heat over a low fire but do not let it boil. Let the soup cool. It can be served either chilled as Vichyssoise or as hot potato soup. If you are serving it as Vichyssoise, chill in the refrigerator and serve icy cold, garnishing the servings with chopped chives and paprika. If you are serving it as hot potato soup—no boiling, please—the garnishing is the last touch, of course. For the hot serving you might garnish with grated cheese or diced crisp bacon.

Onion soup, too, is an American favorite. You will find it on the menu at Maxim's in Paris but, shockingly enough, not on the menus of other equally famous restaurants patronized by epicures. The reason for this as explained to me by Ramon Olivier, one of the great gourmet restaurant operators of Paris, is that the French would never think of having onion soup with a dinner, since it is normally served in a large bowl and, being a small meal in itself, should be enjoyed after the opera or other evening entertainment. And where would the restaurant owner be if his dinner patrons were so nourished that they didn't feel the need or desire for any dinner at all to follow the soup? This is especially true when the onion soup is built up with a topping of rich cheese.

Incidentally, the cheese that is used to roof over the bowl of onion soup in the best places in Paris is Swiss Gruyère, which in the warmth of the soup becomes a luscious stringy, sticky layer, tempting to the spoon. It is then crowned with a sprinkling of Italian Parmesan, grated to powder form. That elevates it to the nobility. Here in America, for the most part, we use an Anglicized version of Parmesan and sprinkle it only lightly over the soup.

There are certainly times when a hostess, like the French restaurateurs, just doesn't want her dinner guests to be so ecstatic over a filling soup that they aren't able to appreciate the dinner that follows. To make sure that they do appreciate that dinner let's consider clear soup— soup that stimulates rather than dulls the appetite, that increases the gastric receptivity for the good things to come.

Just as thick soups are subject to scores of flavor variations depending upon the ingenuity, inventiveness and personal preferences of the cook, clear soups can be made to range a full scale of blended flavors and sub-flavors. It is not only a matter of herbs and spices, it is also a matter of solids, both meat and vegetable, that are added to the original beef or chicken stock—whether that stock is a prepared store-bought bouillon or a rendered home-made stock.

For the cook who likes to pioneer and discover, and has a discriminating palate, there is fun and satisfaction in creating something new. The game does, indeed, call for close watching and frequent tasting to produce a certain wanted flavor or a newly devised surprising flavor. Testing by tasting has been an essential part of the art of soup-making from time immemorial.

In preparing a basic soup stock, whether chicken or beef, there is the possibility that one batch of stock will vary somewhat from another batch, due to the richness and flavor of the original solid ingredients. For instance, a chicken wing or leg from a mature fowl will result in a somewhat different flavor than one from a broiler, and in preparing meat stock a marrow bone from an old tired steer will not have the marrow value of a bone from a prime beef animal. Similar variations may be due to the kind of vegetable ingredients used, garden fresh or from storage, or due merely to the time of year the soup pot is put on to boil. The storage vegetable cannot be expected to contribute the rare delicacy of the newly ripened vegetable.

Simmer, simmer, simmer—but keep an eye on the stock pot and keep a tasting spoon handy. This brewing job needs close attention to forestall the danger of boiling the liquid too far down, leaving you with bare bones, and a small quantity of concentrate. Salted water, to replace that which has boiled away, will restore the bulk without lessening the flavor. When your tasting spoon says that all the goodness has been extracted from the solids and just the right combination of herbs and spices has wielded its magic charms it is time for the sieve, time for the used-up solids to be strained off and the clear soup to emerge.

A really clear soup or consommé must be free from fat, so the big bowl of now-clear stock must cool for a few hours, letting the fat and oils come to the top and form a crust which can then be easily skimmed off. With that last pleasant labor accomplished you have either a wondrously clear soup for cup-serving as a first course at dinner or a soup stock for future use. It should be well refrigerated in capped Mason jars, and it will keep as long as you want.

Perhaps every country in the world has contributed great soups to the international cuisine, the recipes for the most part dictated by the food ingredients that are at hand in the various and contrasting regions of the world. Many of these soups started simply and, through the skill of later chefs, evolved into soup magnificence, emerging from mere nourishing provender to become prized items of the *haute cuisine*.

First, however, an example of a fairly simple soup that had its birth in necessity. Its ingredients were assembled from the rather limited supplies that a new and developing country could furnish, but it was eventually transformed into a notable delicacy. It is Cheddar soup and it originated in its American form as a great favorite in colonial days, a soup that needed no meat, fish or fowl base. Along with American ingenuity, the New England iron foundries and the determination of embattled farmers, you might say it played a part in the establishment of the United States.

Cheddar soup in its earliest and simplest form was little more than a non-stock vegetable soup with the addition of butter, flour and pot milk, seasoned with garlic, pepper, and nutmeg to taste and topped with grated Cheddar cheese which, at that time just as today, was a product of Vermont. But once the lean days of war and postwar were gone, inventive cooks elevated Cheddar soup to an epicurean upper echelon.

Incidentally, if you are eating out on a gala day and lucky enough to be in the general neighborhood of New England, northern New Jersey or eastern Pennsylvania look for Cheddar soup on the menus of small inns and countryside restaurants, the sort of eating places not likely to be found on the big expressways. Just to name an example, there is the Coventry Forge Inn in Pennsylvania, which seats only thirty-two people and is operated by the Callahan brothers, both of whom have a flair for delighting the palate.

Tie on the apron and assemble these ingredients on the kitchen table: half a cup each of finely diced carrots, fresh celery, green pepper, and white onions. These can all be diced at the same time in a big chopping bowl. Other ingredients are four cups of chicken stock (canned will do), four tablespoons of butter and the same of flour, two cups of milk, and two cups of grated Cheddar cheese —the more aged the cheese the better.

Now, over a slow fire cook the chopped vegetables for about thirty minutes. Strain and combine the stock and cooked vegetables in the pot. Add the melted butter and blend in the flour, slowly stirring. Bring to a simmer and add the milk, stirring it in. Bring the mixture to a boil. Because of the milk the pot will need watching and continuous stirring but this you will regard later as a labor of love. Simmer for about five minutes, then, little by little, add the two cups of grated Cheddar, keeping your spoon busy until the cheese is melted. Salt and pepper to taste.

And there you are, ready to serve about eight people. Not much work at all, really, considering the glorious result. You will note that while the primitive recipe included no stock at all, chicken stock is now used and, of course, gives this evolved Cheddar soup an added deliciousness and nourishment.

Would you ever believe that a soup recipe could be the opening wedge to fame and fortune? It may have happened more than once in history but here is one instance of it that I happen to know of personally.

A French chef by the name of X. Marcel Boulestin,

whose genius at the range was unparalleled in his native land, decided to give the British, sometimes derided for their uninspired cooking, a chance to learn what really artistic cooking could be.

Boulestin moved across the English Channel and set himself up as a gastronomical missionary. The result? He attracted not only a devoted local trade but also flavor-conscious travelers from America and all of Europe, for whom his restaurant became one of the "must" places. This pretty much started with a soup called Potage Germiny (sic). Perhaps he did not invent Potage Germiny but he glorified it.

Want to try it? Well, it can't be properly prepared while you're watching a television program but if you really want a treat—not to mention the breathless admiration of your family and guests—stand by for the story of how to produce a masterpiece.

First, prepare about a quart of clear beef soup. This can be done by using either commercially canned bouillon or bouillon cubes. Of course, if you want to be quite professional about it as well as have the satisfaction of creating this great soup from start to finish, you can make your own clear beef stock using almost any kind of inexpensive beef—shin beef, back of rump, back of round or something higher priced if you prefer. There's your basis.

From your herb shelf get down the sorrel and the chervil—both wonderful seasoning herbs that should have a place in every food-lover's kitchen. Melt two or three tablespoons of butter in a saucepan and meld into it, stirring it smooth, two tablespoons of sorrel. Bring your pot of clear stock to a boil then reduce it to a simmer for about ten minutes. Stir the butter and sorrel into the soup as it simmers. From this point on it must not boil.

Next, one at a time, bind in the yolks of four eggs,

making sure they integrate thoroughly, and add a cup of fresh cream. The mixture, stirred constantly over a slow fire, will become smooth and thick—a real potage. Keep the stirring spoon moving gently while the pot simmers for another eight or ten minutes. Put a dollop of butter on the surface and let it float, melt and infiltrate, adding its richness to the soup. Reach for the chervil and add a small dash of it to give piquancy.

It's done—and that wasn't too much of a job, was it? Certainly not, considering the marvelous result! As it is ladled out into bowls or cups add small croutons. Climax! And those at your table will, in spirit, be dining with "The Thirteen Club" in London or in M. Boulestin's restaurant along with the devoted gourmets and epicures of two continents.

Now we come to that fantastic Soup of Soups—bouillabaisse. When that name is mentioned in some circles gentlemen bow and ladies curtsy. Bouillabaisse was humbly born—none more so—and ascended, through skill and talent—not to say the devotion of a world-wide faithful following—to a position of royalty. That is, soup royalty. And it remains there without fear of challenge, revolution or *coup de cuisine*. It does not rule as a monarch but rather dominates as a beloved and inspired leader, a conqueror of all who love glorified food.

For centuries past, Marseilles, France, on the Mediterranean, has been a fishing port, once a small village, now a great seaport. It is still, now as in its earliest days, home port of professional fishermen and one of the great sources of sea food for all of France and beyond. In bringing home the catch and preparing it for market fishermen are always bound to have odds and ends of sea food, both fish and shellfish, that are just not salable commercially. Throw them back into the sea for the gulls and sharks? No fisherman's wife would condone that kind of waste.

Let the sharks and gulls catch their own fish. There were hungry menfolk to cook for and here at hand were the ingredients for a fine soup pot.

Combining the best parts of whatever didn't go to market, some suitable and available vegetables and, judiciously, various herbs, spices and flavorings, bouillabaisse was born. Perhaps you could call it a chowder, since it is thick and hearty enough to be a complete meal in itself. That was how it started, a make-do with tidbits that had no other usefulness and would not bring in a money profit, yet would contribute strength to the hardworking fishermen and health to their children.

Really classic bouillabaisse must, of course, be made with the sea food ingredients available only from the Mediterranean. They cannot be duplicated at any fishing port or market in America. But, take heart. They can be approximated not only along our seashores but from coast to coast, wherever you may live—prairie, forest, desert, mountain. I'll tell you how. But first, I'll describe the way modern Mediterranean bouillabaisse is made by those great chefs who picked up the humble fishpot of long ago and lifted it to royalty.

First, the Mediterranean sea food ingredients—and, mind you, there are many variations of the recipe so I am specifying neither quantity nor procedure. The recipe calls for portions and cuts of mackerel, eel, red snapper, lobster, shrimp, mussels, sea bass and clams. The vegetables are carrots, leeks, onions, tomatoes, and turnips. For flavoring, add garlic bay leaf, chives, salt, pepper, and saffron. That last item, saffron, is most important. It furnishes the dominating flavor of the finished soup, ties together, you might say, the catch-all ingredients of bouillabaisse, unifies it as a distinctive identity among soups. When it comes to serving the lovers of bouillabaisse, either the solids and the liquid may be served together or the solids may be put on a platter for personal selection and the wonderfully flavored liquid served separately.

Does the whole thing suggest a lot of kitchen work? All great results are based on dedicated work. However, if you are not near enough the shores of the Mediterranean to shop around for all these ingredients with their very special regional qualities, unique to those shores, here's a way to make bouillabaisse no matter where you live, as long as it's within reach of a supermarket or a fresh-fish market.

Based on the list of ingredients given above you are hereby elected to be your own boss, that is, you must decide how much and how many of the classic ingredients will go into your version of bouillabaisse. From the deep freeze at the market you may select, according to your own preferences, portions of the following: lobster meat, bass or red snapper, clams or mussels, mackerel, shrimp, bass (sea or fresh water), eel, if available. And if you have any leaning toward other forms of sea food by all means include them.

With those items assembled as the basis of your melange you are ready to start and that start begins with sautéing three or four cut-up onions in olive oil. Next add a tin of tomato purée, stirring it in. Into this thickening mixture, now on the simmer, squeeze some garlic juice from fresh garlic cloves, using as much as your taste for garlic dictates. Now toss into the pot some chopped-up fresh parsley, a dash of fennel, bay leaves and chives, and when all these are melded in add a small amount of hot water, a little at a time, and keep stirring. Now for the sea food—and here let me say that the size of the portions used must be at your own discretion, since this dish is your own concoction and of your own pioneering. Bear in mind that one of the Commandments in cooking is to be resourceful and use your imagination. Those two qualities have gone into every great dish ever put on the table.

After some twenty minutes over a slow fire add the cut-up sea food—bivalves, shellfish, finny fish—and bring to a simmer again for twenty minutes or so. Then add the previously cooked vegetables. Now for the final and distinguishing flavor—saffron. Add it a little at a time, suiting the quantity used to the tastes and preferences of those who are to be served. You have it made.

Speaking of the ancestors of great recipes here's a soup with a lineage that is hard to match—Philadelphia Pepper Pot. In the city of Philadelphia in 1758 or thereabouts there came from the Low Countries of western Europe the first groups of a religious sect known as Moravians. They made settlements in the area of Bethlehem, probably bestowing that hallowed name on their new home. They were, for the most part, Holland Dutch and in morality, cleanliness, industry and frugality—not to say an appreciation of the art of cooking—they were unsurpassed by any immigrants to these shores.

While their descendants over the centuries since have contributed their sturdy qualities to our republic, they have also brought to greater perfection the food conceptions of their forebears. One of their dishes came to be known as Dutch Pepper Pot in rural Pennsylvania and from that beginning, inheriting all the original excellence of Dutch Pepper Pot, came today's Philadelphia Pepper Pot, famous from coast to coast.

Philadelphia Pepper Pot is a soup that can be made for six people, sixty people, or six hundred people, but we'll just talk about the family-size job for the moment. It starts with honeycomb tripe, one of the finest basic ingredients in savor that any soup could have. The first thing to do is to wash the tripe thoroughly in cold water —and do it more than once. This is important.

Buy half a pound of tripe per person, a knuckle of veal and half a pound of beef suet. From your vegetable bin select two Bermuda onions and four medium-size potatoes. Put the well-washed tripe into a pot of water, allowing plenty of water for steaming away. At this point it would be all right to catch your favorite TV shows because the tripe must boil for four hours or more to make it tender and to obtain all of its goodness.

At the end of your boiling time you have a stock pot, although it should not be as concentrated a stock as for lighter soups. Shut off the fire, let the pot cool, take out the tripe, and cut it into small pieces. Wash the veal knuckle and put it into the pot, bringing it up to a simmer and holding it there for two or three hours, skimming frequently. At this point you begin to think that you should have started all this the day before. Never mind. You will be rewarded for your time and attention.

Take out the veal, which has added a very special taste to this energizing soup, and cut from the bone any meat that might be there, now as tender as butter. You have a broth which should be strained and returned to the pot to simmer again. Add the diced potatoes and onions. There should be enough broth to cover. Many cooks using dry pot herbs, such as thyme, oregano, and bay leaf, for flavoring this and other soups, tie the herbs into a little muslin bag and put the bag into the liquor or broth. The flavors are contributed as thoroughly as if the herbs were individually immersed and, of course, they are much more easily removed from the stock.

The pot has already been salted to taste and now, just before serving, comes the touch that gives the soup its name—Cayenne pepper. It must be the real thing and, for best results, freshly ground. Cayenne gives the zestful, hot peppery taste that makes the soup distinctive, the taste that will linger afterward and make everyone want seconds. Of course the quantity of Cayenne can be varied depending upon the individual pepper-loving preferences of the "customers." Cayenne is the magic in this dish. When the soup is poured into cups or soup plates garnish the servings with freshly chopped parsley and your folks will be as thrilled at your table as if they were seated in the best restaurant in Philadelphia.

Here's another way to top it if the gang is really hungry. Make small dumplings by blending the suet—butter, if you prefer—with flour and a little salt and just enough water to make a thick paste and roll into marble-size balls or larger if you prefer. Sprinkle the dumplings with flour and drop them into the soup about five or ten minutes before serving. Allow the dumplings to simmer for five or ten minutes, keeping the pot covered so as not to let the volatile aroma escape. If you cook the soup with the lid off you will find that your Pepper Pot has become a little wishy-washy.

Now for a true luxury soup—oyster stew. There was a day when Americans who lived inland simply couldn't make an oyster stew because oysters couldn't be packed to travel far from their native watery depths. Then some enterprising man developed a way to can them so they could be shipped and stocked indefinitely in grocery stores. This brought oyster stew to the whole continent. While the flavor might not have been quite that of sea-fresh oysters it was still awfully good.

Today, from the deep freeze of your supermarket you can pick up packs of frozen oysters which are so close in freshness and flavor to those that the oysterman brings ashore that, unless you're equipped with superior taste buds, you'll never know the difference when they are used in oyster stew.

Here is a classic recipe for a really classic soup. Assemble the following for a generous serving of six:

2 dozen shucked oysters—
  with the oyster liquor, if
  possible
1 cup of light cream
5 cups of whole milk

¼ cup of butter
Salt and pepper
Freshly chopped parsley for
  later garnishing

If you have a double boiler large enough for a service of six, that's the thing to use. If not, then a pot—but *not* an iron pot—is the next best thing, although it will mean a closer watching to prevent scorching. If you use a pot, go easy on the heat and don't spare the stirring spoon. We'll say you are going to use the double boiler.

Have the water boiling violently in the lower part of your double boiler and pour the milk and cream into the upper. Incidentally, you may vary the richness of the stew to suit the preferences of your tablemates by diluting the cream and milk with a little water or by omitting the water—in short, making it virtually a full meal or merely a soup to precede a meal.

Let the milk and cream come close to a simmer, really hot. Then add the oysters and the water, if any, and stand by to watch the oysters expand and become plump. When the edges start to curl they've had enough. Spoon them out tenderly and, if you wish, add some more milk, cream, or water to give just the consistency you have in mind. Bring up the heat again and add salt and pepper to taste. Put the oysters back in the pot and heat well. Add the melted butter and stir it in.

You have heated a soup tureen and, at your pleasure, you may take the pot itself to the table and pour the stew into heated bowls. Pop some small oyster O.T.C. (Old Trenton Crackers) onto each serving and sprinkle on a garnish of chopped fresh parsley. And there's a bowl to set before a king!

If you have chosen to make a really rich stew it can

be an entire meal, luncheon or dinner, rounded off with some light dessert and coffee. You may consider eight ounces of this oystew stew as a first course, but ten or twelve ounces—well, you've been fed.

On the subject of bland and milky soups such as oyster stew here's one that has both zest and nourishment, the kind of nourishment relished and needed by those who have, perhaps, finicky stomachs, and by convalescents. It is pretzel soup, another gift from Pennsylvania, whose early Dutch settlers had an inventiveness and skill in devising economical and energizing soups.

If you've always thought of pretzels as something to nibble while enjoying a beaker of cool beer here's a new slant on how to use them. For four servings in bowls assemble a dozen or so pretzels, fresh and crisp, six cups of fresh whole milk, a little flour, some freshly chopped parsley and two tablespoons of butter. Melt the butter without sizzling it in the pot over a low fire and stir in the sifted flour. When the flour and butter are blended add the milk very slowly, stirring it in. Bring the pot to a heat just short of boiling and stir in maybe a quarter-teaspoonful of freshly ground black pepper from your pepper mill and the chopped parsley. But no salt; the pretzels will furnish that.

As you see, this soup is a quickie—no long sessions at the range. The job can be done in twenty minutes. You have warmed your serving bowls in the oven and, now, into each bowl break about four pretzels into small pieces. Pour the steaming soup over the pretzels in the bowls and serve. If you wish, add another sprinkling of parsley on top of each serving. It will not only contribute its wonderful flavor but it will also "pretty-up" the bowl.

Speaking of prettying-up a cup or bowl of soup, the art of garnishing calls for some special attention. Garnishing a soup is far more than making it appeal to the eye.

Most garnishes add both fragrance and flavor, contributing those small secondary taste delicacies that make a soup a real creation rather than a mere routine first course.

Here are some garnishings that are both decorative and appetizing. For cream-type soups, of course, a sprinkling of paprika, freshly ground if possible, and a tiny sprig of parsley combine to make a gay, inviting surface, a delightful picture, especially pleasing on clam chowder (cream style), oyster stew, Vichyssoise (with chives), and cream of chicken. Brown croutons and snipped-up chives do wonders for clear soups both visually and gastronomically. Chopped-up toasted almonds give an Oriental touch to such soups as purée of green pea.

A small island of salty whipped cream on a cream of tomato soup adds both flavor and charm. And for lentil soup or split pea soup slice up some small cocktail frankfurters and drop them in together with some old-fashioned oyster crackers. Then, also, there is plain grated American cheese or Parmesan cheese and, if you care to go quite professional, a touch of nutmeg or cinnamon, depending upon the basic soup flavor, and you have produced a taste thrill.

Although flavor and contrasting colors in garnishings contribute appeal to any soup, there are less colorful garnishes that give a soup added piquancy to the palate. One of these is bacon. A few strips of bacon should be fried to crispness and then allowed to cool and dry on paper—a paper towel will do nicely. Crumble the bacon into crisp little flakes and sprinkle them on the surface of the bowl of soup. This can be used on almost all soups except, perhaps, those based on beef stock. Bacon crumbs will go particularly well on cream soups, sea food or vegetable.

Italian-type breadsticks broken up into small bits

furnish another garnish and contribute an added nutritive element to any soup, as well as making an attractive dotted surface in cup, bowl, or soup plate. Remove the crusts and cut the bread into finger strips, then bake in a slow oven until the strips are brown and crisp.

Or try this: Cut half-inch-thick slices from unsliced bread and trim the crusts. Cream a little butter, add to it some grated American cheese and a pinch of nutmeg and spread this mixture on the bread slices. Sprinkle with paprika and put the slices on the broiler, not too close to the fire, until the cheese melts. Remove and trim the slices into shapes such as oval, square, triangular or heart, or even into the initials of those who will sit at your table.

Here's a garnish that will amuse and tempt the children—cheese popcorn. As the corn is popping or, if already popped, warming in a pan, sprinkle some grated American cheese on it. Toss a handful of the cheese-flavored popcorn into the soup tureen or, if the soup is dished in the kitchen, put a few popped kernels on each serving. They will add gaiety to the dish, even if not a great deal of nourishment.

Then there is what might be called a floating island garnish. Beat one egg-white, add two tablespoons of flour and a sprinkle of nutmeg, a tablespoon of grated cheese and a tablespoon of chopped chives. Drop the mixture by teaspoonfuls into the boiling soup. Let simmer for three or four minutes and you'll have delicious cheese-and-chive floating islands, one or more for each plateful.

Another interesting garnish for clear soups is thimble-sized cornmeal dumplings. They are easy to do. Stir enough yellow or white cornmeal into an amount of boiling water to make a thick paste. I'd say, maybe a quarter cup of cornmeal into a half cup of boiling water, and for flavoring, several dashes of Worcestershire sauce, the amount depending upon your appreciation of Worcestershire as a taste or flavor boost.

Cook in a double boiler for twenty-five or thirty minutes until it is quite thick. Watch it closely with stirring spoon at the ready. Now set the top of the double boiler over a low fire and stir in a small amount of finely grated chopped onions and some chives. For further flavor add a little chopped fresh parsley and beat in one egg. Remove from the fire and let the flavory mixture cool in the refrigerator. When it becomes doughy, mold into small, marble-sized spheres. Four or five minutes before serving drop these nourishing little globules into the simmering pot. You will have an interesting, tempting way to present your *pièce de résistance*—and I do mean your soup. You may also deep-fry the tiny dumplings and offer them on a side dish at the same time as the soup is served.

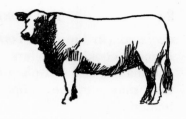

2

Heaven on the Hoof

by Lloyd K. Rudd

America is dotted with steak houses from one end of the country to the other, an indication of the great consuming national devotion to—in some cases obsession with—beef. They are of varying degrees of ritziness; some of the finest food is served in dull backgrounds, proof that the devotees of this substantial food eat at a favored spot not for the decor but because the product is superlatively prepared. They may be pizen-plain or fairly opulent, but they gain a local, sometimes even a national fame by word of mouth for a simply served, perfectly cooked product. You'll find them on the great highways, with a sign out in front saying tersely: Steaks. Or you may encounter them in New York City, Chicago, San Francisco and other big cities.

In France, where the beef is of indifferent quality and a *bifteck* American style is a rarity, those clever French have made sheer poetry out of the serving of beef, by an educated marriage with vegetables in many, many forms. The *pot-au-feu*, which is, as A. J. Liebling recently declared (in the *New Yorker*), "the foundation glory of French cooking," offers a greater joy to gourmets, gourmands, and just plain hungry folk than *bifteck,* since that may not be properly pounded for pre-cooking tenderizing.

It is ironic that the yeomen of the Royal Guard in England are called Beefeaters, since it is quite a feat to get a good piece of beef in the right little, tight little island —as opposed to the lavish availability of American beef.

If you are on a diet, unless your case is special, right now most doctors say—and they mean it—"You need more protein." Most dieting women avoid protein because of the calories involved, and so they miss the important factor: protein is not necessarily fattening, and above all else it supplies energy.

In the United States, if a survey were taken as to favorite foods, most men would say "steak." Broiled steak, which has little but the seasoning added, is perhaps the best way to body-building, furnishing the required nutritional ingredients and supplying a fund from which most systems can draw for a period of days.

Suppose we grant that a good beefsteak, broiled, does supply the greatest amount of nourishment, plus caloric requirement plus energy-building substance, then what do we have to worry about? A number of things.

First: The vegetarians, who do not believe that meat can furnish the substances necessary to preserve health in the body. They believe that George Bernard Shaw, the highly publicized Number One vegetarian, who lived to his almost countless years repudiating meats, proved a point. Perhaps so.

Second: The public-at-large, which does not understand nor appreciate the difference in meats, in their purchase and consumption.

So it seems to me I should set forth a few salient facts.

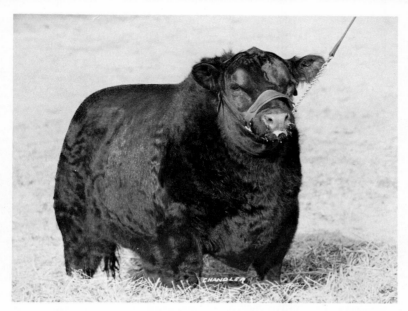

The aristocrats of the cattle world are the Aberdeen Angus breed. This fellow is Ankonian Bombardier, 1959 International Junior and Reserve Grand Champion Angus bull.

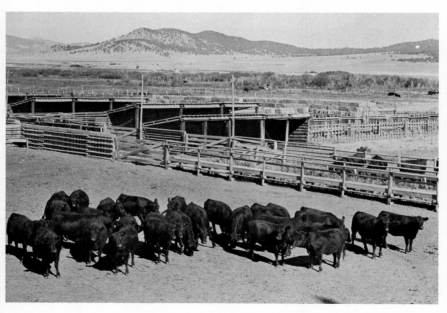

Angus cattle penned at a Montana ranch await shipment to the stockyards.

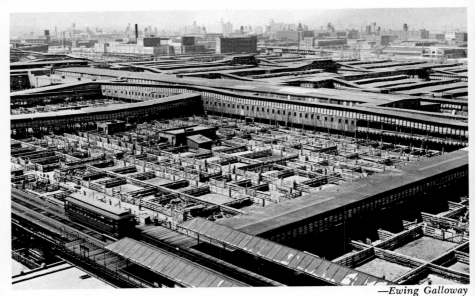

Chicago's famed stockyards. The covered runways make it possible to move livestock from pens to auction center and back in any sort of weather.

An Angus steak is, well . . . need we say more?

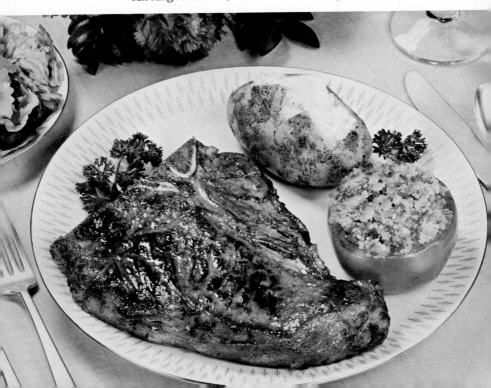

The same amount of steak which would sustain a busy housewife all day long would provide the energy required by a wrestler weighing at least 230 pounds who bangs himself and his opponent around in the ring for a good hour. (All those wrestling holds are not fake, remember.)

In this modern age, the question which comes up most often is that with pre-cut meats, cellophane-wrapped packaging and distribution, how does the housewife know what cuts to select if she cannot apply the thumb test? The thumb test is the real measure of "ripeness" of the beef for cooking, particularly for broiling, steaks. After a fine steak is cut and offered to the customer for approval, he may want to press his thumb in the meat, and if it leaves a dent, it's ready. This implies that the beef has been properly hung and can be cooked right away.

When you select a steak in a supermarket, it is probably already wrapped. Therefore you have to depend on the probity of the butcher, since in the back of the market he has prepared the cuts of meat for wrapping and placing in the refrigerator.

In the best supermarkets, the customer goes to a window and receives a number, then rings a bell to summon the butcher. To him, she describes her immediate need. She tells him the amount of meat she wants, defines the cut, and it is prepared for her just as in the old-time butcher shops, where Mr. Jones knew her every requirement. Many housewives today feel they must accept the cellophane-wrapped parcels, but individual service is just as possible as it ever was.

Although we primarily discuss beef in this chapter, much of the care and treatment applies as well to lamb, veal, and pork. These are all government-graded according to standards set up by the United States Department of Agriculture. The inspector grades the meat carcasses and puts his seal on each one. This testifies to the fact that he has personally (a) inspected it and (b) selected its grade.

However, at the time the animals are brought to market and run on the hoof into the pens in the stockyards they are not graded by the government, but are actually graded, bid on, and purchased by buyers for the packing-house companies. These are the men who poke the stick at the hide of, for example, beef. This is to judge by the springiness whether it has a good layer of white, crisp fat, or whether it has a yellow soft layer of fat or whether it will be marbleized. In the grading of beef, they look at the length of the cow or steer as well as its height. They also consider, for this first-quality beef, which is steer beef, whether it was a young castrated bull, fed on corn for putting on final weight. Corn, of course, is high in carbohydrate content and has a tendency to put weight on the bone. Cattle of this kind are kept in rela-tively small areas, pens, so that they do not get too much exercise and therefore become sinewy and tough. This is a softening-up process so that the muscle-tissue stays firm: it does not get sinewy nor does it bulge and become too tough to eat. The muscle of the steer is actually the meat that is bought and eaten by the consumer. These are elemental facts to those who know about beef-raising, but it is surprising how few people really know anything about the meats they serve or the meats they order in a restaurant.

There are some fine independent butchers still oper-ating their shops, and it is a great help to the consumer to cultivate them, asking their advice about cuts of meat. They buy only the best if they are good exponents of their craft, and they know what goes into the purchase of beef cattle at whatever level.

The cattle buyer has to buy by sight and "feel" and experience in grading. He likes to buy short-legged steers because shin-meat and shank-meat are all waste; he likes to look at the hindquarters, the mid-ribs, and the loin because he looks ahead to the ultimate purchase by that housewife who likes the more expensive cuts—the rumps and the rounds, the rib-roasts, the Delmonicos, the loins, both sirloins and fillets. She is not too interested in the shin, shank, forequarters, neck, or chuck on the forepart of the animal—of course there are exceptions here in certain instances, where recipes call for specific cuts. The steer on the hoof actually is always more desirable when it has deep long wide quarters combined with a wide back, long loins, great spring of rib while being uniformly thick from end to end—providing, of course, it has been aged well or force-fed with corn in a pen.

There are a number of exceptions. If cooks know how to prepare a pot roast, for example, the best cut of meat may be chuck. But to cook a superlative pot roast the essential ingredients are good selection, good preparation, and a knowledge of how the meat may be tenderized by proper cooking after it is sautéed with peppers and onions.

Recipes can be fun-and-games; not drudgery. Here is one which comes from a friend in Connecticut, who for relaxation from his authoring chores, used to cook a magnificent pot roast. He got the recipe originally from a famous amateur cook in Philadelphia. His friends urged him, time after time, to prepare this spécialité. It seemed he never had a failure. Finally he had so many requests for the recipe which was acclaimed as sure-fire that he had a number of copies typed off and sent to friends who had said "How do you do it?"

Pot Roast Magnifique

From your honest butcher—or your equally honest supermarket—you have secured a 3½ to 4 pound treasure of boned and rolled chuck beef and a slab of beef suet. No charge for that last item. Just ask for it when you buy.

Having got it home by car or pushcart you are now entering on an epicurean adventure—not to say emancipating yourself from a lot of daily short-order cooking for days to follow—unless, of course, your family is extra big or extra hungry.

Some three hours before dinnertime reach for that big chef's apron and tie it on snugly. Next, set a half-kettle of water on a rear burner to heat slowly. Rustle out your big cast-aluminum pot with cover and lift out the wire rack that fits so neatly on its floor. Set the rack aside. Give the pot a front burner, toss into it the slab of suet, and adjust the flame to moderate.

While the suet is rendering cut up into smallish pieces one giant-sized green pepper, and an equally large Bermuda onion. Watch the sizzling suet and when an eighth of an inch of fat has been rendered take the suet out and slide in the cut-up pepper and onion for sautéing. For the next few minutes keep an eye on this operation. The vegetables must not get browned, just tenderized.

Now you'd better turn off the kitchen radio because you're going to need to have all your wits about you; anyway you can pretty well guess how today's episode came out by how tomorrow's episode starts. And besides, what you're doing is much more important than whether Maida is going to break her engagement to Charles and be disinherited by her Uncle Robert.

On a platter spread a half cupful of flour, well salted, and place the roast on the platter. With your sharpest small knife cut three cloves of garlic into small wedges. Make incisions in the outer rim of the roast—preferably in the fatty areas—and push the garlic wedges well into the meat. Better take a look at the bubbling peppers and onions about now to see they are not getting browned. Back to the platter. Roll the roast in the salty flour and pat it in on all surfaces.

By this time the sautéing should be done. Scoop out the vegetables, put them back on their plate and leave the suet in the pot for more rendering, giving the pot a hot fire. Do not answer the telephone now ringing in the living room because you've got rather a tight schedule here and it's probably only Janey Peters wanting to tell you all about what happened at the PTA meeting.

Action! Take out the suet for the last time and with a big fork—watch out for sputtering, now—put the roast into the fat, letting it sear, turning it to brown well on all sides. Lift the roast out, put the little grilled rack on the floor of the pot and set the roast on it, flat side down. Turn off the fire under the kettle and pour hot water into the pot around the roast. Let the water come up to ⅔ of the height of the roast as it sits on the rack.

And here comes the seasoning. Distribute the peppers and onions around the roast. Add one large canful of Grade A tomatoes; whole peppercorns, two tablespoons of Chili sauce, one tablespoon of vinegar, a couple of crumpled-up bay leaves and a couple of flourishes of salt. Bring the pot to a simmer, cover it, and, for the moment, your job is done.

Coffee break.

The roast should simmer for perhaps 2½-3 hours, but it must be turned three or four times. The steam in the upper part of the pot is largely what makes the meat tender, rather than the liquid (to be gravy) below. And so while you do other things, the roast is cooking. Try it with a fork now and then to see how it's tendering up. And, maybe a half hour before dinner time, lift it out to a platter and make your gravy. Of course you have filled in your lazy idle moments by peeling potatoes—or maybe you're having bakers—and scrubbing the carrots for boiling. Yes, you've been busy. But when you put it on the dinner table, they'll give you a standing ovation, Cookie!

This author-into-chef came to his selection of a cut of meat through trial and error. The original recipe called for top-of-round steak, but since it is such a hunk of solid meat, he discovered that chuck, being "looser" when tied and rolled, resulted in a better pot roast for him.

Some years ago a retail company issued a promotional brochure entirely made up of famed Rector recipes. It was delightfully illustrated and contained some of the most dramatic of the specialities à la maison Rector. Preserving these was a real service and the booklet had tremendous popularity. Rector recipes were devised in quantities for restaurant serving; the virtue of this booklet was that they were given in family-size quantities, a translation which should have been on every housewife's cookbook shelf.

It is not surprising that there were several recipes involving beef prepared in unusual ways—one of the most popular in this country was Hungarian goulash. This recipe appeals to men. At Rudd-Melikian we make a feature of goulash for our platters. Perhaps you'd be interested in

Goulash by Rector

4 pounds top of round, cut in 2½ inch squares (chuck may be substituted—consult your butcher! Ask for a hunk of suet)

6-7 cloves of garlic (halve these, and use more if you know the garlic-tolerance of your group)

1 teaspoon salt

3 cans bouillon (consommé, if you like) for stock

Bay leaves

Cayenne (a few dashes)

3 tablespoons Hungarian paprika (freshly ground)

3 tablespoons flour

1 large can tomato purée

Fry out the fat, then put in the cloves of garlic, cook until they are brown. This should be done in an aluminum frying pan, or better still, a heavy iron skillet. Brown the meat in the fat and garlic mixture; do it quickly to sear it on all sides. When the meat is browned, transfer it to a cooking pot with cover, add the stock, to which, for each can, you have added a corresponding amount of water, making a total of six cans of liquid.

To the meat, garlic and stock, add the bay leaves (either whole or crushed), then the salt and cayenne. Start the pot slowly, keeping it at low boil or simmer during cooking.

Watch the time: It should not take more than two hours to get it to the next stage. When the meat is partially tender, add the paprika. If possible to obtain, freshly ground paprika gives a special goulash-y flavor; if that is unavailable, canned paprika will do, but you'll need just a little bit more.

Just before you take the meat out to make the gravy, add the can of tomato purée. It is possible to use whole tomatoes, whether canned or fresh, but purée gives a smoothness which is a valued element in goulash. Then make a light flour paste with about four tablespoons of flour, and add to liquid in pot.

In the meantime, you have prepared carrots, onions, and a few potatoes and cooked them separately. When the liquid is thickened, put the meat back in the pot, and add the vegetables, each one lightly salted. Now your main dish is ready, after all the ingredients have been melded.

To serve: Spoon the goulash out on a large platter, surround it with a border of narrow-cut noodles, and sprinkle a lavish amount of freshly chopped parsley over the noodles, which have been lightly buttered. And that's it.

Now to return to the cattle-buyer, left at the post—or the pen—as we digressed.

The buyer picks out the steer and after it has been slaughtered, trimmed and dressed out, the risk is assumed by the packing house, which the buyer represents. By "risk" I mean the condition and quality of the meat have, in a sense, been guaranteed. Then comes the government inspector, generally a resident inspector at the packing house. While in this case he is an expert on beef, there are other experts on poultry, or any meat or fowl which will eventually find its way to the consumer.

Though they are government employees many of them must be reimbursed by the packing houses. Whenever they work overtime, the packing house has to pay the government despite the fact that he is safeguarding the interests of the consuming public and the taxpayer.

Everyone knows that "prime" beef is top grade, but not everyone knows how hard that classification is come by. It has, for one thing, a limited distribution. This is due to the fact that there are few farmers or feeders who elect to keep beef in pens for the extended period of time needed to get the beef up to prime quality. So much more feeding must take place, so much more effort for so little money, it is an example of the law of diminishing returns. Economically the whole process is much less attractive than it should be.

The packing house operator who slaughters this grade of beef finds an inordinate amount of fat which means much waste. This is, of course, the result of vigorous feeding. But what little red meat is left at this point is exceptionally fine and tender, of great quality. There is little left of the actual weight of the steer on the hoof when it reaches the ultimate consumer. No wonder it gets astronomic prices at meat markets and restaurants. Therefore, only certain restaurants, hotels, and clubs are interested in buying and selling prime beef, and then only because they get superlative prices for this premium grade of red meat.

It is obvious from the arithmetic and economics of the

cattle-grower and the packing house operator (or butcher) that to arrive at the limited market of the final purchaser is a long, difficult and sometimes unrewarding circuit. When we talk about prime beef, we are in the economic stratosphere which in women's fashions might be compared to the world of Christian Dior. Those who can afford the wonderful confections at the top must pay the piper. In the area of beef-buying, this is the super-de luxe level.

The responsibility of getting beef into "prime" status is taken by the farmer in the feeder lot on a forced-feeding basis. However, the world over, there is a change taking place, for certain breeds or strains of cattle are lending themselves to breeding programs which are pliant and productive of the best in meats. These are a little heavier in the hindquarters, in the loins and the ribs, where there is depth. They have good bone structure, relatively short legs, short shanks, small forequarters. They have the kind of meat which the discerning say "lays on the bone" and an amount of fat, through a genetic and breeding program, which assures a more tender muscle structure, a more abundant muscle and red meat on the bone—without having too big a bone, which means waste.

The important point is the proper development of this red meat or muscle structure without an overabundance of fat, waste, or trim. This may sound like a technical definition, but the beef-cognoscenti know what it all means, and it is a good idea for the consumer to know, too. It will facilitate shopping. One wonders where all those instructions and drawings which show what is what on marketable steer meat go. In school, I suppose, a few give attention to these facts, but once away from the desk and blackboard, the whole thing seems forgotten. Yet beef, in essence, is important to us all.

I have a special interest in Aberdeen Angus cattle. I learned about them at first hand in Colorado; and during recent years they have captured the imagination of cattlemen the world over, since they are a most rewarding breed.

They are the aristocrats of the cattle world, and breeding them attracts the amateur as well as the professional. Quite recently in a *New Yorker* profile of Eileen Farrell, the singer, the statement was made that the ultimate aim of her husband, Robert Reagan, is to retire to a farm where he can raise Aberdeen Angus cattle. Such an ambition lies at the bottom of the life-plans of many an American—there is an appeal about the superiority of Aberdeen Angus. I think, for instance, of Norman Taylor, author of the authoritative *Botanical Dictionary,* who when he settled in Princess Anne, Maryland, indulged in his lifelong dream, to raise Aberdeen Angus. These are only two examples; there are literally thousands of others.

As for the history of the Aberdeen Angus, they originated in Scotland, near Perth and Aberdeen. In this area there are relatively difficult farming and pasturing conditions, and early in their experimentation with cattle, farmers found they had to breed for quality rather than quantity. After they were satisfied with the product they began to ship their heifers throughout the world. Primarily, they found and developed a fine market in the Argentine.

In Britain, seemingly a logical place to sell this beef, when a steak is served in the best restaurants, it probably will be a Chateaubriand, twenty-eight or thirty-two ounces, sufficient for two or three. The British are not really educated to the virtues of steaks. As opposed to Americans, few British like to eat their beef rare; when it arrives at the table, they consider it underdone or "blue." In our parlance, "underdone" is medium rare, and "blue" is rare, close to blood rare. The wonderful gastronomic experience of a charcoal-broiled steak, with the thick coating of seared meat on the outside and tender forkfuls which require no knife to cut, is almost unknown in Britain. In fact, in many fine British restaurants it is difficult if not impossible to get this kind of beef.

Much of the beef in the Argentine, a famed beef-grazing area, is Aberdeen Angus. I have visited the Argentine and seen on the haciendas the tremendous herds of Aberdeen Angus cattle. I can assure you, from interviews I have had with ranchers of this region, that they do buy some of the finest pure-bred bulls in the world to maintain their standards of excellence in the quality of commercial beef, and even to improve the quality. These breeding programs and their commercial application furnish an outstanding example of superior operation in world agriculture. Their standards are exceptional, as are those of Scotland and America. By America, I mean North America, which includes Canada.

Beef production in Mexico, the northern sections of Latin America, and most of the continent of Europe is relatively poor. I think, for example, of France as where beef comes from cows when they get too tired to live, and were it not for the famous French cooking techniques which produce a tenderized meat, it would be inedible. Such statements are generalities, so I hasten to say there are exceptions all over the world, isolated instances of successful beef-raising. In Australia, for example, there is much interest in Aberdeen Angus, and they are making great strides in up-grading their beef. But it is too early in their program to find Australian beef making much of a dent on the world scene, or even on the local domestic scene.

Since America is looked to to supply much of the beef of the world, it is well to examine where our sources are located. Primarily, I would say, we draw from New Zealand. Many of our less expensive cuts of beef which generally go into the production of ground meat used in canned foods arrive here in the form of boneless, frozen beef. For example, in the year 1958 millions of pounds of this beef found its way here, to be turned into a good quality product which may take many forms when the consumer meets it in the can in combination with other foods. I know of one importer who depends entirely on New Zealand for his supply—he brought in quantities in 1958 in excess of five million pounds. This is the kind of beef which appears in canned stew or canned ravioli and products of this nature. But even face to face with the consumer, it has its uses: it often goes into supermarkets because frozen beef turns to a beautiful red color when it is ground; it is, in appearance, super.

We often refer to "eye appeal" in merchandising, and here is one instance where the eye accepts this product unquestioningly. It seems *right* when it is displayed in a case; better than fresh beef as far as appearance is concerned. I'm not talking now about the virtues of specially ground round or top sirloin with all the fat trimmed off. That is a special order.

The quality of beef in America is as fine as anywhere in the world, and it is more abundant in this country than anywhere in the world. Many elements affect its distribution. Even though we draw on outside sources, even though we protect our consumers, the increase in population and demand for more expensive cuts of beef is altering our over-all picture. Due to the population growth and the constant improvement in our standard of living we are, for the moment, actually running out of beef.

This is the result of several factors. From 1952 to 1957 there was a severe drought through the producing areas of Texas, Oklahoma, Montana, Idaho, Colorado, Kansas,

Nebraska, and other Plains States. It posed a real problem for the farmers: how to bring water in sufficient quantities to the cattle? It was an expensive process to irrigate such parched land with water that had to be transported, and as a result the cattlemen simply reduced the amount of their stock and cut down on their labor. Production from the available pasture land with water was brought down to almost nothing. Many of these stricken areas were pronounced "disaster areas" by the government.

Then the rains came. In 1957 and 1958 the pastures sprang into new life; the water-level table was restored to normal. As a result the ranchers and farmers could keep some cattle for breeding purposes. This meant that importers had a golden opportunity to bring in more beef. With favorable conditions there will be a greater production of beef in the United States, which will force prices down, but we have been faced with the simple fact of economics that with beef off the market the price is high, and in the last twenty months beef has been relatively higher than in the past four or five years.

As a result of less beef on the market, there is more grain available, including corn, which means more for corn-feeding. Since grain and corn are now available in greater quantities the farmer and rancher have been encouraged to purchase them freely and so build up the brood herds. With more of our own calves coming on the market, there is a possibility of restrictions being placed on the importation of beef when we get our internal production up to a high level.

The interim period when our production was reduced because of the drought brought about a number of conditions favorable to our neighbors on the south, notably Mexico. In Mexico beef is not graded, and the farmer gets one price whether he has a prime piece of beef, a commercial piece, or a scrawny piece. By sending his young calves into the United States he is able to get dollars, instead of pesos, and his beef is graded. Therefore he is paid substantially more money for shipping good calves to this country. With the comparatively low labor rate, as well as the low cost of land, it would seem that he might profit by feeding his cattle himself, but in Mexico the technology and status of its Department of Agriculture do not give the rancher much of a break. Any assistance it can render him is not equal to what he can get from this country.

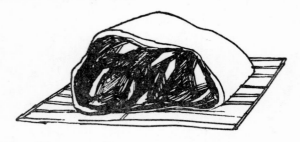

It is true that the Department of Agriculture in Mexico has stepped up its program and taken great strides to help the farmer in the last fifteen or twenty years. There are some serious handicaps, however, to the production of cattle of top grade. There are many areas where cattle cannot be grown because of tic infestation. Tics attack the cattle and may contaminate a whole herd. If they are not controlled, a herd may be wiped out.

But the housewife doesn't need to worry if she is buying her beef in America. Right here I would like to state without qualification that when the housewife puts down her dollars at the check-out counter of a supermarket or buys from an independent butcher shop, she can be sure of the quality of the meat, if it is graded. Later I will quote from the Home and Garden Bulletin Number 1 of the Department of Agriculture about meat buying.

The information is basic and important. (Incidentally, this booklet called "Family Fare" is an invaluable one, in my opinion, and should be in the possession of every housewife and cook. Revised in 1955, it is available at 25¢ to any who send for it to the Superintendent of Documents, U.S. Government Printing Office, Washington 25, D.C.)

In buying "commercial" grade beef, the consumer has to remember that for greatest flavor and an outstanding final result, she must play around with it. This means she may have to use tenderizers, distinctive flavored sauces, even pressure-cook it to break the muscle and fiber tissue down. Its poor condition may be due to several causes, among them that it may be older or that it hasn't been properly fed out, given sufficient grain for an extended period of time and kept restricted, with the result that it gets sinewy and tough. Maybe, as I have suggested earlier, it is a tired old cow or a tired old bull, and perhaps it is just a drought-stricken animal. In this case, it should go to the canners and packers, but if it falls into the hands of the consumer, it may be difficult to cope with in the kitchen.

A cheering thought may be that this is the kind of beef you get pretty much all over the world with some rare exceptions. If it is pressure-cooked, it may come out well from a nutritional standpoint but it may be hardly palatable. It can be greatly improved by sauces—a "dressing-up," proper gravies, proper spicing, the touches which distinguish the cheflike dish when it is served. The cook has to employ more cooking techniques in preparing an indifferent cut of meat than a fine cut of meat. This is what develops the creative instinct in a good cook who values the end result and the appreciation of her guests.

While it may take a bit of skill to broil a steak properly,

it isn't an esoteric difficult-to-learn feat, that is, for the American housewife—she has the protection of her government, whose standards are high. All she needs to know is the grade of her beef and to follow her favorite cookbook's recipes.

As for the trick of broiling a good steak, I've found that some of my good friends, amateur cooks, adopt a routine which produces the ultimate in flavor (provided the guests are not anti-garlic). Using a small brush, after you have rubbed the steak with a clove of garlic, coat the steak with olive oil. Before this, of course, you have slashed the fat at the edges of the meat to prevent curling (if the fat has been trimmed down you're in the clear) and have already heated the broiler. Grease the broiler rack lightly. Place the steak on the rack two inches below the heat, if it is to be rare—three inches, if well done. It is better to leave the oven door open.

When the top side is well browned, season with salt and pepper, then turn and brown the other side. When turning, stick the fork into the fat, not the lean meat. The time table goes like this:

	Total time (minutes)
1 inch thick	
Rare	about 10
Medium	about 15
Well done	20 to 25
1½ inches thick	
Rare	about 15
Medium	about 20
Well done	25 to 30
2 inches thick	
Rare	about 25
Medium	about 35
Well done	45 to 50

For thick steaks, the cuts are rib, sirloin, T-bone, club, top round, and patties (ground beef).

Now for quotes from "Family Fare":

It is not easy for household buyers to judge quality of meat. Best guides for selecting the meat you want are the U.S. Department of Agriculture grades—which most retail stores will use as consumers request graded meat. . . .

The Federal grade name appears in purple on most of the retail cuts of meat. Another purple stamp which may appear on retail cuts is the round one indicating that the meat has been inspected and passed as wholesome food. All graded meat is inspected but not all inspected meat is graded.

Meat packers, wholesalers or retailers may use their own brand names, not to be confused with USDA grades. Letters such as AA and A are never used as meat grades by the USDA.

You may find on your market Federally graded beef, lamb, mutton, veal, and calf. Pork is not usually graded. But *beef* is the meat you will most often find with a USDA grade stamp.

Beef Grades

U. S. Prime: Excellent quality and flavor, tender and juicy, good distribution of fat through the lean meat.

U. S. Choice: Very acceptable quality. This grade is popular because it combines a moderate amount of fat with desirable eating quality. If you find graded beef at your butcher's it is most likely to be U. S. Choice.

U. S. Good: Cuts of this grade are preferred by consumers who desire relatively tender beef with a high ratio of lean to fat.

U. S. Commercial: Most beef of this grade is produced from mature animals. It carries a fairly thick fat covering and lacks natural tenderness. Such Commer-

cial grade meat is often a good buy, but usually requires
a long, slow cooking.

If You Buy Ungraded Beef

You can be reasonably sure of high-quality beef when
the lean meat is light red, velvety-appearing, and
liberally veined with fat, when bones are red, and the
fat is flaky and white.

Thus endeth our beef lesson. But it is really never-
ending, since conditions change all the time and everyone
who likes to eat, cook, or sell beef should be conversant
with the ever-changing market.

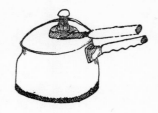

3

Everything Under One Roof

by K. Cyrus Melikian

Most cooks, I am sure, confronted with the never-ending cycle of three meals a day to prepare, feel they cook under pressure—against the deadlines of healthy, hearty appetites, mealtimes, and individual tastes. But in this chapter I am concerned with pressure-cooking in the mechanical sense. Just what *is* pressure-cooking? Many Americans believe it all began only a few years ago when pressure cookers first came on the market. Much emphasis has been given editorially to the virtues of pressure-cooking, with its economy, preservation of flavors, and speed. Promotional material from the companies putting out these excellent utensils stresses the all-important fact that foods cooked rapidly under steam with a small amount of water added will retain all the nutritive elements necessary to health and nourishment.

Actually this method of cooking did not originate with American manufacturers. This is not a new technique for cooking at all. The pressure-cooking method has been employed successfully for hundreds of years in many countries, but perhaps comes to its finest flowering in France. Those dedicated cooks, concerned with both flavor and economy, decided many years ago that here was an answer to a real gastronomic need.

The French, particularly in the provinces, love to keep the essence of food flavors intact. By necessity and by tradition they have long been concerned with keeping the cost low and the food interest high. This has made them inventive and creative cooks, able to take inexpensive cuts of meat and uninteresting vegetables and, with the addition of wine and herbs, turn a prosaic dish into a gourmet's delicacy.

Pressure cooking dates back to the use, in France, of an oval-shaped casserole, defined in America as an oven-baking dish. It is about ten inches long and possibly five or six inches deep, of earthenware material and has a reddish-brown color. There is hardly a good kitchen in this country that hasn't one or more of these wonderful cooking utensils.

The French technique of oven-baking has declined in popularity in the last ten or twelve years, although for the really kitchen-wise cooks, the containers will probably never completely be discarded, no matter what the vogue in utensils. Oven-types of roasting pots and pans—not quite the size to take a turkey—will, I am sure, remain important to good cooks. These casseroles are made of earthenware, not glass, or they may be made of metals finished with enamelware. In France a kind greatly in use has a speckled finish on the outside, brown or red in color. What an uncounted number of delicious viands have been prepared over the years in utensils of this type. Everything from the rarest of delicacies to hearty full meals, but all lovingly tended by the truly creative French housewife or chef.

The utensil comes in two sections: the bottom part of

the pot forms the casserole; this section of the cooking oven utensil may have two homes—on top of the stove, as well as in the oven. It has two handles on the narrow end of the oval and a lid with the handle directly in the center.

This is the universal casserole. I am sure there is no cook who calls herself one who has not used and valued these casserole dishes to the utmost. The dimension of ten by five inches takes care of most domestic needs, but the housewife or cook-of-many-resources may choose other sizes—fourteen by eight inches, for example—to house her culinary triumphs.

You'd need a larger one to prepare, say, a seven or eight pound roasting chicken, with a width of nine or ten inches across. For the experienced cook, a whole series of these oven dishes is standard equipment in her kitchen.

The French casserole can be made a pressure cooker— and this is news to many a modern cook. To seal the utensil, raw dough is put on the outsides of the casserole and the lid. When the casserole is put in the oven the raw dough rises and is glazed on the outside, and a hard crust is formed. The dough acts as a natural seal without any screws, nuts or bolts or other tricky, engineered devices. So modern pressure-cooking has derived from the older, less mechanized times.

There are often problems in this elementary pressure-cooking. There may be too much moisture in the casserole and there is a tendency to boil over because of the excessive steam generated inside the casserole. What does steam ever do but try to escape?

The real reason for casserole cooking is that the substances within the casserole improve in taste with the cooking. This is because, of course, the volatile essences do not go up a flue or become dissipated in the steam from an open kettle. Therefore the flavors are retained and are melded in the cozy interior of a casserole. Take any flavorful meat or poultry rich in fats or oils or indeed in any of the esters and the casserole becomes the best home for preparation, in combination with vegetables. Also, a well-prepared casserole dish usually made up of a number of ingredients not only may serve as an initial meal, but can be successfully used as a leftover. It is almost better the second day.

A casserole dish has more chances for success than many straightaway entrees prepared in other ways. In your experience, how many people, even expert cooks, can produce a perfectly timed and broiled steak? How many roast beef dinners have fallen flat on their roast beef faces because they were overdone or improperly cooked? But the even slightly careless cook can scarcely ruin a well-planned casserole dish. Served with a tossed salad and a simple, light dessert, you get credit for being the best and most thoughtful cook in your group. Only don't forget the perfect coffee!

I don't want to sound complicated about the laws of physics involved in the daily cooking job which confronts most women several times a day, but pressure is measured by pounds per square inch; liquids turn to gas when the temperature rises; the higher the temperature rises the more pressure is generated. In our experimental kitchen we are much concerned with practical ways of feeding the multitudes. We try out recipes on a small, domestic basis, then we must adapt them for feeding hundreds of people. We work with any number of combinations of food, combined with heat. While it may mean little to a housewife that she is dealing with chemical properties and laws of physics, as we are, there are some basic facts she must, if not consciously at least instinctively, observe.

Water starts boiling at 212 degrees Fahrenheit—all those little bubbles come up like fury. The liquid state turns to gas and steam at a higher temperature. As the temperature increases, the pressure increases. As a result of the pressure increasing, the steam forces its way through and into whatever your solid substance is.

Right now seems a good time to introduce a fine recipe for a casserole dish which has a long and important history and is distinguished on two counts: economy and savor.

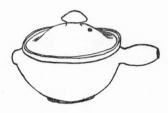

Oxtail Casserole

If you are economy-minded and have a hungry family to feed week in and week out, here's a dish that not only will bring cheers from those who sit at your table but will also be so easy on your budget that you'll want to make it at least a once-a-month regular. Oxtail casserole can be made for as little as twelve to fourteen cents a serving. How's that for keeping a watchful eye on the family funds? Because it is such a boon to the domestic purse as well as such a really glorious main dish, I am going into detail as to its preparation.

First a word on its basic ingredient—the oxtail. Oxtail is one of the most delicious and savory of meats and also one of the most inexpensive. The meat that is tucked between the joints of an oxtail is sweet and tender. Good oxtails can be had at any time of the year and, in your deep freeze, will keep and keep. Also, being a nonmuscular cut of meat, oxtail can always be counted on for tenderness.

All right, here's what to assemble for oxtail casserole:

1 oxtail	1 teaspoon of sugar
1 teaspoon of salt	1½ cups of tomato juice
Dash of fresh-ground pepper	2 medium-size onions
2 tablespoons of flour (biscuit flour preferred)	1 bay leaf
	6 stalks of celery
2 tablespoons of light olive oil (or a light salad oil)	½ teaspoon of thyme
	1 can sliced mushrooms (or fresh if available)

Now with a good steel kitchen knife, cut the oxtail into pieces approximately one and a quarter inches long. Roll the pieces in a mixture of the flour and salt. When coated, sprinkle a little pepper on the top. Heat the oil in a casserole on top of the stove or in a frying pan for transfer later to the casserole. Sprinkle the sugar on the nuggets of meat and let it cook for a few minutes until the sugar has caramelized into a brown coating. Now, to the casserole add the tomato juice, slowly, and the sliced-up chips of the onions. Add the bay leaf, crumpled up into bits in the palm of the hand, the chopped-up celery, and the thyme.

Bring the casserole to the boiling point, then cover and simmer over low heat for two hours or so. About twenty minutes before serving time stir the casserole with a *wooden* spoon and add the sliced mushrooms. If you are using fresh mushrooms they should have been previously cooked until tender. Now with everybody wanting to know when that fragrant dinner will be ready, dish the contents of the big casserole into small individual warmed-up casseroles in which you have spooned a good-sized helping of hot buttered noodles. That's it—and will you get admiring glances from your appreciative family.

Now let's see how this is adapted to a banquet such as a church or club supper—and the same mass production technique can be used by the housewife who has freezer storage space and is thinking of high-speed, low-cost dinners, ready almost in a jiffy. Here's how to prepare some 850 servings at one time, whether for one big dinner or to be served on oxtail-casserole days to the family.

Simply multiply the ingredients by 24. Start with 24 oxtails, twenty-four teaspoons of salt, forty-eight table-spoons of flour, etc. The cooking process can be essentially the same and there is no need to use a restaurant-type giant-size casserole. It can be made in three or four batches. Here's the difference in procedure between the one-shot casserole and the big job, either for storage or for dining hall banquet: Instead of cooking over low heat for some two hours, bring it to a boil in thirty-five to forty minutes then pop it into the oven, which has been brought to a steady heat, just enough to keep it simmering. If you want to use the original casserole for another batch empty it into a large roasting pan, cover tight, let the oven heat finish the cooking while you are preparing the next batch in the casserole on top of the range. And remember, don't add the mushrooms until the final cooking is almost done.

Here's a thought in regard to the mass production of oxtail casserole for storage in the freezer and family use in installments. The flavors—meat, vegetables, herbs, spices—blend and enhance one another through their longer residence together; they "marry" you might say (quite polygamously) and produce an exquisiteness of flavor that could be had in no other way. Yes, it could be compared to the aging of vintage wine, gaining in flavor-value through a period of storage.

Casserole cooking has been elevated by many cooks to a high art, and even the most usual of foods such as macaroni and cheese with tomatoes can be varied with flavors to make poems of everyday gastronomy. It may be thought of in an infinite number of ways: as the *pièce de résistance* of a buffet supper; or as dinner-in-a-dish, with the accompaniment of a crisp tossed salad and coffee; or as a quick method of serving many people who suddenly appear at your table without much warning. The high-speed recipes are what the impromptu hostess values, since they can be just as delicious as more elaborately prepared viands taking hours to cook. Not that they are as satisfying to the creative cooking soul. No. The cook, male or female, who loves to test, potter and fuss, won't appreciate to the full the virtues of the rapid-fire dish.

But no more than thirty minutes of cooking time is an element to be cherished and many a frenzied housewife will want to seize upon a last-minute remedy in emergencies. Take, for example, a frankfurter casserole supper, using tomatoes, frankfurters and green peppers, some onions, grated cheddar cheese and seasonings and spices such as cloves and garlic. It can be done in a great hurry, and is an invariable hit with hungry guests, or even your own family, when you come back from a cocktail party and find those hors d'oeuvres weren't filling enough.

Sea food, especially, has a distinct place in casserole cooking. There are tuna puffs, and tuna lima-bakes and shrimp peek-a-boo, salmon-olive casserole, oyster scallops, tuna-cashew casseroles, fish-bake casseroles—all good Lenten and Friday variants of the usual fare. People who observe days of abstinence for religious reasons get more bored, in my observation, by their restrictions than they might if catered to by sympathetic and intelligent cooks. If you cannot have meat on Fridays for fifty-two weeks of the year, then the substitutes must be imaginative enough to whet the appetite.

Casseroles in industrial feeding have many advantages. They provide a maximum of taste pleasure at a minimum of expense, except in the ingenuity of the cook. Just to name a few possibilities: Swedish meat-ball casserole; baked shrimp-and-cheese casserole; hamburger casserole; creole-barbecued chicken casserole; beef-and-eggplant casserole; macaroni, tomato, and cheese casserole; beef stew casserole; or the prime old-fashioned favorite—lamb pot-pie casserole. Lamb, of course, isn't the only form of meat or poultry; the pot-pie can be made with pork, chicken or even beef.

One of the advantages of casserole cooking is that the dishes really freeze beautifully; the only problem might be if your dish requires a topping. After the mixture is cooked and cooled in the refrigerator, it can be quickly frozen, especially if you use an aluminum container, a Pyrex-type casserole, or a plastic freezer compartment container. I always advise people not to keep their casseroles in the deep freeze for more than two months, although you might be safe up to four months. The reason for this is that most casseroles are highly spiced, or fairly so, and these spices have a tendency to marinate even at low temperatures; this will change the characteristics of the mixture and, therefore, its flavor.

Consider the virtues of a casserole dish of Swiss steaks with vegetables; or a complete turkey dinner as a casserole; or lobster creamed with macaroni; or pork with spaghetti or baked lentils; eggplant Parmesan, Yorkshire hot pudding—the variety is endless—even stuffed rolled cabbage can be done excitingly in a casserole. Meatloaf ring in a casserole is also an appetite-tempter. On a rainy Saturday night, baked beans with ham is both filling and delicious, and as an alternate a smoked butt of ham with vegetables, or spaghetti-stuffed peppers. There are so many delightful ways to serve casserole dishes that the ingenious cook could provide a different one for every night in the year, without too many repeats.

For main courses or for buffet suppers, once more the casserole is supreme. For a special occasion such as a New Year's Eve party, consider the taste sensation of a barbecued chicken in casserole. Or, the universally appreciated shrimp Creole served as a casserole. For entertaining a large mob of people, pork-and-rice (in an enormous dish from which the guests serve themselves) goes with many things.

I have a favorite recipe: an Armenian casserole. As you know, the Armenians are fond of lamb, and with good reason—since there is little beef in their native land, they can't enjoy the marvelous flavoring of good steer beef, but they have become the world's experts (I maintain!) in cooking lamb. Here's my formula for a wonderful lamb dish:

Lamb-and-Eggplant in Casserole
(A serving for eight)

3 pounds boned lamb shoulder, cut into small cubes
½ cup good light-grade olive oil
1 cup onions, minced and chopped
1 cup green peppers, chopped

1 cup raw, regular white rice
3 pounds eggplant (about two medium eggplants)
½ cup grated Parmesan cheese
cinnamon to taste; salt; garlic salt

For this recipe, I recommend a Dutch oven type of casserole. Brown lamb thoroughly in the olive oil, add onion and green peppers, sauté, cover and let simmer until tender (if you are using pre-cooked lamb, omit the simmering). In accordance with the directions on the package, cook the rice but *don't* use water, use chicken broth. Next, pare and dice the eggplants, cook in an inch of boiling salt water for about five minutes. Drain well. Into the rice, stir the lamb, the eggplant, tomatoes and the rest of the ingredients. Let it cool off in the refrigerator for about an hour. Then put into the oven at about 350 degrees Fahrenheit. Turn the mixture into a two-quart casserole, top with Parmesan cheese and bake for an hour until it starts to bubble. I like to think of this dish being served with string beans, hot French bread or pumpernickel, and a nice, cool salad.

This is a good place to mention the cooking skills the Armenians have brought to bear on the preparation of eggplant, which is so good in the lamb casserole dish. They do so many things with eggplant—they fry it, slice it, stew it, extract the juice—no Armenian cook worth his salt fails to have some eggplant recipes. It is even served pickled, the pickling process much the same as for dill pickles. The tiny eggplants are pickled before they mature, and can be quite delicious: it's a popular way to serve them in the Mediterranean area and the Near East. I am of the opinion that eggplant does not have much appeal to the American palate, perhaps because it has been conspicuously left off menus, and American cooks are not too familiar with its virtues, or its exotic aspects.

The Italians have an eggplant Parmesan, which combines two taste sensations—it's as if you were eating meat with cheese on it. In fact, the Italians are also past masters of casserole cooking. Partly this is due to the expert use of their magnificent cheeses, which they often combine with veal; they also have a wide, pasta-type of noodle which they use effectively in casserole dishes designed for the main course of a dinner. They have been wise in discovering that casseroles not only provide elegant taste treats, but are rich in nutrition. Good casserole dishes are prepared to blend and marinate the flavors of meat, vegetables, and cheeses and offer a base for the addition of herbs and spices, of cognacs and wines, red or white, dry or sweet. When vegetables are cooked separately, the nutritional value often is lost in the juice which is poured down the drain. When cooked in a casserole, this juice is preserved and serves to thin out the gravy. In Italy and France, particularly, a piece of French or Italian bread or a hard twist roll is eaten with the dish, and this makes for a completely balanced meal. It's quite the thing to "sop up" your gravy with a hunk of bread—even Amy Vanderbilt won't object.

Right now I'd like to tell you of one of our Armenian dishes, called "dolma." Dolma is a pickled, green, young and tender grape leaf, which may come from the vine of any kind of grape. Around Memorial Day my mother and her friends go out to pick the succulent young leaves from the vines, subsequently to pickle them in a brine solution of salt and water. They are put up in an earthen crock and later stuffed with rice, celery and ground lamb, sautéed onions, green peppers, and parsley. All this is cooked in a casserole with some stewed tomatoes to which a little water and a little chicken broth have been added. This is simply delicious, especially if served with yogurt on the side.

To digress a moment on the subject of yogurt. It is, as you know, an old Middle East dairy product—I like to eat rice with yogurt, dolma with yogurt, and I like just plain yogurt. Recently I had the opportunity to meet Mr. Metzger, a member of the board of the Dannen Yogurt Company. He has a beard like Commander Whitehead, which seems these days to be a fine way of being remembered in a promotional way. We talked about yogurt and he asked, "Would you like to have some?"

"I'd love some," I said.

"How would you have it—with strawberries or prunes, or pineapple?" he asked.

"No, I like mine plain," I answered.

Then he said, "Well, you are really and truly a yogurt eater."

"Why?" I asked.

"Well," he said, "we flavor yogurt because yogurt does not have appeal to people without some recognizable flavor. They become yogurt eaters because there is a predominately strong taste of strawberries, or something else in it."

I was impressed by the promotion-minded approach to their marketing, but more impressed by Mr. Metzger, because if you think Gaylord Hauser is a yogurt fan, he is really *the* yogurt fan, and makes its acceptance a real religion.

As I say, this was a digression. In casserole cooking, which was our topic, there are innovations taking place every day, conveniences, new technologies which will, it is to be hoped, improve and refine the business of daily cooking. The Casserole is King, no doubt about it. First on the list for picnics or cold-weather nights, great for midnight snacks, indispensable for buffet suppers, cocktail parties, and big, populous wingdings.

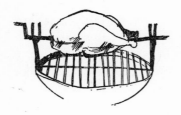

4

Man, King of the Coals

by Lloyd K. Rudd

In the last few years a new dimension has been added to the world of men. In the past the male animal, caged for a week end at home, puttered around doing chores. But things were to change. Out of a new-born interest in food and cooking emerged the outdoor barbecue, at which man could be King of the Coals. So his favorite indoor sport of grousing has turned, in innumerable instances, to his favorite outdoor sport of astounding and amazing his friends—some of whom he summons from vast distances to partake of his excitement—and neighbors, who couldn't bear the smells that drift across the well-tended lawns and stone walls without being included.

Because it is a well-established fact that when a man gets interested in cooking, he goes all out—all outdoors, that is—he doesn't have to think of it in terms of putting three meals on the table every day; his is a precious, esoteric contribution which brings into play all the

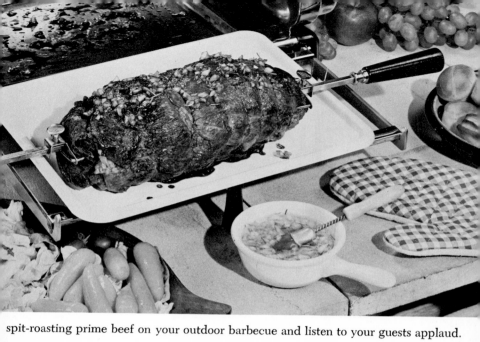

spit-roasting prime beef on your outdoor barbecue and listen to your guests applaud.

those skewers to use. Shish-kabob tastes even better grilled outdoors over charcoal.

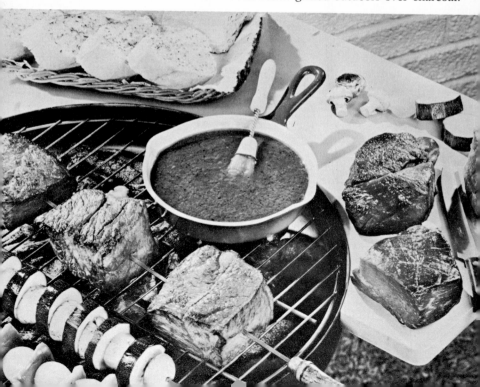

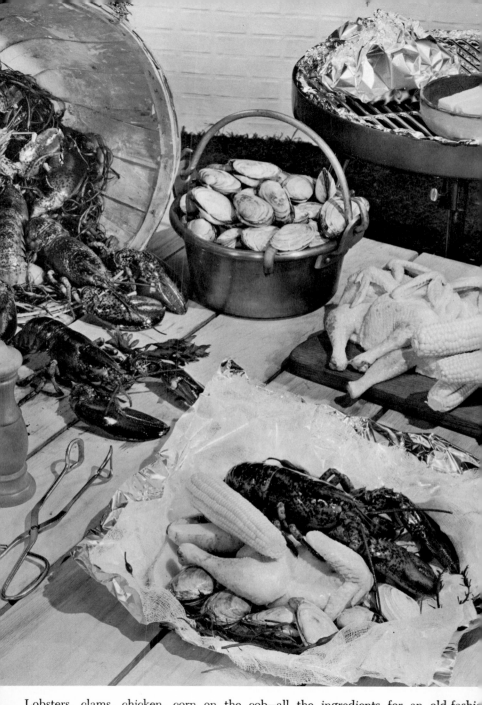

Lobsters, clams, chicken, corn on the cob—all the ingredients for an old-fashi‹‹
clambake that you can barbecue in your back yard.

imagination and zest of an Escoffier, plus the ham actor and the showoff who exist in many of us. He can revel in a recipe which may have taken many days in the experimental stages before it is mastered, and finally deliver it as a triumph of skill and taste. So a new outdoor sport has been born.

The outdoor barbecue is not an unmixed delight. There are as many difficulties in achieving a perfect result as there were on the old-fashioned picnic, but the patience of hard-headed manufacturers of equipment has resulted in a number of fool-proof devices, so that the actual cooking has become simplified.

When the women's magazines show the perfect setting —the arched trees overhead, the sunlight dappling the flagstones, the orderly arrangement of plates, glasses, napkins and tasteful small bowls of flowers on the glass-topped serving table—they omit the smoke, the grit, the confusion which may attend the male cook-out, where the chief object on the grill may be the host.

But as things are developing, more and more men and *women* are getting so expert they are contributing a whole new set of procedures and recipes to the outdoor scene— in some parts of the country now a year-round performance. They have mastered the efficient way of starting a fire of charcoal; they have discovered the quickest trick in setting up a grill; they know that coals are ready for cooking when they are covered with a fine gray ash. They have even found out about a sizzling action foam which lights the charcoal in a second, clings to each briquet, and turns the bed of coals into even-burning heat in a matter of minutes. They have learned how to cook roasts or fowl on a spit, and have borrowed a number of "tenderizer" aids from their kitchens to help build their reputations as discriminating cooks.

Your Grill and Building the Fire

Charcoal briquets, the most readily available fuel, give a long-lasting, steady cooking fire. Shake them into the grill and ignite with a charcoal starter (available at food markets, hardware stores), wait thirty minutes until all the briquets are burning. They will show small gray ash spots. Hickory chips may be added before cooking to give flavor to the food.

Wood, especially oak, hickory, fruit woods such as apple and wild cherry, make excellent aromatic fires. When building a wood fire, start with small dry sticks and paper. When this is burning, add larger logs. Wait until these burn down to a good bed of coals (about one hour) before cooking.

When you buy or build a barbecue, be sure that the draft and ventilation can be controlled, so that the fire will burn properly. Check the prevailing winds and locate the barbecue grill where the smoke will not blow toward your dining area, patio, or house.

Safety is a factor in planning and precautionary measures should be taken in advance. Equipment needed includes a pair of asbestos gloves, a bucket for water, and a place to store wood, charcoal, and briquets where they cannot catch fire.

Special caution: Starting a fire with gasoline or kerosene is dangerous because of their explosive nature.

A cardinal rule in outdoor cooking is to be patient when you start your fire: allow one to one and a half hours before you begin cooking. This will give you time to take care of any necessary preparations and get the right bed of hot coals for the right cooking temperature.

Hard woods such as fruit woods burn much slower than soft woods, and are more aromatic. They add flavor and spice to your barbecue cooking. Hard woods have a tendency to throw sparks and safety precautions should be taken.

Controlling the temperature of your fire is important in determining how long it will take for meat to achieve the desired degree of doneness. Approximate temperatures are, for grilling, 350 degrees F.; for spit barbecuing, 275 degrees to 300 degrees F.; for skewer barbecuing, 275 degrees to 300 degrees F.

There are many simple ways to control the temperature. The easiest is to have an adjustable device to lower or raise your grill or spit. Learn to read temperatures using a meat thermometer. The size of your fire and the amount of coal and the kind of cooking vessel used—a cast-iron fire pot or a light gauge aluminum fire pot, etc.—also should be taken into consideration. If you use aluminum foil to line the fire pot, it will reflect the heat and increase the temperature.

If you are buying a portable grill for barbecuing keep these things in mind: (a) The size of the grill. (b) Whether you will want a larger size for occasions when you have guests. (c) Is it portable and easily moved to be protected from the weather? (d) Is it top-heavy or well balanced? (e) Is the weight of metal of which the fire box is made heavy enough not to burn out quickly or melt from the heat? (f) Is the grill easy to clean? (g) Does it have an attachment for skewer and spit cooking? (h) If it has an electric motor for skewer or spit cooking, is the motor heavy enough and sufficiently insulated so that heat or water will not harm it?

If you decide on a permanent grill and barbecue, careful thought should be given to the design. Does it incorporate, in addition to the grill, an attachment for spit and skewer cooking? A Chinese oven? A warming oven where rolls and dishes may be kept warm? Also consider such conveniences as electrical outlets, storage compartments for charcoal, wood. Do not incorporate an incinerator as part of the grill.

Additional Equipment

Equipment for a cook-out can be simple or elaborate depending upon one's individual standards and requirements. It can include an automatic dishwasher and hot and cold running water, or it can consist only of the simple necessary items.

Some of the basics that I find helpful are: (a) Tongs for handling food on the grill, or charcoal. A pair of good work gloves can be used in case of emergency. (b) Several sharp stainless steel knives of different sizes. (c) Pepper mill. (d) Two sizes of metal skewers, preferably with wooden handles—one size skewer to be used for large pieces of meat like shish-kabob; the other, for such small items as chicken livers and oysters. Metal skewers should be square, not round or twisted. Food on square skewers will not slip or rotate when food is turned, but on a round skewer or twisted skewer, some things like tomatoes or shish-kabob may slip and not turn around properly. (e) Wire hinged grill for fish and sea food, hamburgers, etc. (f) Wire hinged basket grill for poultry and larger size foodstuffs. (g) A long-handled fork. (h)

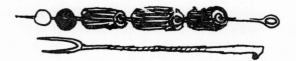

A long-handled basting brush. (i) Heavy apron (preferably without pictures or fancy sayings on it; your friends will give you those).

If you plan a sit-down dinner outdoors, you should have a simple durable serving table with wheels, and a chafing dish or hot plate to keep vegetables and food warm and convenient for serving. This serving table can also be used for china and silver to eliminate many trips back and forth from the kitchen. Ice buckets, coffeepots, napkins, etc., can be kept on the serving table.

A large deep tray for taking dishes and silver back to the kitchen for cleaning should also be on hand.

There are several methods and ways of cooking foods outdoors. They are grilling, skewer cooking, spit cooking, and Chinese oven cooking. In addition, there are modifications of spit cooking which utilize a pit in the ground. This is ideal for camp-outs or cooking extremely large pieces of meat, such as a steamer roast of beef, sometimes referred to as ox-roast; a suckling pig or a whole hog, weighing from fifteen to one hundred pounds; a festive lamb roast using a whole spring lamb. In pit roasting, if you have a temporary pit, build a fire of a large and deep bed of charcoals. Such a fire could take four or five hours to build and to get the right consistency of heat in the coals. It is important to have large smooth rocks in the pit fire. The rocks will get hot and radiate a steady heat for a substantial period of time.

The size of the pit depends on the size of what you are cooking. If you have a permanent pit, it should be approximately three feet wide and five feet long on the inside, and should be lined with fire brick. You can use a protective metal screen on one length of the five-foot side. This should be about three feet high and preferably of aluminum or stainless steel to reflect some of the heat, which would normally be lost in the air, on the food being cooked on the spit.

Fifteen-pound Suckling Pig

After it has been dressed, eviscerated and washed, the suckling pig should be wiped down with a weak soy-sauce inside and outside, allowed to dry, and then at least an hour before cooking rubbed with lard or olive oil. After it has been placed on the spit the pig should be rotated constantly and basted either with melted lard seasoned with salt and pepper or with olive oil and salt and pepper. Garlic juice or crushed garlic-marjoram might also be added to the latter. This coating will keep the skin from cracking or blistering while the pig is cooking.

It will take about three and a half hours to cook a 15-pound suckling pig; a 30-pound one about four hours and 40 minutes.

Many cooks stick an apple in the pig's mouth. They do this not just for the sake of appearance but to determine when the roast is done. The steam that builds up in the pig cooks the apple, and, theoretically, when the apple is cooked, so is the pig. This, however, is not a sure method of determining degree of doneness. Apples, of course, vary in size and texture and so does the size of the mouth of the pig.

In the Caribbean Islands and countries where pit cooking of pigs goes on every day, the cook has the pleasure of knowing the pig is done when the eyes fall out of its head.

For the more squeamish barbecuer, though, there is no substitute for a good meat thermometer. 160° indicates the pig is done. Insert the thermometer in the thigh or loins, the fleshiest part of the pig.

The ears are the most brittle part of the pig. They can be covered with muslin, basting periodically with olive oil or lard.

Suckling pig is good with sauerkraut cooked in a pot with a few spareribs, some pork chops, thyme, and a slice or two of apple. Suckling pig is also good with freshly made apple sauce. A barbecue sauce with suckling pig is not recommended. It is, however, quite acceptable with an 80-pound hog that has been pit roasted. With a large hog you can use the following sauce, which is a modification of french dressing:

3 cloves of garlic crushed or their equivalent in garlic juice	crushed peppers to taste
	½ cup olive oil
	½ cup tarragon vinegar
Fresh ground pepper	¼ cup lemon juice
Chili powder or red hot	2 teaspoons salt

Mix well, heat and serve warm on pork.

Barbecuing Steak

Beef is still the favorite meat for outdoor cooking. There are many kinds and cuts of steaks from the most expensive filet mignon to flank, round, and hip steaks. Here is how to cook it:

Sometimes steaks should be marinated before you grill or broil them in a barbecue. If you buy meat in advance and freeze it, regardless of the quality, it has a tendency to be a little dry or to lose some of its flavor. Marinate these frozen steaks in a sauce of olive oil, lemon juice, fresh-ground pepper, and salt and let stand for at least one hour after thawing. This will make the steak meat more juicy and flavorful and will revive the fresh taste.

After the steak is cooked, put a little melted butter on it. The natural juices will drain to the bottom of the dish on which you serve it.

If you are using lower cost cuts of meat, add some wine vinegar or some white wine to the sauce described above. This will have a tenderizing effect. A little commercial tenderizer could be used on the meat before marinating.

There are many ways to grill steak. Large pieces can be cooked and cut finger-size across the grain so that people who want medium to well-done steak can be served the outside cuts and those who like their meat rare can get the inside cuts.

Do not punch a steak with a fork to turn it over. Prongs are the proper things to use, or you can use your hand protecting it with an asbestos glove. Press your thumb on the top of the steak. If the meat is soft, your steak is cooked rare. If the meat is reasonably firm, the steak is medium. And if it is quite hard, it's well done.

Following are two timetables for grilling a steak:

One-inch Steak

Very rare	8 minutes	Medium	12 minutes
Rare	10 minutes	Well done	15 minutes

Two-inch Steak

Very rare	14 minutes	Medium	25 minutes
Rare	18 minutes	Well done	30 minutes

These time requirements are approximate. They will vary with closeness of the steak to the heat; size of the fire; and moisture content of the meat. Use these values only as a guide and not as an ironclad rule.

Other Cuts of Beef

Prime rib of beef may be cooked on an outdoor barbecue by two methods:

1. You may spit roast it 20 minutes to the pound. Use a meat thermometer and check the meat; at 140° F. it is cooked rare.

2. You can use a Chinese oven*, which employs a technique of hot smoke cooking. Hang meat on hooks or in a basket hanging in the Chinese oven, allowing it to cook

* For explanation of the Chinese oven, see pages 76 and 77.

20 minutes to the pound, again checking with a meat thermometer.

Hamburgers are always popular for barbecuing, either on the grill or on a stick. The meat should be ground fine and can be extended with fine cracker crumbs, one egg for every pound of ground meat, and perhaps some evaporated milk (three or four ounces for every pound of ground beef). Salt and pepper, of course, and you may add mustard or Worcestershire sauce, chopped parsley, sautéed onions, etc. You can cook the hamburgers on a rotating skewer, or make patties and put on the grill, using a spatula for turning. You may paint them with a little butter as you grill them.

Four for the Skewer

Shish-kabob. "Shish" means skewer. "Kabob" is anything cube-shaped that goes onto a skewer—lamb, beef, sea food, vegetables, and a variety of other things.

The word "shish-kabob" has been spelled in many ways, and it has been interpreted in many ways. Almost everyone has his own recipe for shish-kabob. Being an old shish-kabob cooker myself, I think you will like these ideas.

Lamb shish-kabob is considered the most authentic of the Oriental shish-kabobs. Lamb of good quality should be used. The fat around the kidneys should be light and flaky, and firm, and the color of the meat should be red. The meat itself should be firm. Young lamb should be eaten shortly after it has been dressed.

The best lamb is spring lamb. Spring lamb is small and tender and it can be used for shish-kabob without marinating first. When the lamb is older it requires more attention before cooking. It should be skinned and then marinated. The older the lamb is, the longer it should be marinated. Put the cubes of lamb into this marinade:

1 cup of wine
1 cup of olive oil
¼ cup of vinegar or lemon
   juice
1 tablespoon grated onions

Crushed garlic clove
¼ teaspoon freshly ground
   pepper
Salt and oregano to taste

The most popular cut of lamb to use for lamb shish-kabob is the leg. The loin is the tenderest part and equivalent to the filet or sirloin of beef. The leg also provides more usable meat, has less waste, and is therefore more economical. The shoulder of the lamb is quite usable for shish-kabob.

Here's the procedure for cooking it: Have the butcher bone a leg of lamb and remove all fat and gristle. (You can, of course, follow this procedure at home.) Cut the meat into one to one-and-a-half inch squares and marinate for a few hours, or longer if the meat is from an older lamb.

Put the meat on square skewers and alternate with the other ingredients as follows: cube of meat, mushroom cap, cube of meat, small tomato, cube of meat, slice of onion, cube of meat, green bell pepper, cube of meat, small tomato. The vegetables will add delicate flavors to the lamb. However, shish-kabob may also be made with plain lamb or with any other combination of vegetables you like. Eggplant is an interesting vegetable to use.

Shish-kabob is not only an outdoor barbecue treat, but if the weather is cold or inclement you may prepare it indoors if you have an electric rotisserie, or you may be fortunate enough to have a built-in barbecue in your kitchen.

For those who would rather use beef instead of the lamb, the top of the round or side of the round should be chosen. It is important, however, that round steak, which is lean, be marinated in olive oil.

To prepare *chicken shish-kabob* cut three pounds of boned chicken into one and a half inch cubes. Thread them on a skewer. Dip skewer into mixture of one cup of chicken stock, one teaspoon of lemon juice, three-fourths teaspoon each of minced garlic and some powdered cumin, one-third teaspoon of salt. Place the chicken over the charcoal for about 15 minutes, or until done.

To prepare *spit barbecued duckling*: Using a four- or five-pound duckling, skewer it compactly from just in front of the tail, through the backbone, diagonally to the point near the wishbone, and again through the backbone. Spit roast the duckling for approximately one and a half hours over a low barbecue fire.

Baste frequently with the following sauce: ½ cup of orange juice; ¼ cup of soy sauce; 1 teaspoon of honey; ½ teaspoon of monosodium glutamate; some freshly ground pepper.

Heat sauce on the side of the grill and brush it warm on the bird. Use poultry shears to cut duckling into quarters to serve.

This will serve four.

To prepare *wild mallard duck* split a two to three-and-a-half pound Mallard duck up the backbone with poultry shears. Place it breast-side down on a cutting board, and press down breastbones using another board, or pound gently with a meat tenderizing mallet. Insert duck in hinged wire grill and broil over a hot charcoal fire until done to taste, about 10 to 15 minutes each side, basting it at least once on each side while cooking it, using the following sauce: 1 cup of prepared French dressing; 1 teaspoon of dry mustard; 2 teaspoons of Worcestershire sauce; 2 teaspoons of grated orange peel; 1 teaspoon of grated lemon peel.

Divide duck and breast bone into portions.

Will serve two to three.

A Popular Recipe for the Grill: Barbecued Spareribs

This recipe is for four to five pounds of spareribs. If they are too wide they should be cracked in half with a meat cleaver or sawed. Salt the ribs and grind fresh pepper on them. Brown on both sides on the grill over charcoal. When they are partly done, start to baste with the following barbecue sauce (remember that pork must be cooked thoroughly):

½ cup honey
⅔ cup soya sauce
⅔ cup ketchup
1 teaspoon of dry mustard
1 teaspoon of paprika
½ teaspoon tabasco sauce

4 or 5 drops of garlic juice
1 clove of garlic, finely mashed
1 teaspoon of salt
1 cup of orange juice
1 cup of wine vinegar

Combine all the ingredients over a slow flame in the kitchen.

This is an especially good dish for outdoor consumption, because people love to eat the spareribs with their fingers. It's fine too, though, for cooking indoors in the broiler.

Grilling Fish and Sea Food

Fresh fish: All fish used for grilling should be fresh. The eyes should be clear and bright, the gills pinkish red, the scales bright and firm.

Fish should be scaled and eviscerated. A small hole pricked on one side before fish is cooked will prevent it from puffing and losing its shape. Fish heads, if left on during cooking period, enhance the flavor of the fish. Don't handle the fish too much, or it will not stay whole. If your fingers and utensils pick up a fishy odor, they may be cleaned easily with a little ammonia and water or a couple of tablespoons of vinegar or lemon juice in water.

Fish comes in two categories, fat or oily, lean or dry. Most fish are lean or dry and need butter or sauce to supply the oil. A few fat or oily fish are: butterfish, sea herring, mackerel, salmon, shad, catfish, lake trout, whitefish.

All fish should be seasoned with butter, herbs and/or spices. If you season with flair, you will make many new flavor discoveries.

Some tips for grilling fish: use a hinged hand grill, so the fish will be held firmly and not fall apart while cooking, and so they can be turned easily. It is also wise to preheat the hinged grill until it is hot enough to mark the fish when you place it on the grill.

Flour and oil the fish and baste with oil several times during the grilling process.

Insert a toothpick or a small fork in the fish. If the fish flakes, the fish is done. Remember it is always better to have it slightly undercooked than overcooked.

Charcoal broiled trout: Dip the trout into seasoned flour, then into melted butter. Broil over charcoal, brushing frequently with melted butter for 10 minutes, or until fish is cooked. Serve with lemon and your favorite butter sauce. If you want to improvise, wrap one piece of bacon around the trout before grilling.

Barbecued haddock: Dip haddock fillets in soy sauce, salad oil, and sherry wine, mixed in equal proportions. Roll each fillet in sesame seeds. Heat oiled hinged broiler and arrange the fillets in it. Broil until fish flakes easily when tested with fork and sesame seeds are golden brown. Fillets usually cook in five minutes. With a lean or dry fish, try marinating the fish for one hour before barbecuing.

Marinating sauce for fish: With a fork, combine one-half cup each of olive oil and dry wine; add two cloves of garlic, finely chopped; one tablespoon of crushed pepper corns; one teaspoon each of salt, Worcestershire sauce, and paprika.

Skewered oysters: Be careful not to overcook these. Thread oysters on square skewer. Brush with butter. Put on rotary grill, or, if you like, wrap oysters in partially cooked bacon strips. Thread the bacon strip with the oyster on a skewer. Place a mushroom in between every oyster that is wrapped in bacon. Cooking time—about 5 to 10 minutes.

Lobster

Lobsters come principally from Maine and Nova Scotia. The only lobster to use in cooking is a live lobster. A live lobster is greenish, brown and black in color. When the lobster is cooked the shell turns red. Never overcook the lobster, or it will become tough.

Lobsters are male and female. The female has coral roe, which is a real delicacy. Lobsters have two different-sized claws and whichever is the largest claw determines whether the lobster is a right-handed lobster or a left-handed lobster. As a rule, the two claws are never the same size. If the lobster loses one of his claws, it has the amazing ability to grow another one.

Lobsters come in four different sizes: chicken (one pound in weight), medium, large, jumbo (four pounds in weight). Anything over a jumbo should be used only for lobster salad because it becomes too stringy and tough when boiled or broiled.

Lobsters are best when served with butter. Drawn butter is butter that has been melted in a double boiler over water, and not directly over the heat in a saucepan. With drawn butter try a couple of drops of Worcestershire sauce for variety. Five sauces for lobster follow:

Butter Sauce: In a saucepan melt three-fourths cup of

butter, pour clear butter into heated serving dish and add a few drops of lemon juice to taste.

Anchovy Butter Sauce: Rinse 10 to 12 anchovy fillets in cold water, or let them stand in cold water for 30 minutes to an hour. Chop finely. Add them to the butter sauce with one tablespoon each of chopped parsley and chopped chives.

Black butter (or *beurre noir*): Three-fourths cup of butter in a saucepan over high heat. Melt butter until it begins to turn brown. Add three tablespoons of chopped parsley, a few capers and one teaspoon of wine vinegar.

White butter sauce (or *beurre blanc*): One-fourth cup of white vinegar. One tablespoon each of finely chopped onion and parsley. Salt and pepper. Simmer in a sauce-

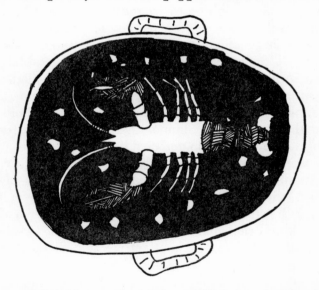

pan until liquid is reduced by half. Remove from heat but keep warm over hot water and gradually beat in three-fourths cup of butter. Serve hot and foamy.

Try *mustard butter* with lobster salad: In a saucepan

melt one-half cup of butter. Remove the pan from the heat and add one teaspoon of lemon juice and one-fourth teaspoon of salt. Beat in gradually two and one-half teaspoons of prepared mustard and continue beating the sauce until it is thick and cool. Serve slightly chilled with lobster and other shellfish.

Grilled Lobster (Half and Half)

For outdoor grilling of lobster I like to parboil the lobster and then finish it on the grill. Thus, I am assured the lobster is properly prepared in advance and there is no last minute cutting or cleaning to do. Boiling the lobster makes it more tender but grilling it makes it more flavorful.

To parboil a lobster I suggest this court-bouillon recipe: Melt three tablespoons butter in a saucepan. Add one large onion, one large carrot, three stalks of celery, all finely chopped. Cook until vegetables are brown. Add two quarts of water, one bayleaf tied with two sprigs of parsley, six peppercorns, two cloves. Add two tablespoons white wine vinegar. Bring to a boil and cover the pan tightly. Simmer the court bouillon for 30 minutes or longer. Strain and cool before using.

Plunge the live lobster into the court bouillon.* Boil for five to seven minutes, depending upon the size of the lobster. Remove with tongs, let cool at room temperature and split lobster lengthwise, removing the dark vein along the back and the small sack behind the head. Crack the claws. (Lobster may be kept refrigerated or on cracked ice until ready to be grilled.)

To grill, place the lobster first with the meat-side exposed to charcoals for approximately one or two minutes.

---

* Substitute recipe for court-bouillon: two tablespoons vinegar, two quarts of water, two tablespoons salt and seaweed. Bring to a boil and plunge lobster into boiling solution.

Then turn over with the tongs and place the shell-side on the grill until the shell starts to discolor to a dark brown, or black. While lobster is cooking baste with your favorite lemon and butter sauce recipe.

An Outdoor Favorite: Corn

When buying corn be sure to check it by examining the husks. The ears of the corn should have fresh green husks, the kernels should be plump and well filled, and should be soft and milky. Soft, small kernels indicate immaturity, while hard, glazed kernels without milk indicate the corn is overripe. Sweet corn in the yellow or white variety is preferred to the so-called field corn.

Because corn is so perishable, if you must store it leave the husks on, wrap the ears in cellophane, put them into a plastic bag, and refrigerate them. If you do not have cellophane or a plastic bag, a wet towel will do. Wrap it around the corn and put into the refrigerator. Keep at about 40 degrees Fahrenheit.

If you are going to prepare the corn by cooking it in water, be sure it has been properly cleaned and the silk and husks taken off. Place corn in the pot in a criss-cross fashion so that the ears on the bottom and on the top will be cooked to the same degree. Salt added to the water will make the corn tough. If the corn is a little old, add some sugar to bring back the sweet flavor. When corn is old its natural sugars start to turn to starch, and corn becomes old three or four hours after it has been husked and cut. One teaspoon of sugar for each six ears is approximately the correct amount to use. Use a 12-quart pot for about eight ears of corn. Bring the water to a boil and pour over the corn, which has been placed in a separate pot. Bring the water to a boil again and let boil for about four minutes.

If you want to cook corn on a barbecue grill, leave the

husks on but remove the silk. After you have wet down the husks so they won't dry out too fast, place the ears on top of the grill. Corn will cook fast and should be watched to avoid burning. Turn every 30 seconds to a minute.

Corn is always best when served with butter, salt, and freshly ground pepper. Furnish corn-eating bibs and corn-cob holders if you like.

Here is a marvelous herb butter which goes very well with corn:

1 tablespoon of chopped chives	½ teaspoon of tarragon
1 tablespoon of chopped fennel	½ teaspoon of marjoram
	a few bread crumbs
1 teaspoon of chervil	1 pound of butter

Cream the butter. Crush all herbs with mortar and pestle, adding a couple drops of brandy. Blend mixture of creamed butter and herbs together. Put mixture in earthen crock and chill in refrigerator. This may be prepared in advance and kept in the refrigerator until you are ready to serve your corn, or may even be frozen for future use.

A Cook-out Specialty, Fine too for a "Cook-in"

Swiss cheese fondue can be enjoyed in a cook-out and also indoors during the winter or inclement weather. It is probably the most ceremonial of all cheese dishes. There is quite a bit of tradition about the making of Swiss cheese fondue, and the utensils needed are somewhat different than you would normally find in the average kitchen.

To make fondue you should have the following:

1. An earthenware casserole that can withstand high temperatures and that is approximately 2½ quarts in capacity.

2. Long slender wooden-handled tin forks.
3. An alcohol or a Sterno burner, or an electric or L. P. Coleman type stove that can be placed in the center of the table around which you are going to eat.

The eating of Swiss cheese fondue is a community participation. The bread—and it should be French bread, lightly toasted, or Swiss rolls cut into small cubes and lightly toasted—is placed on the end of long wooden-handled tin forks. Everyone has his own fork and swirls it around to coat the bread with the fondue in the communal pan.

There is an interesting story that, if a cube of French bread falls into the fondue pot from your fork, then you owe a treat at your home or at some suitable place for another fondue dinner.

The ingredients you need for making Swiss cheese fondue for five are:

1 clove of garlic
1¾ cups of dry white wine, preferably Fendant Swiss Wine or Neufchatel
¾ pound of grated Swiss Emmentaler or an equal amount of Swiss Emmentaler and Swiss Gruyere

cheese, totaling ¾ of a pound
1 teaspoon of arrowroot or 2 teaspoons of cornstarch
3 tablespoons of Kirschwasser
Freshly grated black pepper

Rub bottom and sides of the heat-proof casserole with garlic. Add wine and heat it at a low temperature. *Do not let the wine boil.* Add the cheese a small amount at a time, stirring it constantly with a wooden (*not* metal) spoon.

When the cheese is smooth and creamy and barely simmering, add the arrowroot or the cornstarch which has been blended with the Kirschwasser. Stir the mixture until it starts to bubble just a little bit, then add pepper to taste and, if you want, a little nutmeg. Place the casserole over low alcohol flame. Keep the fondue hot, but not simmering. If it becomes too thick, add white wine, a little at a time, and stir.

The most important things to remember about making Swiss cheese fondue are that you cannot use a high temperature and you cannot rush the process. If you use too high a flame the cheese will become stringy and the white wine will lose its flavor by evaporation.

You may substitute Cognac or applejack or a little white rum or Calvados for Kirschwasser. However, you must use a genuine Swiss Emmentaler cheese or Swiss Gruyere cheese.

The Swiss customarily eat a boiled potato with some horse-radish and a dill pickle with the Swiss cheese fondue, and serve with it the rest of the slightly chilled Swiss white wines.

Chinese Oven Cooking
(Also called Smoke Cooking)

The smoke-oven technique is probably one of the oldest cooking methods. It involves suspending the food on hangers supported by steel rods on the top of the oven, or placing the food in baskets and suspending the baskets inside the oven. The best type of wood to use is hickory or fruitwood charcoal. Proper oven temperature is determined by the size of the fire in the fire box; a thermometer registering the temperature is most important, as the temperature varies depending upon the thickness of the walls. With a portable Chinese oven of sheet metal, there is a high loss of heat, but if the oven is made of brick it retains the heat. The temperature range in the oven is from 300 to 500 degrees F. Chinese cooking is best using the higher temperatures.

To cook a prime roast of beef, allow approximately 20 minutes to the pound in order to have the prime beef cooked rare. You will need a cooking thermometer to determine doneness, and it should read 120 degrees F. in the flesh of the meat if you wish to serve it rare.

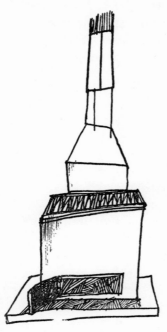

Spareribs cooked in a Chinese oven are ideal as an appetizer or as hors d'oeuvres. Paint them with a weak solution of soy sauce and hang in the oven. Allow to cook to a degree of doneness you like. Cut in small pieces and serve with an appropriate Polynesian or Chinese sweet and sour sauce.

When cooking poultry in a Chinese oven, have the heat low enough so that the poultry will not absorb a smoky taste.

Fish is particularly good prepared in a Chinese oven,

both salt-water and fresh-water varieties. Place the fish in the basket and hang in the oven. Check with a fork or toothpick to see if the fish is flaky, at which point it will be done.

Try experimenting with the Chinese smoke oven, using different combinations of food. Keep a record of the time and temperatures for future guidance.

If you enjoy the smoke cooking technique you might even consider building a smokehouse and smoking your own hams.

Closed-Pit Cooking

When I was a young man working for a contract farm team in Oklahoma during the summers, there was a rancher whose specialty for cooking for the farm team was to cook in a closed pit.

This is an interesting method of cooking, which probably started when utensils were not available. It was a useful method during the prairie schooner and covered wagon days, when a large number of people had to be fed. There is also a special flavor to food cooked in a closed pit.

The rancher in Oklahoma used pit cooking for boneless cuts of beef approximately 10 to 12 pounds in weight. He would get a number of pieces of this boneless beef and marinate them in a large bucket, using various and sundry mixtures of red wine, vinegar, water, olive oil, or peanut oil. The recipe is approximately as follows for a small quantity:

1 bottle of red wine   1 cup of water
1 cup of vinegar   1 cup of olive oil

Season with salt, crushed garlic, thyme, and plenty of freshly ground pepper and Cayenne pepper and chili powder, if you like the chili flavor.

Remove the meat after it has been marinating for at least one hour and wrap it in cloth that has been dipped into the marinating solution. It seems to me the rancher used burlap in three or four layers, redipped in the marinating solution, and tied it tightly. Nowadays we would wrap with aluminum foil, which will permit the marinating solution to penetrate into the meat.

The closed-pit is approximately the size of the open-pit fire, and rocks are used in it as in an open-pit fire. About four or five hours are required to get the coal bed to the right temperature.

Before placing the meat in the barbecue pit, move the bed of charcoal to one side and line the bottom of the pit with wet corn husks. Then place the meat that has been marinated and wrapped in cloth and aluminum foil on top of the husks. Place more wet corn husks on top of the meat. Add hot ashes as the fourth layer of the closed pit. Put some earth on top of the hot ashes and let cook for from four to six hours.

It is difficult to determine the length of time or the degree of doneness in this type of closed-pit cooking. The meat should be checked periodically, testing one of the wrapped pieces to ascertain this degree of doneness.

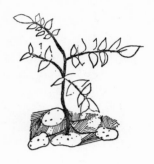

5

Underground Magic

by K. Cyrus Melikian

Remember the first potato you ever baked? The kids had built a bonfire, out back somewhere or in a vacant lot. After it got to burning pretty well someone said, "Let's bake potatoes!" and everyone scattered to raid the potato cellar. They came running back with the biggest potatoes they could find and tossed them around the rim of the blaze in the hot ashes. Then, with a stick in hand, each kid watched his special potato and the bakers were prodded and turned to get a good toasting on all sides. Swirling smoke made eyes stream and cheeks got tingling red from the heat. Finally all the potatoes were done. You raked them out and broke their charred skins. And there inside was a mealy little feast—yes, even without butter—much, much more delicious than any potato you'd ever had at your home dinner table. Or that's the way it seemed, anyway, because you had baked it yourself. Or was it because of the healthful open air, your youth, the adventure of cooking, the fun of doing things on your own?

Those bonfire-baked potatoes duplicated, in a way, the first potatoes ever cooked by man. The long-ago ancestor of all the various kinds of cultivated potatoes we have today was a small, wild primitive tuber that came from— no, not Ireland—from what is now Peru in South America. Possibly it got into an Indian's campfire by accident, but through the good fortune of that accident all the world fell heir to one of Nature's great gifts of deliciousness and food value.

Those first little South American potatoes and their aristocratic descendants were destined to travel far and contribute greatly to the nourishment and epicurean pleasures of man. Potatoes were introduced into Europe by Spanish and English explorers of the sixteenth century. Nearly another century was to pass before the potato was generally accepted and cultivated as an almost universal food. Indeed, for years in various parts of Europe potato plants were grown in flower gardens for their dainty and colorful blooms.

Agronomists, working toward the improvement of the potato, took them in hand, civilized them and fleshed them up and started them on the way to popularity. But it was not until 1621 that a shipment of English-grown potatoes was brought to North America, by way of Bermuda, landing in the sparsely settled colony of Virginia. The soil there proved good for them and the colonists came to use potatoes as a regular food. Another century passed before a group of Irish settlers brought potatoes to New England. Today the state of Maine produces almost twice the tonnage of potatoes as the next largest potato-yielding state. Maine is gifted with a most felicitous soil for potato raising.

So what is called an Irish potato is far from Irish in origin. But once it was introduced into Ireland the soil and the climate were more than suitable. In Ireland, probably more than in any other farming section of the world in those early days, the potato not only flourished but also provided an economical, strengthening food—as witness in the heartiness of the Irish people.

Incidentally, the word "spud" for potato comes from the word "spade." In Ireland a small-fingered spade was used to dig the potatoes from the ground. This spade came to be called a spud—a warping of the pronunciation through the mixture of Gaelic and cockney English—and gave its name to the vegetable for which it was devised.

In some parts of Ireland the potato is known as a "Spudsy-Murphy," for the numerous agricultural Murphys on the island. Thus we have in America the casual words "spud" and "murphy," both designations for the potato.

What is a potato? That may sound like a silly question but in chemistry and food value a potato is a complicated little gift package from Mother Earth to her children.

A potato is more than 75 per cent water, which is close to the percentage of water in the composition of the human body. The next most valuable elements are calcium, phosphorus, iron, thiamin (vitamin B_1), riboflavin (vitamin B_2), niacin (a member of the vitamin B complex), and, as if those ingredients were not enough, a potato contains small amounts of sulfur, manganese, chlorine, copper, silicon, boron, fluorine, iodine, aluminum, sodium, and magesium.

Perhaps you think of iodine as something to put on a cut finger, but it is also an essential element in the chemical balance of the body, both for man and animal. The richest percentage of iodine is found in potatoes grown near the seacoast. These soils contain iodine-rich ocean water that has seeped in, an action that has been going on through the centuries as a result of the rise and fall of ocean water levels and the rise and fall of continents.

Thus, the potato grown in almost any seacoast area

such as Maine, Long Island, the Carolinas, California, and states bordering the Gulf of Mexico will bring to the table a gift of iodine far surpassing that of potatoes from the Central States such as Ohio, Michigan, and Wisconsin where ocean water with its ingredient of iodine has never had much of a chance chemically to enrich the soil. The lack of natural iodine in the Central States led to adding it to table salt for general use, but particularly for use in the inland sections of the country. The result? A marked decrease of goiter in those states, where it once was so frequent.

One medium-sized potato contains one hundred calories, 2 per cent protein, 19 per cent carbohydrate, and a high percentage, depending on the variety, of ascorbic acid (vitamin C). That last item is most important. One average-weight newly dug potato, boiled in its jacket, supplies about one-fourth of the ascorbic acid recommended by the National Research Council as a day's requirement for a man or woman twenty-five years of age. Could anyone ask more than that from a vegetable?

Right here I should explode a myth—maybe a couple of myths. Way back in the sixteenth century when the potato was first introduced into Europe—a period in which strange superstitions abounded—the absurd notion was whispered about that potatoes were the cause of leprosy, a disease fairly prevalent in many European countries at the time. It was strictly a case of trying to pin the blame on some villain. Lacking any scientific medical knowledge on the subject, the fearful populace had to find a culprit no matter how ridiculous their suspicions now seem to us. But were their suspicions any more ridiculous than pointing the finger at decent old ladies in Salem, Massachusetts, and calling them witches? Stupid prejudices die hard, and it took many years for potatoes to live down that most gross of slanders.

Now for exploding a more modern myth, one that is still believed by thousands. Potatoes are *not fat-making* for reasonably normal persons. They do not cause obesity. Further, they do not need to be avoided by persons who have a tendency toward overweight. These are the verified conclusions of Dr. J. H. Kellogg, Superintendent of Battle Creek Sanitarium in Battle Creek, Michigan, who is recognized as an eminent authority on foods and their effect on human health.

To quote from Dr. Kellogg's article, "The Special Dietetic Virtues of the Potato":

> The potato is truly a most remarkable product. It contains within its aseptic covering a rich store of one of the most easily digestible of all forms of starch. The observations of Mossé, Von Noorden and others have shown most conclusively that the starch of the potato is more easily digested and appropriated by the body than the starches of wheat, corn, rice, and most other starchy cereals. In laboratory tests made by the writer it was found that potato starch digested in less than one-sixth of the time required by cereal starches. The experience of hundreds of physicians in the treatment of diabetics has shown that in many cases the starch of the potato is more easily assimilated or better utilized than other forms of starch.

That just about blows to pieces the myth that the potato is the culprit in ballooning up the human figure. Except in those extremely rare cases where obesity is an individual chronic tendency, the cause of overweight is simply overeating. And so the potato as prepared in all of its varied forms gets a clean bill of health. As for the dieting person who is counting calories the rule would be simply measure your potato intake as you would with any other form of food.

The potato family—an enormous one still increasing—could be said to be somewhat like the races of the human family. From the small tender little thin-skinned marbles, so sweet and delectable either creamed or simply boiled and buttered, to the solid, rugged, dry-fleshed bakers from Idaho and the rare and fancy Red McClures grown only in a small section of Colorado, they are all closely akin and of much the same composition. Red McClures, a "sport" cross pollination of Perfect Peachblow, have a ruddy skin and tinted flesh and are most fastidious as to the sort of soil in which they will grow and prosper. When procurable they command extra prices from discriminating epicures.

All varieties of potatoes, however, are highly selective as to the terrain in which they will reach their finest development. They specify their favorite farmland, it might be said, and there is just no use expecting a Nittany Cobbler of Pennsylvania to feel at home and develop its best qualities in the soil that produces the Luscious Burbank of California.

Perhaps the most notable trait that all potatoes have in common is the nutritional value of their skins. The valuable mineral content of potatoes is largely in the skin. And although these priceless and necessary minerals infiltrate, to some extent, the mealy center of the potato, the skin, whether the potato is boiled or baked, contributes the most concentrated and variegated mineral values. Hence a loss of value occurs when potatoes are peeled, although, of course, for certain potato recipes, the skins cannot be used. Many nutrition-wise people eat the skins of baked potatoes for the wealth of the needed minerals they contribute. Besides, they taste so good.

It should be said right here that the white potato is no relative at all of the sweet potato or yam, although they are both tubers and grown underground. But also grown underground are the root vegetables—carrots, turnips, beets—and for that matter, peanuts. But each is of a different genus, each, by its mysterious nature, taking different components and flavors and chemical elements from the soil. The only thing they have in common is their wondrous ability to derive from Mother Earth various and special nutriments for man and animal. Each is unique, as the potato is unique. Each adds its special wealth to the physical welfare of its consumers.

The potato lovers at your house have every right to expect potatoes at their best. That means that potatoes must be selected and bought with the same care and attention as beef and poultry or any other perishable food. As in all food buying there are times when the purchaser should find herself hearing a voice from within saying, "Not good enough." Here are some tips on how to choose really prime potatoes at your market.

In appearance potatoes should have smooth, clean surfaces. Don't hesitate to pinch them to test their firmness and skin quality. Refuse to accept wilted, leathery or spongy potatoes. They may have been frozen or victims of improper storage and thus have lost flavor and color as well as their mineral values and will be spongy when cooked. Insist upon shallow-eyed and regular shaped potatoes. Avoid those showing a green color on the surface. They are likely to have a bitter flavor. Dark brown spots are evidence that they have been scarred and bruised, predicating decay. Small black-lined holes are clues that wireworms have been at work. Turn away from the freakish outsize potato because it is likely to have a hollow heart.

If you have storage space and buy potatoes in quantity for use over weeks or months give them housing in a cool, moist, darkened place that has an average temperature of 50 to 60 degrees Fahrenheit. Under these conditions a late-crop, mature potato should remain firm and usable for as long as three months. Be sure that any defective ones are discarded before storage; they would contaminate their hibernating fellows. Warning—if you have a heating plant in your basement place your storage bin as far from it as possible. A plywood storage closet built in a remote corner of your basement, far from heat-waves, would provide an ideal place to tuck away apples, oranges, carrots, rutabagas, cabbages, and other vegetables and fruit—and also save you from too-frequent trips to the market.

The stored potato, however, even under ideal temperatures and storage conditions will change somewhat in chemical content. When a potato of whatever breed is first harvested it has its highest percentage of starch content and if cooked soon will be at its best and will taste its best. As storage time passes the starch content gradually diminishes and the sugar content increases. This change is related not only to the age of the potato but to the variation of storage temperatures.

Stored potatoes before they are used should be taken out of storage or the refrigerator and kept at room temperatures for a week or ten days for conditioning, even to the point when they start tiny white sprouts. This brings up the starch content and restores the potato virtually to its harvest-day nutritional value. Actually a potato which has just started to sprout is the perfect candidate for French frying. Mind you, no sprouting should have started at the time when potatoes are first bought and put into storage. At that time their eyes should be just dimples.

One great difference between the busy housewife, shopping list in hand as she approaches the grocery store, and the United States Department of Agriculture is that the latter is able to scour the potato-growing areas from coast to coast and bring back some 160 varieties of potatoes to test and analyze and cook in various ways whereas the housewife has only three or four choices at the most in making her purchase. However, if it is possible for the home shopper to make a wider selection, here are some interesting things that have been discovered by your government about the suitability of different tribes of potatoes for home cooking.

For boiling it has been found that the following family names ranked highest in general desirability, flavor, chemical values, and economy: Chippewa from Maine and Michigan, Irish Cobbler from Maine, Katahdin from Maine and Pennsylvania, Russet Rural from Michigan, Sebago from Maine and Wisconsin, and Triumph from Nebraska. These same potatoes, the Department reported, were also best for hash-browning and salad making.

Are you thinking of mashing? Here are the varieties found to be the best mashers based on their high degree of mealiness: Russet Burbank, White Rose, Green Mountain from Maine and New York, and Irish Cobbler from Maine. Incidentally if you don't really feel the need of the arm exercise that goes into mashing and prefer the quicker and easier way offered by the packaged dehydrated mashed potato powder, for which the skilled processors of this item mostly use Idaho bakers, you'll get the same result or even better.

If you're tuning up your oven for a roast—turkey, beef, leg of lamb—and have planned to put a hot baked potato on each plate, here are the beauties that will turn out the best: Russet Burbank, White Rose from Idaho, Green Mountain from New York, Irish Cobbler from Wisconsin, and Sebago from Washington. Notice how some of the varieties are repeated as "best of breed" whether for boiling, mashing, or baking. They may be called the aristocracy of the potato world. In buying potatoes for the home table your grocer or vegetable-man should, if you insist, be able to tell you by name just what potato he is offering you.

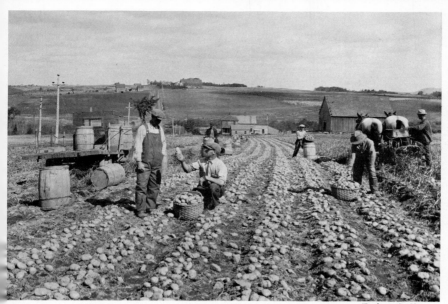

Potato harvest time in Maine's famed Aroostook County.

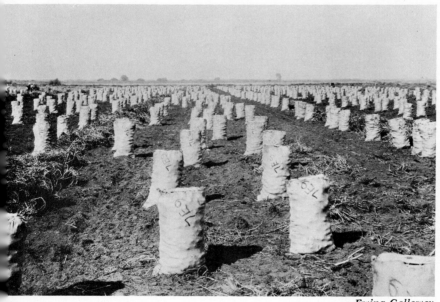

This acre of land on California's San Joaquin River delta produced 962½ bushels of spuds in one season.

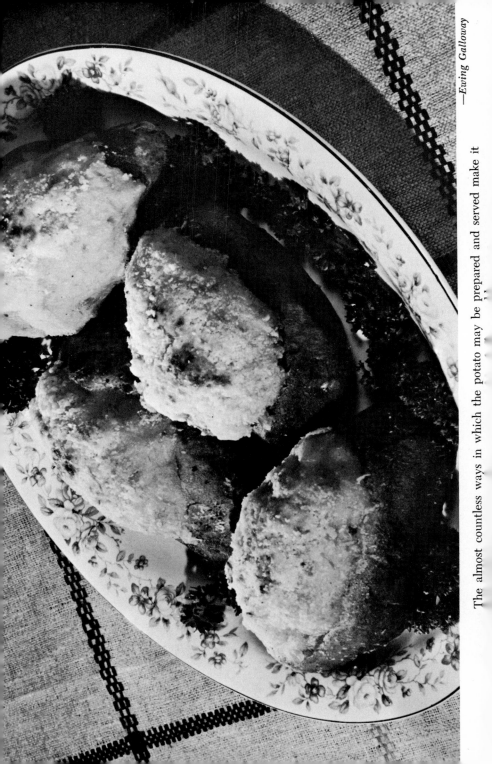

The almost countless ways in which the potato may be prepared and served make it

Speaking of aristocrats here's one that is so high-hat it seldom if ever leaves its native state. I have mentioned it earlier. It is the Red McClure of Colorado. It doesn't mean to be supercilious, it's just that travel and storage do not agree with it. It is grown at altitudes of 4500 to 9000 feet in the San Luis Valley, a small south-central section of Colorado where there is little rainfall. Hence the potato fields have to be irrigated with water from the mountain streams, fed by immaculate snows. The soil in the valley is unusually rich in the minerals it contributes to the Red McClure, making it a veritable gold mine of nutritional values. It is medium in size, mealy in substance with a reddish, almost auburn skin and delicately tinted flesh. Although smallish for a baker, the Red McClure bakes wonderfully. If you're lucky enough to live anywhere near the San Luis Valley you can buy a potato that is denied to most other people. Perhaps a way will be found to ship Red McClures, but up to now this ruby-like jewel refuses to be transported very far and remain at its usable best. However, a close relative, Red River Reds, with quite similar appearance and attributes—and with less objection to going places—are produced in Minnesota and North Dakota. They thrive in the northern counties adjacent to the Red River and, if you wish, will come right into your shopping bag and your home.

To get back to run-of-the-mill potatoes, the dependable domestic standby among vegetables, one of the most delicious ways to prepare them is French fried. In restaurants, all the way from lunch counters to hotel banquet tables, French fries represent some 50 per cent of all potatoes served. Since they are that widely called for, the housewife shouldn't dream of letting her admirers escape to the corner diner or sandwich counter. It takes only a small amount of equipment to compete with the best French-frying chef in town—a pot for the fat (which can be used again and again) and the wire basket in which the potato segments achieve their crisp perfection. That perfection consists not only in the crunchy toothsomeness of the French fries but in their fragrance and their inviting looks, light tan to golden brown to deep brown, depending on the tastes of those for whom you are cooking. The one necessary thing is to dip them out of their hot fat at the very last moment before serving. That's the point at which they are supreme. Here's an important consideration if you are maintaining a food budget: don't discard your slightly sprouted potatoes— French fry them! Don't hold back just because French frying seems to involve more work than boiling or baking. Actually French frying, so far as cooking time is concerned, is the fastest route from raw potato to dinner plate. In many homes it makes the greatest hit among all potato preparations.

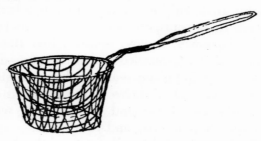

As to the potatoes you should choose for French frying: they should be firm under your thumb and finger, have solidity. After peeling, cut shallow slabs from four sides and both ends, making the potato a quadrilateral in shape. Cut segments lengthwise into uniform sizes, perhaps three-eights of an inch by four inches. This will insure each segment getting the same degree of cooking and browning —no rawness in one and crustiness in another. For good results in the home kitchen the cutting-up should be done immediately before the segments are put in the basket and immersed in the hot fat or oil. Next best, they should be kept ready in a bowl in the refrigerator. They should not be immersed in water. Watery segments not only will sputter when immersed in fat but will cook more slowly than if dry and will lower the temperature of the oil or fat and thus delay frying and browning. The ideal temperature of the fat in the pot when you immerse the basket of segments is approximately 380 degrees Farenheit.

There are two procedures at your choice in preparing French fries—the one-stage method and the two-stage method. The latter is probably the more propitious for the home-kitchen cook because it helps her get the plate on the table more quickly. The two-stage method of French frying is widely used by professional short-order cooks as a help in serving the customer promptly, and it also enables the home cook to get the French fries to the table crisp, fresh and piping hot as they should be. Well in advance of your dinner hour heat your pot of fat or oil to 360 or 380 degrees and lower the empty fry basket into the pot. Next raise the basket, put in the amount wanted of raw potato strips and lower the basket gently into the hot fat. Let the strips cook for about four minutes or until they are tender to the fork but *not brown*. Lift the basket and put the partially fried strips on paper towels. If you are cooking for a crowd repeat the process with other batches of raw strips.

If you wish, this pre-frying could be done the day before since these half-fried strips will keep perfectly in a covered container in your refrigerator and even longer in a deep-freeze compartment. As the dinner hour is closing in and your soup and meat are about ready for the table heat your pot of fat again, leaving the empty basket in. Watch that kitchen clock because here goes with the last-minute-before-serving detail. Gently place the par-

tially fried strips in the lifted basket and fry for about
one minute or so—or until golden brown. Serve immediately.

After the frying is done the oil or fat in the pot when
cool but not congealed should be strained through muslin
before putting aside for the next using so as to catch
small potato scraps and crumbs that may have accumulated during cooking.

Speaking of French fries the question is sometimes
asked—mostly by housewives, skilled with the paring
knife but somewhat tired of using it day after day—who
is it that peels all the tons of potatoes for restaurants,
institutions, catering services, frozen food packagers, canners, and dehydrated potato processors. Well it's all done
by the commercial potato peeling industry which had its
birth in a small way in 1931. Since then it has grown to be
a nation-wide service, not only available to the large
wholesale processors but also to domestic users. Today the
housewife can buy at her grocery store packaged, peeled
potatoes in units as small as twelve ounces.

Of the millions of pounds of commercially peeled potatoes some 85 to 90 per cent of the total are eventually
prepared as French frying sticks, ready in an instant for
the pot and, of course, a large demand is for crinkle-cut
slices. There are three methods used in commercial peeling—abrasive, caustic, and steam. A recent survey shows
that the abrasive method plants were the most numerous
and peeled the most potatoes although the caustic method
plants, less numerous, peeled about twice as many potatoes
per plant.

Have you always thought of potatoes as either boiled,
baked, creamed, mashed, fried, or as a salad? Perhaps
for most domestic cooks that's about all the reasonably
convenient ways to prepare them what with a thousand
other urgent things to do around the house. Actually there

are some 500 ways to use this great vegetable—more than merely hash-browned or potato pancakes to go with a pot roast. You might try a few of them if you are planning something special for a dinner and want to feel that warm glow that comes from hearing praise and appreciation from those at your table.

Incidentally, if you are entertaining any guests who are on a diet and avoiding butter and rich gravies you might substitute a large scoop of cottage cheese to nest in the opened, steaming spud, mixed with freshly chopped chives and parsley. Your thoughtfulness will make a real hit.

If you really want to create a great treat out of a baked potato, try this: Scoop out the two halves of the baked potato (previous to baking having brushed its skin with butter or oil) and empty the mealy innards into a bowl. Mash well, add milk, salt, pepper, one beaten egg, and a teaspoon of butter. Beat well until the consistency is that of heavy mashed potatoes. Put the mixture back into the skins, brush the top with cream, sprinkle with paprika and put the halves back into the oven to heat thoroughly. At the last minute before serving put the halves under the broiler to brown on top.

Here's another treatment of the baked potato that merits a standing ovation at the dinner table. This one is credited to the Pennsylvania Dutch. It calls for fresh, ground country sausage, the kind you make into patties. Sauté the sausage, allowing about one tablespoon of sausage meat for each potato, for three or four minutes before your potatoes, baking in the oven, are fully done. Baste the potatoes with the sausage grease while they are still baking. It gives a better conductivity of heat to the innermost core. When your fork tells you the potatoes are done, cut them lengthwise and scoop out the mealy contents. Into the potato skins place a mixture of the partially cooked country sausage and the scooped-out potato, packing it in tightly.

Return the potato halves to the oven at a temperature of about 375 degrees Fahrenheit for ten minutes or so, giving a chance for the sausage juices and flavors to infiltrate the potato. If you wish, put the halves under the broiler for a little browning. One might almost say you have a complete meat-and-potato meal with the addition of a fresh vegetable salad and an appropriate sweet for dessert.

For another version, remove the fully baked core of the potato and, after making it malleable with a fork, pack it back into the skins between layers of Cheddar cheese. Brush the skins with butter to keep them tender and chewable and put them back in the oven for perhaps fifteen minutes to give the cheese and potato time to meld. Before serving, garnish with paprika, add a sprinkling of salt and freshly ground pepper from your pepper mill.

Is there another vegetable beside the potato—or for that matter any fruit or grain—that can be used and enjoyed as an ingredient of each course of a single dinner, and without the diners feeling a surfeit of the recurrent ingredient? Probably not. Yet the potato can be a delicious component of every dish served, from soup to dessert. Want to try such a dinner? You could look upon it as just a culinary stunt or an amusing conversational topic—or maybe you'd like to give your family and guests an extra physical uplift by putting before them a truly generous shower of those great riches the potato contributes to human health.

First, before the guests get to the table, potato chips as nibbles with the sherry or cocktails. Potato chips served before dinner with tempting "dips" such as cream cheese and chopped chives or moist shrimp paste in bowls will not take the edge off the appetite—in fact they are likely to stimulate it.

Next, depending upon the time of year, you have a choice between hot potato soup or chilled Vichyssoise. For a recipe for both these see Chapter 1.

Now, the main course. Potatoes here can take a dozen different forms—baked, mashed, French fried, creamed, hash-browned, potato pancakes (with pot roast), or choose your own, whichever is suitable to go with the meat you are serving. To go with this course you can whip up a panful of potato muffins. Here's the way to do that. If you have some leftover mashed potatoes in the refrigerator so much the better. This recipe will give you a dozen tender, delicious muffins, hot from the oven. Assemble four tablespoons of shortening, two of sugar, one well-beaten egg, one cup of mashed potatoes, one cup of milk, two cups sifted flour, three teaspoons of baking powder, one-half teaspoon of salt, three slices of crumbled crisp bacon. Cream the shortening and sugar and blend in the potatoes and milk. Mix and sift the flour, baking powder and salt, add it to the creamed mixture, stir until smooth, then fold in the crumbled bacon. Fill the greased muffin tins two-thirds full. Bake at 400 degrees for 20 to 25 minutes. Voila!

That brings us to the salad course. You have two choices here, cold potato salad and hot potato salad. First, the cold. Boil four medium-size potatoes in their skins, peel and dice. When cool mix in two tablespoons finely chopped scallions, one teaspoon salt, two tablespoons chopped green pepper, one-fourth to one-half cup of finely cut celery, the same amount of diced cucumber, two hard boiled eggs, chopped. Stir gently one-half cup mayonnaise or thick salad dressing into the mixture, blend in one-half teaspoon of prepared mustard. Chill three or four hours before serving.

For hot potato salad, five or six servings, take three cups of diced raw potatoes and cook in a small amount of boiling water until tender. Crisp four slices of bacon, remove from pan and chop. Take two tablespoons bacon fat and fry one-fourth cup chopped onions until brown. Blend into the fat one tablespoon of flour, one teaspoon dry mustard, one teaspoon salt, one tablespoon granulated sugar. Add one cup of water, stir and boil for two minutes. Add two tablespoons of the hot mixture to a beaten egg, then stir this combination into the rest of the mixture. Add one-fourth cup of vinegar and reheat. Pour the hot dressing over the hot diced potatoes, mix in the chopped bacon and serve hot.

Is everybody ready for dessert? It is potato custard pie —and don't think of it as a heavy, pasty dessert. It is light and fluffy as a dessert should be to top off a hearty dinner and has no suggestion of potato flavor. Peel a medium-size perfect potato, boil it until tender and mash it smooth. Stir in two tablespoons of butter, one-fourth cup of sugar and let the creamy mixture cool. Add the beaten yolks of two eggs, one-half cup of milk, the juice and grated rind of half a lemon and blend the mixture well. Fold in the stiffly beaten whites of two eggs. Pour this filling into an uncooked pastry shell and bake in a 400 degree oven for about 25 minutes or until the crust is baked. That's it. Serve warm along with a demitasse of after-dinner coffee. At this point you can tell those at the table that they have been benefited with more Vitamin C than by any other dinner they ever sat down to—not to mention all the other healthful elements that abound in that quite magical tuber, the potato.

Now for those who like to experiment in the kitchen, here are some really challenging, off-beat recipes, fully tested, fully successful and at the same time real tests for you as a chef.* Attendez-vous!

Devil's Food Potato Cake

You'd never know there's potato in this luscious chocolate confection, but because it's there the cake stays moist longer. For a rich, smooth devil's food, try this recipe.

½ cup milk	2 cups sifted cake flour
3 squares chocolate	3 teaspoons baking powder
1 cup hot mashed potatoes	¼ teaspoon salt
1 cup shortening	1½ teaspoons vanilla
1¾ cups sugar	¼ cup sugar
4 egg yolks	4 egg whites, stiffly beaten

Heat milk and chocolate together. Stir until melted; add to potato and blend well. Cream shortening and sugar until light and fluffy; add to chocolate mixture. Pour in egg yolks and beat well. Mix and sift together flour, baking powder, and salt. Stir into chocolate mixture slowly, then add vanilla. Make meringue by gradually beating ¼ cup sugar into egg whites. Fold into cake batter and pour into three 8-inch layer cake pans lined with wax paper. Bake in moderate oven, 350°, for 25 to 30 minutes. When slightly cool invert on rack and remove wax paper. After cake is cold, spread frosting between each layer, over top and sides.

Stovies

4 large potatoes	½ teaspoon salt
2 medium onions	⅛ teaspoon pepper
¼ cup butter or meat drippings	

* Recipes from *State of Maine Potato Cook Book,* published by Maine Potato Committee.

Pare and cut potatoes and onion in ⅛-inch slices. Melt butter or meat drippings in heavy frying pan (4 slices of salt pork may be tried out and fat used, as well as crispy meat). Add potatoes, onions, salt, pepper, and water to cover partially. Use tight lid to cover closely and cook until vegetables are tender and water absorbed. Serves six.

Potato Acadia

An artist who creates beautiful pottery at his Frenchman's Bay studio introduced this recipe to his Maine neighbors. It comes from the Isle of Jersey and blends two vegetables for a distinctive flavor. It is something different in a potato dish.

4 medium potatoes
2 parsnips
3 tablespoons butter or margarine

¼ cup milk
1 tablespoon chopped chives or parsley
salt and pepper

Pare potatoes and cut in half. Pare and cut parsnips lengthwise in quarters. Boil together until tender. Mash well; add butter or margarine, milk and chopped chives or parsley. Season with salt and pepper to taste. Serves six.

Potato Puffets

Delicately crisp outside, light and tender inside, each puffet is just a little larger than bite size. In Maine they're usually served with fish, broiled halibut, for instance.

5 large potatoes
¼ cup butter or margarine
½ teaspoon salt
few grains cayenne pepper

2 tablespoons cream or top-milk
1 egg yolk
1 cup fine bread crumbs

Boil potatoes in jackets; peel and mash. Add remaining ingredients; beat until smooth and free from lumps. Spread on platter to depth of one inch. When cool, mold into balls about the size of walnuts. Roll each ball in flour; then dip into egg mixture* and roll in bread crumbs. Fry in hot deep fat, 390°, for five to six minutes. (If desired, sauté in butter instead of deep fat.) Serves six.

Potatoes Chantilly

Outdoors or in, this delicious dish will "bring down the house." It's a hit cooked over campfire or your own kitchen range.

3 large potatoes	salt and pepper
3 tablespoons butter or margarine	1 tablespoon chopped parsley
½ cup heavy cream	½ cup grated Cheddar cheese

Pare potatoes and cut in slender strips, as for French fries. Place potatoes in center of large square of aluminum foil. Carefully add cream; sprinkle with salt, pepper, parsley, and cheese. Bring aluminum foil together and "drug store" wrap, sealing or folding all edges to make a tight package. Place package on cookie sheet or shallow pan and bake in hot oven, 425°, for 40 to 50 minutes. Unfold foil; serve potatoes from foil or slide onto hot platter. Makes four generous servings.

Delmonico Potatoes

Maine people aren't the only ones who enjoy Delmonico potatoes. This recipe has won acclaim in restaurants and homes everywhere. Full of nourishment, the creamy mix-

---

* Egg mixture.

2 eggs, well beaten	few grains pepper
¼ teaspoon salt	2 teaspoons salad or cooking oil

(Mix all ingredients thoroughly)

ture is a tasty supplement to any cold meat supper or luncheon.

2 tablespoons butter or margarine
1½ tablespoons flour
1 cup milk
½ teaspoon salt
¼ teaspoon pepper
4 cups sliced boiled potatoes

3 hard-cooked eggs, sliced
½ cup cubed Cheddar cheese
2 tablespoons chopped pimiento
salt and pepper
¼ cup shredded Cheddar cheese

Prepare white sauce with butter, flour, milk, salt, and pepper. In buttered casserole, arrange layers of potatoes, eggs, cubed cheese, pimento, and white sauce. Sprinkle each layer with salt and pepper. Cover top with shredded Cheddar. Bake in moderate oven, 350°, for 30 to 40 minutes, or until brown and bubbly. Serves six.

New Day Potato Scallop

Sharp Cheddar cheese, a reminder of the cracker barrel days, plays a part in this up-to-date recipe. The tangy flavor of the scallop perks up a plain meal. Try it with meat loaf and sliced ripe tomatoes for budget-conscious, good eating.

4 cups cubed raw potatoes
½ cup chopped onion
½ teaspoon salt
1 cup heavy cream

few grains pepper
⅓ lb. Cheddar cheese
2 tablespoons diced salt pork

Mix potatoes, onions, salt, and pepper; place in buttered 1½ quart casserole. Cut or shred cheese and scatter over potato mixture. Fry pork until crisp; add cream, stir well, and pour over contents of casserole. Cover and bake in slow oven, 300°, for two hours or until done. Serves six.

Baked Potato Aroostook

An original recipe from Maine's big potato county, Aroostook, this baked dish is a delicacy enjoyed by those who grow the crops. Easily prepared, it's crusty and delicious with any roast.

6 medium potatoes
1 cup finely grated bread crumbs

½ cup melted butter or margarine

Pare potatoes and dry well on a towel. Roll each potato in butter or margarine, then in crumbs. Repeat rolling process in butter and crumbs. Place potatoes in baking dish and bake in moderately hot oven, 375°, until cooked —about 50 minutes. Serve at once. Serves six.

Pat's Potato Candy

"A far cry from potatoes in the role of the world's number one vegetable, but wonderful if you want to pamper your sweet tooth." Pat says Maine people seem "to go for" the bitter-sweet combination of smooth dark chocolate and chewy coconut fondant. The mashed potato base keeps the candy moist and delicious.

¾ cup cold mashed potatoes
4 cups confectioners' sugar
4 cups shredded coconut, chopped

1½ teaspoons vanilla
¼ teaspoon salt
4 squares baking chocolate

Mix potatoes (plain mashed, no butter, milk or salt added) and confectioners' sugar. Stir in coconut, vanilla, and salt; blend well. Press into one large or two small pans so that candy will be about ½-inch thick. Melt chocolate over hot water. (Do not allow water to boil. If

chocolate gets too hot it may be streaky when hardened.)
Pour chocolate on top of candy. Cool and cut in squares.
(For variation, make haystacks by forming white mixture
into cones 1-inch high. Allow to stand uncovered for 20
minutes. Dip base of each cone in melted chocolate; place
on wax paper until chocolate hardens. Yield—about 100
small haystacks.)

Potato Doughnuts

State of Mainers have a highly developed taste for
doughnuts, served at breakfast or any other meal. The potato doughnut is warmly regarded by these connoisseurs
of deep fat cookery. Here's a new version of an old
favorite.

1½ cups mashed potatoes	2 teaspoons vanilla
1½ cups sugar	¼ teaspoon cinnamon or nut-
1 tall can evaporated milk	meg (optional)
(1⅔ cups undiluted)	5 cups sifted all-purpose
3 eggs, beaten	flour
1 teaspoon salt	3 teaspoons baking powder

Pare and boil potatoes; mash while hot. Add sugar and
allow to stand in hot potatoes until sugar melts. Pour in
milk, eggs, and vanilla. (Nutmeg or cinnamon may be
used in addition to vanilla.) Mix and sift flour, baking
powder, and salt together. Add to liquid mixture to form
dough firm enough to roll, but keep as soft as possible.
Roll into ¼-inch thickness and shape with doughnut cutter.
Fry in deep fat at 370°, turning to brown on both sides.
Drain on paper towel or napkin. Makes about 36 doughnuts.

Potato pancakes are classic, and here is how to prepare
them. Take six medium-sized peeled and grated potatoes

(or cut them into very small pieces). Put them into an electric blender until they are reduced to a thick purée. Spoon off as much as possible of the potato liquid and beat in two eggs and salt and fresh-ground pepper. Add some fine cracker crumbs until the batter is firm enough to hold its shape. Fry the batter by tablespoonfuls in a generous amount of hot fat until the cakes are browned and crisp on both sides; add a little grated onion or minced parsley to the batter if desired.

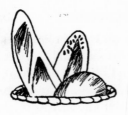

6

All Mankind Salutes this Kernel!

The Story of Bread

by Lloyd K. Rudd

The subject of bread is so vast that even to embark upon it takes courage. Into its story are woven elements which include Wheat in History, Wheat and Civilization, wheat products, kinds of wheat. There are three hundred varieties of wheat grown in the United States, and thirty thousand throughout the world; they all belong to one of fourteen species, only seven of which are grown here.

With the introduction of enriched self-rising flour, hardly more than twenty years ago, the whole picture of baking was changed. It is not possible to do more than touch on the highlights, but for the consumer, the highlights are what matter in turning out a good home-baked product, which may be anything from a macaroni casserole to Boston brown bread.

The history of wheat is a fascinating continuing story and follows the development of civilization. In 1948, an archaeologist uncovered a village in Iraq believed to be about 6,700 years old. In it were found two kinds of wheat similar to that grown today. Chinese historians record the growing of wheat some 4,700 years ago. The Bible is full of references to wheat growing, storing, uses and diseases, especially in Palestine and Egypt. Even further back in recorded history, ten to fifteen thousand years before Christ the virtues of wheat as a food had been discovered by man.

Many a war has been waged over land valued for its wheat-producing properties, and in this present state of world crisis, wheat is used by the United States as one of its greatest weapons for peace, in feeding hungry peoples the world over.

It is thought by anthropologists that primitive man was forced to wander over the surface of the earth in search of food; once he discovered that wheat was good to eat, he started to save it. Then followed his discovery that when a kernel was dropped in the ground it would grow and produce more wheat, so he could then settle down in one place to live, and this inevitably led to more leisure time, and experimentation with the development of new skills.

What a discovery it was when man found he could grind wheat between stones and make flour! This was the first flour milling. Flour was mixed with water and baked over fire. It is believed that the first loaves of bread were dark pancakes. About 2600 B.C. the Egyptians experimented with processes of fermentation and discovered the way to make dough rise, and stay light.

The methods of milling have been developed and improved over the centuries. Flour was first milled by pounding the grains of wheat between two stones—in time the lower stone became hollowed-out and the upper one more rounded, which resulted in the first mortar and pestle. This hand-operated mill was called a saddlestone, from the shape of the lower stone. For a period of about 1,700 years this method of milling was practiced, until 300 B.C., in Chaldea, Egypt, and Palestine.

From this method it was a long step to the rotary mill, or quern, made by fitting two large, flat stones together. Wheat was poured through a hole in the upper stone and allowed to trickle down to the lower stone. A stick acted as a lever to turn the upper against the lower stone, grinding the grain. Once this revolving-type mill had been developed, any number of them were put into use, some so large they were dragged around by slaves or horses, hitched to a lever arm.

Milling changed little in principle for centuries; the improvements came in the sources of power for turning the millstones. About 100 B.C. the Romans were using water power to turn the large millstones. Wind and water cut down the manpower and made it possible to increase flour production. It is believed the first mill in North America was built by the French in Nova Scotia in 1605. Gradually machinery to handle the grain entered the picture, and volume flour production was assured.

The invention of the steam engine in 1769 by James Watt made possible the next important step in milling, the development of the roller mill. Although it had long been known that steel rollers were superior to millstones for milling flour, wind and water power couldn't turn the rollers fast enough. Steam power proved effective. The first successful roller mill was used by a Swiss, Jacob Sulzberger, in 1834.

Edmund La Croix developed the middlings purifier in Minneapolis in 1870. The purifier is a machine using strong currents and bolting cloth to separate the outer coat of the wheat, the bran, from the endosperm, the inner portion from which white flour comes. Bolting cloth makes a sieve or mesh with openings to allow particles of a certain size to pass through. The purifier improved flour immensely. Because La Croix failed to patent his own device, however, he was involved in much litigation, which was finally settled against him. But the better flour produced became known as "Patent" flour, so called to this day.

Many types of power are used today to make flour. Electricity generated by water, steam, or Diesel engine is most widely in use, but sources of power from Diesel, steam, and gasoline engines are directly used in some mills.

Many prominent personalities have been identified from the beginning with wheat growing and flour milling. One of the most famous wheat-growers and millers in early American history was George Washington, whose mill was located in the Allegheny Mountains. So excellent was the quality of his flour, it was accepted in the West Indies and other markets with little or no inspection. It was enough for buyers to see the stamp, "George Washington, Mount Vernon," for them to buy eagerly.

The testing of flour is important. Laboratory tests for determining the composition are not regarded as enough. So after sample lots of flour are provided, bakery and family flours are checked in actual production, through testing kitchens where home economists bake a variety of products. Only after the miller, chemist, baker, and home economist have given approval is the flour ready for market.

Before we get into the actual flour-to-bread processes, a word should be said about the classes of flour. The various types of wheat from which the flours are milled are durum wheat, hard wheat, soft wheat, and combinations or blends of hard and soft wheats.

Following are the uses for which the flours are milled:

Macaroni flours. Those milled especially for making macaroni, spaghetti, and noodles. These flours are chiefly milled from durum wheat, which is high in protein. Properly speaking, macaroni flours are not bread flours and perhaps do not belong in this chapter, except that a large percentage of such flours are made from wheat.

Bread flours. Milled for bakers, made from either hard spring or hard winter wheat, or a combination of the two. These make good yeast breads, are somewhat granular to the touch.

All-purpose, general purpose, or family flours. Flours blended for all household cooking. Depending upon the area where the wheat is grown they may be of hard wheat or soft wheat, or a blend of both. Lower in protein than bread flours, family flours contain enough protein to make good yeast breads, as well as quick-type breads.

Pastry flours. Usually finely milled from soft wheats, low in protein especially for making pastry and chiefly used by bakers.

Cake flours. These are the most finely ground of all flours, milled for the lightest cakes, from soft wheats. These represent the most highly refined flour streams of the mill.

Years ago, nutritionists were becoming alarmed at the deficiencies in the American diet, and clamored for changes in standards which would make up for these lacks. Because bread is eaten by practically everyone in some form or other every day, flour was chosen as the best means to add the necessary elements to the nation's diet, including vitamins.

This led to the introduction of *enriched flour*—white flour to which specified B-vitamins, the food mineral iron and often calcium have been added in prescribed amounts. The required ingredients for enriched flour include thiamine, riboflavin, niacin (formerly called nicotinic acid), and iron, and the optional ingredients are calcium and Vitamin D. For enriched self-rising flour, all of these ingredients are required except Vitamin D, which is optional. Self-rising flour, both white and wheat, is flour to which have been added the leavening ingredients, bicarbonate of soda and monocalcium phosphate or sodium acid pyrophosphate or both, and salt for seasoning.

There are almost countless varieties of bread, varying from the molasses-drenched brown bread of Boston to the "reducing loaf" so thin you could read a page of print through it. By the way, bread is now on most reducing diets; it has been demonstrated that the nourishment it affords may well be a necessity in any diet requiring calorie-counting. The average slice of white bread contains only 65 calories.

In large supermarkets, you may find as many as fifty to seventy-five varieties, sometimes more. Every day, experiments go on in the research organizations of the bakers of America, to produce more and different breads with exotic or familiar flavors. How would you like a raisin loaf, flavored with mint? You may have it. Or does your taste run to rye bread with lemon peel? Without too much searching, it is available. In 1958, a baker in Fallbrook, California, Virgil Wedeking, perfected a formula using half an avocado (about three ounces) to a one-pound loaf of bread. The result is a product with a rich, nutty flavor and a delicate green color. Users were enthusiastic about it, especially when it was toasted.

You may even have variety in plain white bread. The loaves may be hearth-baked—placed directly on the oven floor instead of in pans (Arnold breads, for instance)— furnishing them with a golden crust and a delicious aroma of wheat and yeast. Or they may be pan-baked and raised to such a degree that each slice seems gossamer-light and quite removed from wheat. Or there are loaves so packed with milk, butter, eggs, and sugar—compact and delicious —each slice a full meal.

The history of the discovery of raising bread is attributed to an indolent Egyptian slave who let his fire go out when he was baking the usual flour-water paste to make the flat cakes he was supposed to turn out. In the morning he found that the dough had, surprisingly, puffed up several times its original size. But he shoved it in the oven, anyway, and today's bread was born. It became the national custom to let dough stand overnight before baking it. Louis Pasteur gave the world the reason for this phenomenon, after observing bread dough under a microscope. Spores of yeast settled in the dough, multiplied at a furious rate, and gave off carbon dioxide. Tiny bubbles of the gas permeated the dough, gathered into little pockets expanding it. Baking expelled the gas, leaving the baked bread light and delightfully flavorsome.

The raised loaf is produced predominantly from wheat (in some degree by rye) flours, which is why wheat has been, since earliest recorded time, man's favorite grain. Even in countries where rice is a more important crop, such as India, China and other nations of the Orient, wheat is so important that its crop failures have resulted in national food shortages.

The United States alone in 1955 produced approximately a billion bushels, on some seventy million acres, in the Great Plains and North Central States, some areas east of the Mississippi, and in the Columbia River Basin and uplands of Washington, Oregon, and Idaho. Kansas leads in the number of bushels, but North Dakota and Montana are not far behind.

Great storage elevators dot the country and contain some billion and a half to two billion bushels of surplus. While that is sufficient to keep the United States from famine for a long time, it also permits this country to extend foreign aid as a means of insurance for world peace.

You may always think of the old song "Down by the

Old Mill Stream" as an image of bucolic charm, but the term *millstream* now affords a completely different picture. This is the endless, sibilant river that is the flow of wheat in the process of becoming flour. The nation has 1,799 flour mills throughout some 45 states, and they grind out more than twenty billion pounds of flour a year.

Wheat pours into the mill on belt conveyors from giant elevators, steel and concrete cylinders which hold as much as fifty thousand bushels of wheat apiece. In the mill it flows up and down by means of pneumatic tubes through floors packed with processing machines. At the very center of the process are pairs of steel rollers with progressively finer corrugations. Revolving toward each other the pairs of rollers pulverize the kernels more and more finely. Between each set of rollers the stream passes through flour bolters which sift off the bran and wheat germ. So automatic has this process become that a huge mill may be run with a minimum of workmen, and these only check on the flow of the millstream.

Few millers do any commercial baking, since milling and baking are two separate businesses. In a modern bakery great storage bins hold many tons of flour, which is flowed to sifters, and conveyed to a floor where it is joined with water and yeast to become the preliminary "sponge." In this giant mixer, capable of taking many hundreds of pounds, great steel arms beat away at the mass for some minutes until it is dumped into a steel trough and wheeled into a moist fermenting room. It is allowed to rise for five hours, then returned to the mixer where other ingredients are added, and again it is tumbled into the trough and sent to the fermenting room for another hour.

Next the dough is trundled to a divider, which, with uncanny precision delivers exactly one pound of dough to a bite and hurries the ensuing hunks to the rounder.

This whirls to roll the bits of dough into balls which are allowed to rise briefly, then are flattened into cylinders and plumped into pans. The pans are passed through a highly steamed atmosphere, much like that in a Turkish bath, where the yeast does extra work, and on to a traveling oven. The length of this oven may vary, usually it is about one hundred feet or more long. When the loaves are expelled from the oven they have been baked in passage and are delivered to the cooling racks at the far end, some four thousand per hour. As soon as they are cooled, they go to automatic slicers-and-wrappers and then, on to the grocers and to the ultimate consumer.

Never let it be forgotten that one of the things built into the modern process of baking is the wonderful, satisfying aroma. It is said, however, that sad though it is, bakers early lose the sense of smell, since they get so used to it. But in the baking, it is there, just the same.

To revert for a minute to the nutritional revolution in flour and bread. The reason bread today is so vital to the health of the nation dates back to the 1930s, when one of the great discoveries was that of B-complex vitamins. B-vitamin deficiencies resulted, it was proved, in uncounted cases of pellagra. For every one properly diagnosed, there were innumerable others. In May, 1941, the National Nutrition Conference for Defense was convened in Washington by President Roosevelt. Not too long thereafter, under the leadership of Dr. Russell M. Wilder, the Mayo Clinic's nutrition specialist, with the aid of experts from the National Research Council, the American Medical Association, and the American Public Health Association, the conference launched the Bread Enrichment Program. From the beginning, millers and bakers cooperated enthusiastically. Today, a majority of the states have laws making enrichment mandatory. Even without a national law governing the introduction of the required ingredients, 75 per cent of our bread now carries the extra nutrients.

The Army will vouch for the success of this program. Formerly there were thousands of clinical cases of pellagra, but it has almost disappeared from this service. It is admitted that enrichment of bread is responsible for almost eliminating the disease in America.

The story of the invention of America's favorite contender in the consumption of bread dates back to the eighteenth century, when that dissolute rake, The Earl of Sandwich, wanting to gamble and eat at the same time, ordered his dinner served between two halves of a loaf of bread. This legendary approach to the sandwich is brought up to date by the hero sandwich which may be almost as large and thick as the English earl's. Hundreds of thousands of sandwiches are made and sold every day; by far the greatest number are made of white bread, though there are classic choices of ham or Swiss cheese on rye, and cream cheese on diet breads. Not long ago, I visited the self-service cafeteria of one of America's great women's magazines, and the employees, I noticed, almost to a man, munched happily on sandwiches. The scene was typical of thousands repeated throughout the country— at luncheonettes, school cafeterias, drugstore counters, industrial plants, department store lunchrooms—in short, just about everywhere in a civilization that wants to eat in a hurry, but needs to derive nutrition at the same time. Statistics show that during the picnic season we eat nearly half again as much bread as during the other months of the year. There are innumerable ways of putting nearly every known fish, meat, dairy, and vegetable product from artichokes or anchovies to zucchini between bread slices. There are whole books published about new sandwich treats, probably of value chiefly because they try to stimulate new taste sensations, but at a guess it is likely that the trusty standbys of ham-and-egg, egg salad, the robust Western, and hamburger with onion will continue in top rating.

The standard white loaf is a universal favorite throughout the country, though there are sectional preferences in bread consumption. I learned that in Washington, D.C., and in Southern California, there is a great deal of moist, crumbly whole-wheat bread in the local diets. These breads are made of a flour which may be from 10 to 60 per cent whole-wheat flour, the rest white flour—the average is about 40 per cent whole wheat. On the other hand, the three great port towns of New York, New Orleans, and San Francisco consume great quantities of French and Italian breads. The distinction is that French breads are long and thin, and Italian breads are short and fat or round. One of the simplest of recipes, Italian bread is made with flour, water, salt, and yeast, and while delicious when freshly baked, it is likely to go stale only a short while out of the oven. It's a bread that can best be baked at home to insure freshness, but few housewives are willing to turn the clock back to the slavery of home bread-baking, alas! Consider the statistics. Fifty years ago, 95 per cent of America's bread was baked at home. Now commercial bakeries produce 95 per cent of all the bread eaten.

In some places rye breads are popular. Rye flours, like wheat may be refined to eliminate the bran, or they may consist of the whole grain which produces the bread called pumpernickel. But even pumpernickel, a great favorite with certain German-influenced sections in towns (i.e., Yorkville in New York) and Milwaukee as a city, is made with only 20 per cent rye and 80 per cent wheat, because rye dough if pure will rise only slightly.

Milwaukee goes for the darkest, solidest pumpernickel; coupled with Limburger cheese it couldn't be fuller of calories or, indeed, nourishment. In some areas of the Middle West, such as Minneapolis, rye bread is served Swedish style—its color comes from molasses and it is tinged with a faint flavor of orange peel. If you go for sour rye, your spot is Philadelphia where it is made with a starter rather than ordinary yeast. It tastes like a delicate cheese. And all across the country is a small loaf of salty rye which carries the tang and sharp recognizable flavor of caraway seeds.

While raisin bread is a prime favorite, it finds its most compatible home in St. Louis. There it is baked in a number of ways, including cinnamon raisin and raisin nut. It is also available in an iced loaf, which is close to cake and is a wonderful ladies' choice for club doings and bridge teas.

There is hardly anything in the food line which cannot be added to bread to produce an edible product. Whether it will be everyone's dish is another story. In California there is a bread which includes dates, oranges, lemons, apricots, peaches, and prunes. Can you ask for more? Well—in Chicago not too long ago, a loaf was turned out which was made of whole wheat, rye, soya and barley flours, oatmeal, sesame seed, plus dehydrated spinach, celery, lettuce, pumpkin, cabbage, carrots, parsley, and sea kelp.

Speaking of soya, these breads as well as potato breads have had acceptance in certain parts of the States. The percentage of these flours is usually five to the whole. Banana, cheese, tomato, peanut, and sweet-potato breads have been enjoyed here and there throughout the country.

Commercial baking processes have undergone some drastic changes in the past few years. In 1953, there was introduced to the market a new bread-making principle called "continuous mixing." This is achieved by a process with the Baker Do-Maker. (Long *o*, please.) Automation of the whole bakery is complete with this process. It is, so its sponsors claim, the missing link between raw ingredients and fast, automatic baking and handling equipment, and provides the needed automation ahead of the continuous oven, fast depanners, modern slicers and wrappers. First the dry ingredients are mixed, and the soluble ingredients mixed into them, which produces a texture of bread substantially smoother than the usual commercial bread. There are several advantages: in appearance the bread is light and appetizing due to evenness of grain and softness of texture. The process eliminates flour streaks in the bread and hard flakes in the crust because no dusting flour is used. It toasts more uniformly because the grain is more uniform. It holds sandwich filling better because of the compact structure and absence of holes. And because it stays fresh longer, it increases shelf-life.

From the consumer point of view, less butter is needed to spread the surface because the slices have no holes, and in using spreads such as marmalade and mayonnaise, savings of up to 30 per cent are effected.

Many discoveries in baking have been made quite by accident, but one of the most dramatic is the story of the "Brown 'n Serve" rolls which burst on the market to the delight of harried housewives. In the town of Avon Park, Florida, a baker named Joe Gregor was also a volunteer fireman. A fire broke out just as he had a batch of rolls ready for the oven, so he rushed away to do his civic duty, pulling the rolls half-baked out of the oven. Returning from the fire, he found the cold, unappetizing rolls sitting pallid and waiting, and he debated about throwing them out, but had a second thought and put them back to bake. This resulted in a major baking triumph, because it didn't take long to work out a foolproof formula. He began in a small way, locally, and was soon selling more half-baked rolls to be finished in the customer's own oven than fully baked ones. Mr. Gregor found out, much as the Egyptian slave had, centuries before, that there is always something you can learn about bread-baking.

A salesman from one of the big flour-milling companies (General Mills) visited him, and with the cooperation of the salesman's boss, the company acquired the idea and perfected it for mass-production use, and something very new had been added to baking. Many a hostess takes full, complacent credit for the piping hot rolls which come fresh from her oven, but who cares about such a minor deception?

We haven't paid nearly enough attention to yeast, the greatest of all leavening agents, insofar as bread is concerned. It is known as a biological leavener and is a tiny plant which multiples rapidly under proper conditions and requires moisture, food, and warmth for growth. Sugar is necessary for the yeast plant, and while wheat flour has some sugar, it is not enough for the yeast requirements. A small amount of sugar, therefore, is added in making yeast-raised breads. As the yeast grows, it generates carbon dioxide gas, which bubbles through the flour mixture to make the dough light and porous. Active dry yeast is not nearly so perishable as compressed yeast; both, however, may be used satisfactorily in baking bread.

Other leavening agents include soda, a chemical leavener and baking powders, which may be tartrate, phosphate, or combination-type. The labels on commercial powders are self-explanatory. This may seem elementary information to the experienced cook or housewife, but it is surprising to many home economists how little many in the present generation know of bread-baking, and they find many cooks are downright frightened of the responsibility of turning out a palatable loaf or any one of the quick breads. There are those who see poetry in bread-making, and one of those is Richard Blake, a well-known television executive, and a fine, experienced amateur chef. He has a recipe in which he uses cornmeal, and when asked for it sent in the following:

Bread-making is a dandy hobby. The process involves pleasure of several kinds: physically, kneading is a pleasant, relaxing sensation (page Freud, or put it down to merely an outlet for tension), punching down the risen dough is fun, and smelling the stuff baking is strictly an aesthetic delight.

Fresh-baked bread tastes pretty special. But it slices easier when it's staler. All things considered, you're about as well-off financially in buying the stuff, and probably better off nutritionally.

Basic bread recipes can be varied quite a lot, as fancy, experience or taste wills. I've found this a satisfactory recipe:

Start by dissolving two packets of yeast powder in a quarter-cup of tepid water in a large bowl. Add to this two cups of warm, but not hot, liquid. This can be either water (if you're a skim-milk fan, in which case the proper amount of skim-milk powder is mixed in with the flour) or scalded milk. Raw milk, pasteurized and/or homogenized, kills the yeast action. Evaporated milk doesn't. Two tablespoons of sugar should have been dissolved in the liquid to speed the yeast fermenting action, and one of salt. Also two tablespoons of shortening. I think lard tastes best. Butter or margarine is okay. And for those off on a non-cholesterol kick, make it corn oil.

My variant to the original recipe is to add one-half cup of corn meal, which has been cooked five minutes in water as per package directions for mush: pour the meal mixed with one-half cup of water into one cup boiling water, stir until thick. Put aside until this next step is finished:

Sift, a cup at a time, three cups of flour into the yeast-liquid mixture. Mix with an egg beater or an electric job. Then the cornmeal. Then, add about three cups more of flour, stirring with a heavy spoon until it gets too thick to stir.

At this stage, dump the dough on a floured board and let it set—"rest"—for about ten minuites. Then begin kneading, with frequently floured hands. Add more flour from a shaker if necessary from time to time until the mass is no longer sticky as you fold and knead. Keep this up until the surface is satiny. That means that everything is distributed properly and the yeast is going into action.

Put it back in the bowl, by now rinsed out and greased. (Some people believe in a non-greased bowl, but the dough's apt to stick.) Put in a warm place and cover with a wet towel or plastic film—something to keep out the drafts. Let it rise until doubled in size— about two hours. Punch down, knead again slightly and divide into two loaves for the first baking, another loaf to go in the freezer for another day's baking, and what's left over (a scant half) for rolls.

Put into well-greased bread pans (rolls into muffin tins) and let rise again until doubled. A good place for this rising is in the oven, unlit, of course. Otherwise, cover them over with wet towels. Brush the top with melted butter or margarine for a good crust, and with milk for a darker crust.

Start baking at about 400 degrees. After about twenty minutes, lower heat to 250 degrees and let bread finish at that. Should take about another half-hour. Bread is done when it sounds hollow when thumped. Cool on racks. (Rolls take only about twenty-five minutes all told.)

The dough you've put in the freezer will rise again when defrosted. It will rise some if just tucked in the refrigerator.

Batters for pouring griddlecakes, waffles and popovers, or drop batters, which include muffins, quick coffeecakes, corn breads, cream puffs, fritters and dumplings, and soft doughs, for biscuits, scones and doughnuts—all need a bit of study before they are attempted by the novice. If directions are carefully followed, there should be few failures, though many things have to be watched, from overmixing or underbaking to an overly stiff batter, or improper use of eggs.

A basic sweet dough may be used for any number of yeast bread recipes and to make everything from hot cross buns to French peasant rings. Here's how it's made (recipe supplied by Wheat Flour Institute):

Basic Sweet Dough

2 packages yeast, compressed or dry
¼ cup water (lukewarm for compressed yeast, warm for dry)
1 cup milk
½ cup sugar

2 teaspoons salt
¼ cup shortening
5 cups sifted enriched flour (about)
2 eggs
1 teaspoon grated lemon rind (if desired)

Soften yeast in water. Scald milk. Add sugar, salt, and shortening. Cool to lukewarm. Add flour to make a thick batter. Mix well. Add softened yeast, eggs, and lemon rind. Beat well. Add enough more flour to make a soft dough. Turn out on lightly floured board and knead until smooth and satiny. Place in greased bowl. Cover and let rise in warm place until doubled (about one and a half hours). When light, punch down. Let rest 10 minutes. Shape into rolls or coffeecake. Let rise until doubled (about 45 minutes). Bake in moderate oven (350° F.) 20 to 30 minutes.

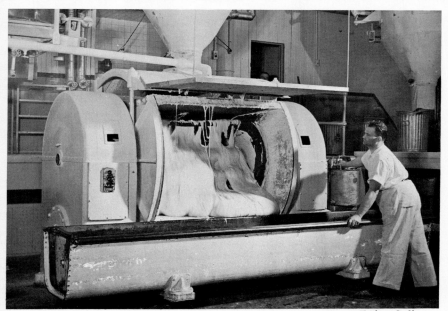

In modern commercial bread baking, machines like this one thoroughly mix the dough.

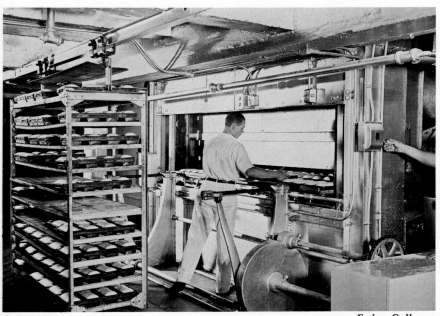

Pans of dough go into this moving oven which bakes over 4,000 loaves of bread an hour.

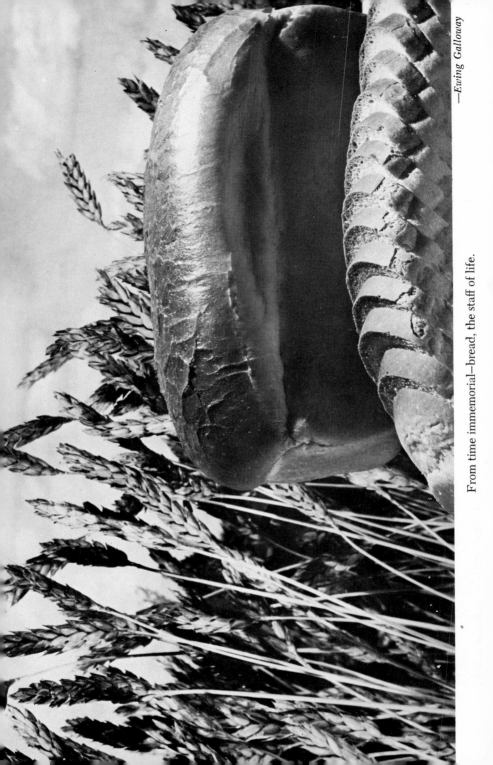

From time immemorial—bread, the staff of life.

Makes two or three coffeecakes or about three and a half dozen rolls.

There is a twin recipe for basic beaten batter which is yeast-leavened (also courtesy Wheat Flour Institute), and this is part and parcel of such confections as a syrupy coffeecake, crumble squares, apricot puffs, orange marmalade swirls, and many others. Here is how it goes:

Basic Beaten Batter (Yeast-Leavened)

1 package yeast, compressed or dry
¼ cup water (lukewarm for compressed yeast, warm for dry)
1 cup milk
¼ cup sugar
1 teaspoon salt
½ cup shortening
3¼ cups sifted enriched flour (about)
1 egg (use 2 eggs for richer batter)
½ teaspoon vanilla extract (if desired)

Soften yeast in water. Scald milk. Add sugar, salt, and shortening. Cool to lukewarm. Add two cups flour and beat well. Add softened yeast, egg, and vanilla extract. Beat well. Add more flour to make a stiff batter. Beat thoroughly until smooth. Cover and let rise until bubbly (about one hour). Use with different toppings to make coffeecakes and puff rolls. Let rise until doubled (about 30 minutes). Bake in moderate oven (375° F.) 20 to 30 minutes.

Makes two 8-inch square or 9-inch round coffeecakes or about two dozen 3-inch puffs.

I suppose there is no general rule about home baking except the most dependable of all: when you have found the recipe you want to use, follow it carefully, and do not improvise as your more experienced grandmother might have done, since now you are supplied with plenty of accurate equipment for baking, including measuring cups, measuring spoons, mixing bowls of proper sizes, spatula, flour sifters and sieves, rolling pins, and baking pans of proper sizes either of glass or aluminum. There are innumerable other convenient devices in a completely stocked kitchen, but cooks learn to know what they depend on for their best results, and these become chiefly a matter of individual choice.

There are many ways in which baking may turn out successfully at home by observing certain basics. For example, take the matter of baking pans. Many recipes specify the size and shape of the pans to be used. If such directions are given, the home cook is wise to follow them. The rate of browning desired influences the kind of pan to use. A bright, shiny pan reflects the heat and slows down the browning of the crust. Biscuits are best baked on this type of sheet. A dull, dark pan absorbs the heat rapidly and browns the crust faster. Muffins are best cooked in such pans, as well as yeast breads. Glass baking pans are good for loaf breads. Since glass tends to hold the heat, oven temperatures should be reduced about 25 degrees.

Pans give shape to bread, and many breads are recognized by their distinctive shapes or textures. An experienced eye can tell when popovers, for instance, have been baked in a heavy iron popover pan, with cups deeper than they are wide.

There are certain essentials to remember: some breads are cooked by frying in deep hot fat, that steamed breads and puddings are cooked in a steamer, a deep-well cooker or a deep kettle; a heavy hot griddle turns out the best griddlecakes or hot cakes; the waffle baker gives distinctive shape and texture to the batter that is dropped on it.

That brings us to the three basic mixing methods. Wheat

Flour Institute says: "To bring about those qualities that make yeast-leavened products such favorites, three steps are necessary. First, the ingredients must be combined in the right proportion. Second, the dough must be fermented properly. Finally, the bread must be baked in the correct temperature."

Yeast bread recipes follow one of three basic patterns: Most homemakers prefer the straight-dough method because it is simple and provides consistently good results. The sponge-dough method is used today chiefly by commercial bakers and is the oldest method of making yeast dough. The third, the batter method, eliminates the steps of kneading and shaping.

You may see by this skeleton outline how breads are brought into being, but for sound advice to achieve the best results, pick your authority and depend on its counsel, because a bread-baking session is just as successful as the marriage between the cook and her cookbook. There are so many intrabaking steps before that perfect loaf or coffeecake or batch of Parkerhouse rolls is ready for the table that too much attention cannot be paid this absorbing business of bread-baking.

Quick breads, so called because they may be mixed and baked faster than yeast-leavened products are popular for home baking. The leavening agents in quick breads do not require the long fermentation period needed by yeast. They are the prime favorites of Southern cooks, but they have general national acceptance, too. Some of them, like griddlecakes and waffles are round-the-clock choices; they begin the day with breakfast, are often served at luncheon with other foods, and may end up an after-theater party in a midnight snack.

Quick drop batters may produce such delights as quick coffeecake, orange upside-down coffeecake, strawberry surprise (which gets a real tang from the use of cinnamon), cherry-filled coffeecake, blueberry coffeecake, butterscotch coconut coffeecake, applesauce loaf, date-nut bread—the list is so long and tempting that the adventurous cook would never leave the kitchen; she would have her nose pressed either to the recipe file or the oven indicator from dawn to dusk. It is known that there are any number of people—of both sexes—whose idea of a good time is not to spend their leisure hours over whodunits and suspense stories, but who acquire a collection of cookbooks and read them through time after time, savoring their favorite recipes in fantasy. Whether this is a positive urge to increase their cooking repertoire, or simply to stimulate their taste buds in a gastronomic— if literary—orgy, is hard to say. I can only admit I am one of these.

Breads of the Wide, Wide World

To skip lightly over the treasures of our domestic scene seems positively un-American, but since wheat and therefore bread belong to the universe and America is an amalgam of so many nationalities and race-strains, it seems fitting to include here some typical breads of countries which have contributed so much to the palatability of our foods.

Each country has produced typical breads, some of which have been incorporated into our national diet, introduced by second- and third-generation cooks who inherited the recipes. Such a one is the following—I think it is suitable to start this section since it begins with "A"— Armenian Thin Bread. It has a long and dignified history as a ceremonial bread. It is sold commercially in gourmet shops, and is a featured item at Trader Vic's and New York's Plaza Hotel. Served in these places, it is about four or five inches in diameter and is covered with sesame seeds. This is the cocktail size, but the same bread is available in a large, flat round, thin, and cracker-like. It is often confused with matzoth or unleavened bread, but actually it is not.

Armenian Thin Bread

The recipe I have calls for five pounds of flour, two tablespoons of salt, one tablespoon of sugar, one cup of melted butter, four cups of lukewarm water, and one yeast cake, dissolved. To make this dough, in a large mixing bowl combine two cups of lukewarm water with two tablespoons of salt and one tablespoon of sugar dissolved together. At the same time, dissolve the yeastcake and the other two cups of lukewarm water in another mixing bowl. Then stir well with the mixture of salt and sugar, add some of the flour, and work the dough until the flour is completely incorporated with the mixture. Then knead well, and because of the large quantity I would cut the dough into pieces and press out all the air. You will then be kneading the equivalent of one pound at a time, which is easier than handling the whole mass. Next allow the dough to stand covered in a warm place for about four hours, giving it time to rise.

Now divide the dough into about sixteen round balls the size of an orange, and roll out each ball with a little flour to prevent it from sticking. Use a long-type rolling pin and roll out to the width of the oven you are using. With the dough on the rolling pin (hanging over) take it to the oven, heated to about 350 degrees, spread it out on the bottom plate, and bake. The baking is over when it's slightly brown, or the way you like it best. It comes out hot and dry and crisp, a fine thin bread which may be stored indefinitely but will be fresh whenever you choose to serve it. Add sesame seeds, sprinkled generously by hand, to give just the right fillip to its taste.

It might be mentioned here that an important tip about kneading is to lubricate your hands. Put a light—very light—coating of shortening on them, or a little olive oil. Caution here: go easy on the olive oil, since it might penetrate the dough and make it too fat. Also, whenever the dough stands, cover it with a damp cloth to prevent drying, or getting a crust on top.

Weather, in my opinion, has little to do with the condition of the dough. Perhaps when the weather is damp, it may be more stiff, and when dry, more soft. But I doubt it.

French Bread

French people call this slender, crusty bread *pain ordinaire,* or "every day" bread. If you were to visit New Orleans, you would see great stacks of these loaves in grocery stores, some of the loaves two feet long. When Frenchmen settled in Louisiana, they brought with them their recipes for this delicious bread.

2 cups warm (not hot) water	1 tablespoon sugar
1 package active dry yeast, or 1 cake compressed yeast	2 teaspoons salt
	5¾ cups sifted flour
	1 egg white, unbeaten

Measure warm (not hot) water into warmed bowl. Sprinkle dry yeast over water. (Crumble compressed yeast into lukewarm water.) Stir until dissolved. Add sugar, salt and three cups flour. Stir to mix, then beat until smooth and shiny. Stir in two and a half cups more flour. Sprinkle remaining one-fourth cup flour on bread board or pastry cloth. Turn dough out on flour and knead until satiny smooth, five to seven minutes. Shape into smooth ball. Rub bowl lightly with shortening. Press top of ball of dough into greased bowl, then turn dough over. Cover with waxed paper, then clean towel. Let rise until doubled (about one hour). Punch down. Divide into halves. Shape each half into a ball. Cover and let rest five minutes. Rub a little shortening on palms of hands. Then roll each ball of dough under the hands to form a long slender loaf about three inches in diameter. Start rolling at the center and gently work hands toward ends of loaf. Do this several times to make well-shaped loaves. Place loaves four inches apart on lightly greased baking sheet. With sharp knife cut diagonal gashes about three-fourths inch deep about one and a half inches apart into top of each loaf. Cover and let rise until a little more than doubled (about one hour). Bake in moderately hot oven (425° F.) 30 to 35 minutes. Remove from oven. Brush with egg white. Return to oven for two minutes. Remove from baking sheet and cool on rack or across tops of pans.

Yields two loaves or one loaf and twelve rolls.

Swedish Limpe

Swedish people make a variety of rye breads, but *limpe* is one of the favorites. It is often baked in plump round loaves, but it may also be baked in a regular loaf pan.

1½ cups water
¼ cup brown sugar
2 teaspoons caraway seeds
2 tablespoons shortening
2 teaspoons salt

½ cup warm (not hot) water
1 package active dry yeast,
    or 1 cake compressed yeast
4 cups sifted white flour
2 cups sifted rye flour

Into small saucepan measure a half-cup water, brown sugar, caraway seeds, shortening, and salt. Bring to boil and simmer gently five minutes. Remove from heat and pour into large mixing bowl. Add one cup cold water.

Into cup or small bowl measure a half-cup warm (not hot) water. Sprinkle dry yeast over water. (Crumble compressed yeast into lukewarm water.) Stir until dissolved. After yeast dissolves, stir two cups white flour into liquid in large bowl. Add dissolved yeast and mix well. Stir in remaining two cups white flour. Mix well. Stir in one and a half cups rye flour, reserving remaining half-cup rye flour for kneading. Sprinkle one-fourth cup rye flour on bread board or an pastry cloth. Turn dough out on floured board or cloth and knead until smooth and satiny. Use the remaining one-fourth cup rye flour if dough feels sticky and too soft. Place ball of dough into greased bowl, first pressing top of dough into bowl to coat it lightly with fat. Turn ball over. Cover and let rise until doubled (about one and a quarter hours). Punch down. (For a finer-grained bread, let dough rise a second time until doubled.) Divide dough into halves. Shapes each half into a ball. Place on lightly greased baking sheet about four inches apart. If desired, make three or four cuts a half-inch deep with sharp knife across tops of loaves. Cover and let rise until doubled (about one hour). Bake in moderate oven (400° F.) 45 to 50 minutes. Remove from baking sheet and cool on racks or across tops of bread pans away from drafts. For a shiny crust, brush tops of loaves with milk or egg white when done, and return to oven for two minutes. If preferred, dough may be shaped in regular loaves and baked in bread pans.

Yields two loaves.

Sally Lunn

This bread is named after a young woman who lived in Bath, England, in the eighteenth century. Her bread is said to have been so good that the most fashionable people bought it from her.

¾ cup milk
2 tablespoons sugar
1 teaspoon salt
2 tablespoons shortening
1 package active dry yeast,

or 1 cake compressed yeast
¼ cup warm (not hot) water
2¾ cups sifted flour
1 egg

Scald milk. Add sugar, salt, and shortening. Stir to dissolve. Pour into mixing bowl. Cool to lukewarm. While milk cools, sprinkle dry yeast into warm (not hot) water. (Crumble compressed yeast into lukewarm water.) Stir until dissolved. To cooled milk add two cups flour. Mix well, then beat until smooth. Stir in dissolved yeast. Add egg and beat at least one minute. Stir in remaining flour and beat until smooth (about two minutes). Scrape batter down from side of bowl. Cover and let rise until doubled (about one hour). Stir down and turn batter into greased 9-inch round cake pan 1½ inches deep, or into loaf pan 4½ x 2¾ x 9 inches. Let rise until doubled (about one hour). Bake in moderate oven (350° F.) 45 minutes. Turn out on rack. Cool slightly. Serve warm, with margarine or butter and marmalade. Separate pieces with two forks instead of cutting with knife.

Yields one loaf.

Grecian Feast Bread

Feast bread was most often baked at Easter and sometimes at other church holidays. Since it is like a coffeecake, it is good for breakfast or brunch. Slices spread with margarine or butter, and served with glasses of milk, make delicious afternoon or evening refreshments.

1 recipe basic sweet dough
½ cup currants
¾ cup confectioners' sugar

1 tablespoon milk or cream
15 blanched almonds
¼ cup sliced candied cherries

Make basic sweet dough. Stir in currants before mixing-in last cup of flour. Then finish mixing dough and knead. Shape dough into smooth ball and place in lightly greased bowl. Cover and let rise until doubled (about two hours). Punch down. Divide dough into three equal parts. Shape each part into smooth ball. Place balls on lightly greased baking sheet so that they form a three-leafed clover, about one-half inch apart. Cover and let rise until doubled (about one hour). Bake in moderate oven (350° F.) 40 to 45 minutes. Remove from baking sheet and cool on rack. When cool, mix confectioners' sugar and milk or cream to make a soft frosting. Pour over each of the three "loaves," letting frosting drip down sides. Arrange almonds and sliced cherries in three-petaled flower shapes on frosting. Cut into thin slices.

Yields one loaf.

Kulich

From Russia comes *Kulich*, a sweet bread baked in tall, slender loaves. *Kulich* was originally a holiday bread, but it is appropriate the year around. Its round slices add interest to any meal, whether they are served fresh or lightly toasted.

1 recipe basic sweet dough
¼ cup raisins
¼ cup chopped almonds

1 teaspoon grated lemon rind
Frosting

Make basic sweet dough. Stir in raisins, almonds, and lemon rind before mixing-in the last cup of flour. Then finish mixing dough and knead. Shape into ball. Place in lightly greased bowl. Cover and let rise until doubled (about two hours). Punch down. Divide into halves. Shape into balls. Press each ball into greased one-pint can (such as fruit or juice cans), or one-pound coffee or shortening cans. Cover and let rise until doubled (about one and a quarter hours). Bake in moderate oven (350° F.) 30 to 35 minutes. Turn out of cans at once. When cool, frost tops with confectioners' sugar frosting and decorate with almonds and sliced candied cherries, or sprinkle with small colored candies.

Yields two loaves.

Frosting

½ cup sifted confectioners' sugar

2 teaspoons top milk or cream

2 tablespoons slivered almonds

2 candied cherries, sliced

Mix sugar and milk to make smooth, thin frosting. Pour over tops of loaves. Decorate with almonds and sliced cherries. To serve, cut slices from top to bottom so each slice has a bit of frosting.

Viennese Striesel

Almost all European cooks make braided loaves. Sometimes the loaves are made from plain basic sweet dough. Sometimes they are filled with fruits and nuts. Some are served plain, some are glazed, some are frosted and sprinkled with chopped nuts. Some of the loaves are made of only two braids, one placed on top of the other. Some of them have layers of three and even four braids. In Austria all braided breads are called *Striesel*, but Swiss,

German, and Scandinavian cooks have other names for
them.

1 recipe basic sweet dough
¼ cup seedless raisins
¼ cup chopped candied
cherries
2 tablespoons chopped candied orange rind

⅛ teaspoon mace
½ cup confectioners' sugar
1 tablespoon top milk or
cream
¼ cup chopped nuts

Make basic sweet dough. Stir in raisins, cherries, orange
rind, and mace before mixing-in the last cup of flour. Then
finish mixing dough and knead. Shape into ball. Place in
lightly greased bowl. Cover and let rise until doubled
(about two and a quarter hours). Punch down. Divide
into nine pieces. Shape each piece into a ball. Cover and
let rest five minutes. Roll each piece under the hands to
form strands about 15 inches long. Weave four strands
into a loose braid. Lay the strands on a lightly greased
baking sheet, overlapping them at the center. Braid from
the center toward each end. With the sides of the hands
make a "trench" down the center of this braid. Now
braid the next three strands loosely, again braiding from
the center toward each end. Lay this braid on top of the
first one, placing it in the "trench." Last of all twist the
two remaining strands loosely around each other. Lay this
twist on top of the loaf, bringing the ends of the twist
down over the ends of the loaf. Tuck the ends of the twist
under the loaf. Cover and let rise until doubled (about
one and a half hours). Bake in moderate oven (350° F.)
40 to 45 minutes. Remove from baking sheet to rack.
When cool, make frosting by mixing confectioners' sugar
with milk or cream. Spread on loaf. Sprinkle with chopped
almonds or walnuts.

Yields one large loaf.

Danish Coffee Twist

1 recipe basic sweet dough	or butter
3 tablespoons sugar	Honey glaze
½ teaspoon cinnamon	¼ cup slivered blanched
1 tablespoon soft margarine	almonds

Make basic sweet dough. When dough has doubled, punch down. Shape into ball. Cover and let rest five minutes. While dough rests, mix sugar and cinnamon. Flatten ball of dough, then roll out to form long narrow sheet about six inches wide and one-fourth inch thick. Spread with soft margarine or butter. Sprinkle with sugar-cinnamon mixture. Roll up to make long, slender roll. Seal edge by pressing firmly. Twist roll by pushing ends in opposite directions. Lift to lightly greased baking sheet and shape into a large pretzel. Tuck ends of roll under edge of "pretzel" to keep dough from untwisting. Cover and let rise until doubled (about one hour). Bake in moderate oven (350° F.) 25 to 30 minutes. While coffee twist bakes, make honey glaze (see below). Brush hot glaze over twist as soon as it comes from oven. Sprinkle with slivered almonds. Remove from baking sheet to cooling rack.

Yields one cake.

Honey Glaze

2 tablespoons sugar	1 tablespoon margarine or
¼ cup honey	butter

Measure ingredients into small saucepan. Bring to boil, stirring constantly. While still hot, brush on baked Danish coffee twist.

Stollen

Stollen are traditionally served in Germany for Christmas breakfast. Often thin slices are served with coffee or a glass of wine to guests or callers during the holiday season, as fruitcake is served in England. But this sweet fruited bread is suitable as a special treat at almost any meal.

1 recipe basic sweet dough
½ cup chopped blanched almonds
¼ cup finely cut candied citron
¼ cup finely cut candied cherries
1 teaspoon grated lemon rind
1 tablespoon soft margarine or butter
2 tablespoons sugar
½ teaspoon cinnamon
Frosting (see next page)

Make basic sweet dough. Stir in almonds, citron, cherries, and lemon rind before adding last cup of flour. Then finish mixing dough and knead. Shape into smooth ball. Place in lightly greased bowl. Cover and let rise until doubled (about two and a quarter hours). Punch down. Cover and let rest 5 to 10 minutes. With palms of hands press dough into oval shape a scant half-inch thick. Spread half of oval with soft margarine or butter. Mix sugar and cinnamon. Sprinkle over margarine or butter. Fold unspread half lengthwise over sugar and cinnamon, making edges even. Lift to lightly greased baking sheet. Curve the ends slightly. Press down the *folded* edge (*not* the open edge). This helps the loaf keep its shape as it rises and bakes. Cover and let rise until doubled (about one and a quarter hours). Bake in moderate oven (350° F.) 30 to 35 minutes. Remove from baking sheet. When cool, frost and decorate.

Yields one loaf.

Frosting

¾ cup sifted confectioners'
  sugar
1 tablespoon top milk or
  cream

3 candied cherries, sliced
2 tablespoons chopped or
  slivered almonds

Mix sugar and milk or cream to make a smooth thick
frosting that will just pour. Pour it over top of loaf, letting
frosting drip down sides. Decorate with sliced cherries
and sprinkle with almonds.

Guglhupf*

Rich, festive and cake-like is *Guglhupf,* made from a
batter instead of a dough. In Vienna, where Guglhupf was
perhaps most famous, this cakelike bread is frequently
served for dessert, or as refreshments on special occasions.
It is delicious with fruit salad or with bowls of stewed
fruits and glasses of milk.

½ cup milk
1 package active dry yeast,
  or 1 cake compressed yeast
¼ cup warm (not hot)
  water
½ cup sugar
½ teaspoon salt
2 eggs
½ cup melted margarine or
  butter
2½ cups sifted flour

½ cup chopped raisins
1 teaspoon grated lemon
  rind

For Pan:
1 tablespoon margarine or
  butter
2 tablespoons fine bread
  crumbs or finely ground
  almonds
15-16 whole blanched
  almonds

* From brochure "Breads of Many Lands," by Clara Gebhard Snyder,
distributed by Educational Service, J. Walter Thompson Company.

Scald milk. Pour into mixing bowl and cool until it is warm (not hot). While milk cools, sprinkle dry yeast into warm water in cup. (Crumble compressed yeast into lukewarm water.) Stir until dissolved. To milk in bowl add sugar, salt and one and a half cups flour. Mix well. Add dissolved yeast and beat until smooth. Add eggs and beat thoroughly. If you prefer, beat the eggs first in a separate bowl. Add melted and cooled margarine or butter, about a tablespoon at a time, mixing it in well before adding more. Stir in remaining one and one-fourth cups flour. Then beat batter about five minutes. (An electric mixer set at moderate speed is good for this.) With rubber scraper scrape batter down from side of bowl. Cover and let rise in warm place until doubled (about one and a half hours). While batter rises prepare baking pan. Use either a fancy mold that holds a quart or two one-pint molds, or a seven-inch angel food cake pan. Rub the inside of the pan generously with margarine or butter. Then sprinkle the fine bread crumbs into the pan. Shake it to coat the whole inside of the pan with crumbs. Arrange almonds in a design in bottom of pan.

When batter has doubled, stir it down. Mix in the raisins and lemon rind. Carefully spoon the batter on top of the almonds so as not to spoil your design. When all the batter is in the pan, cover and let rise in warm place until doubled (about one and a quarter hours). Bake in moderate oven (350° F.) 45 to 50 minutes. Look at the cake after it has baked 15 minutes. If it is turning brown, lay a piece of clean brown wrapping paper over the top for the rest of the baking period. This is a rich batter and browns easily. When done, turn out of pan on wire cake-rack. If you wish, dust lightly with confectioners' sugar. To make a design on top of the cake, lay a scalloped lace paper doily on the cake and sift confectioners' sugar over it.

Lift the doily carefully and pour the extra sugar back into the container.

Yields one cake.

Italian Christmas Bread

2 packages yeast, compressed or dry
¼ cup water (lukewarm for compressed yeast, warm for dry)
1 cup milk
⅔ cup sugar
1 teaspoon salt
¾ cup soft butter or margarine
7 cups sifted enriched flour (about)

4 eggs
1 egg, separated
1½ teaspoons vanilla extract
½ cup golden seedless raisins
⅓ cup finely chopped blanched almonds
⅓ cup chopped candied citron
⅓ cup finely chopped candied lemon peel
1 tablespoon water

Soften yeast in one-fourth cup water. Scald milk. Add sugar, salt, and butter or margarine. Cool to lukewarm. Add two cups flour and beat well.* Add softened yeast and mix well. Cover and let rise in warm place until mixture is bubbly (about one hour). Stir down. Beat four eggs and one egg yolk, reserving one egg white for glaze. Add eggs and vanilla extract to flour mixture. Beat well. Add enough more flour to make a soft dough. Turn out on lightly floured board or pastry cloth. Gradually knead in raisins, almonds, and candied fruits. Continue kneading until smooth and satiny. Place in greased bowl, cover, and let rise until doubled (about one and a half hours). When light, punch down. Divide dough into two equal portions and let rest 10 minutes. Shape each portion into round

* Because of the volume of this dough, preparation will be easier if you beat in the flour with an electric mixer at low speed. Use it again for the second addition of flour as long as possible. As the dough becomes stiffer, the last one and a half to two cups of flour must be mixed in with a wooden spoon.

loaf and place in well-greased eight-inch round pan. Combine egg white and water. Brush tops of loaves generously with egg white mixture. Let rise until doubled (about one hour). Brush with egg white mixture again and bake in moderate oven (350° F.) 35 to 40 minutes. Makes two eight-inch round loaves.

Irish Soda Bread

3 cups sifted enriched flour†
⅔ cup sugar
1 tablespoon baking powder
1 teaspoon soda
1 teaspoon salt

1½ cups currants or dark seedless raisins
2 eggs, beaten
1¾ to 2 cups buttermilk
2 tablespoons melted shortening

Sift together into a large bowl flour, sugar, baking powder, soda, and salt. Stir in currants or raisins. Combine eggs, buttermilk, and shortening. Add liquid mixture to dry ingredients and mix just until flour is moistened. Turn batter into greased loaf pan 5¼ x 9½ inches. Bake in moderrate oven (350° F.) about one hour. Remove from pan immediately. Allow to cool thoroughly before slicing. Makes one loaf.

Belgian Carmique

1 package yeast, compressed or dry
1 cup water (lukewarm for compressed yeast, warm for dry)
1 cup milk
½ cup sugar
1 teaspoon salt

1 teaspoon ground cardamon
⅓ cup butter or margarine
7 cups sifted enriched flour (about)
1 cup seedless raisins
2 eggs
1 egg, beaten
1 tablespoon water

Soften yeast in water. Scald milk. Add sugar, salt, cardamon, and butter or margarine. Cool to lukewarm. Add

† If using self-rising flour, omit baking powder and salt.

two cups flour and beat well. Add softened yeast, raisins and two eggs. Add enough more flour to make a soft dough. Turn out on lightly floured board or pastry cloth and knead until smooth and satiny. Place in greased bowl, cover and let rise in warm place until doubled (about one and a half hours). When light, punch down. Divide dough into two equal portions. Let rest 10 minutes. Shape each portion into round loaf. Place in greased nine-inch round pans. Let rise until doubled (about one hour). Mix egg and water. Brush lightly over tops of loaves. Bake in moderate oven (375° F.) 40 to 45 minutes. Makes two round loaves.

Italian Bread*

2 packages yeast, compressed or dry
½ cup water (lukewarm for compressed yeast, warm for dry)
2 cups boiling water
2 tablespoons shortening
2 tablespoons sugar
1 teaspoon salt
6 cups enriched flour (about)
1 egg white
1 tablespoon water

Soften yeast in half-cup of water. To boiling water, add shortening, sugar, and salt. Cool to lukewarm. Add two cups flour and beat until smooth. Add softened yeast and about two cups more flour. Beat well again. Cover and let rise in warm place until light and bubbly (about 45 minutes). Beat down and add enough more flour to make moderately stiff dough. Turn out on floured board or pastry cloth and knead until smooth and satiny. Place in greased bowl, cover and let rise until doubled (about one and a half hours). Punch down. Divide dough into three equal parts. Cover and let rest 10 minutes. Combine egg white and water. Roll each portion of dough to rectangle about

* Wheat Flour Institute, Test Kitchen.

one-fourth inch thick and 13 inches long. Roll tightly like a jelly roll and place on greased baking sheet. Tuck ends under slightly, sealing edges securely. Using scissors or sharp knife, make diagonal cuts across top of each loaf about one-eighth inch deep. Brush top with egg white mixture. Let rise in warm place until almost doubled (about 45 minutes). Brush with egg white mixture again. Bake in hot oven (425° F.) 35 to 40 minutes. Makes three loaves.

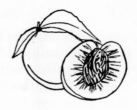

7

Blushing Beauty with Stony Heart

by K. Cyrus Melikian

The next time you serve a peach shortcake with all of its syrupy and ecstatic sweetness you might, if you wish, give a big measure of credit, or perhaps make a low bow, to the East—both the Far East and the Middle East. You owe them both an appreciative gesture in return for your present pleasure.

Like so many of today's good things to eat, peaches have come a long way to our modern table, in time and distance and evolutionary progress from their forebears, improving with each generation through the help of the hand of man and his intelligence.

Primitive peaches were grown some three thousand years ago, historians say, in ancient China—where the word for peach was *tao*—but they were little like the velvety fruit that cuddles into your cupped hand as you shop at your grocery or market today.

Like many of the races of man, peaches moved westward. As they migrated, they gained flavor and beauty. When they reached Persia, now known as Iran, they got their family name—peaches. Perhaps even the early Persians used the word to describe a gorgeous girl.

Early Persian traders and travelers brought peaches to ancient Greece and they were written of as early as the year 322 B.C. as a delicious Persian fruit. Their westward trek continued. They won their way to Italy where they became a prized and expensive item on the menu of Roman feasts around the beginnings of the Christian era. As the centuries crept by peaches invaded and charmed all of Europe—first France and Spain and North Africa, then little by little, all of the countries of western Europe. By the thirteenth century peaches had leapt the Channel and peach trees were growing in England. Through all these years orchardists with skill and patience had cultured and improved peaches to such a degree that a Spanish peach would not have been recognized by an early Chinese peach grower as even a distant relative of the small, tough fruit he had enjoyed.

The climate and soil of Spain offered perhaps the best conditions for the cultivation of peaches and early Spanish explorers and discoverers brought peach pits from their best orchards to the New World for planting and introduced the fruit into Mexico and Florida. By that time settlers from many countries were forming colonies on the American continent and Captain John Smith in 1629 reported "peaches in abundance" in the Jamestown colony. Peach stones from England were being sent to Massachusetts for experimental planting. From then on peach pits were being hopefully nested in the various soils of all North America. Today some thirty-five of our fifty states produce peaches in commercial quantities, not to mention the isolated back yard family pets that bloom and produce fruit for a single household and perhaps the juvenile raiders of the neighborhood. In quantity, the most important peach-growing states are California, Georgia, South Carolina, and Michigan.

There are two basic varieties of peaches: freestone and clingstone. The former are used mostly in season as a table delicacy and eaten uncooked. The latter are largely used in canning or frozen for the market, although they are also used for home pickling, cooking, and pie-making. To quote from a U. S. Department of Agriculture pamphlet (AIB No. 54), "Either clingstone or freestone may be white-fleshed or yellow-fleshed. Clingstone varieties may be further classified into those of melting-fleshed (soft-fleshed) or non-melting fleshed (firm, as California melting clingstones). Most of the peaches that ripen earliest are melting-fleshed clingstones. Many of the older varieties that ripen early are white-fleshed. The non-melting cling-stones are grown primarily for commercial canning. They hold their shape well when canned. They are also a desirable type for home pickling."

Here are a few things to keep in mind about buying peaches for home consumption: To assure best flavor— not necessarily highest content of vitamins A and C— select the mature peach, and remember that the most beautiful surface is not the best indication of maturity. Sniff them to get the unmistakable fragrance of the fully ripe fruit. Hold them in your hand and give them a gentle press to test their ripeness, but never pinch them with thumb and finger. That will merely form a mushy spot. Peaches, ripe or unripe, are more sensitive to pressure than any other fruit. Most peaches grown for shipment must be picked before they are fully ripe, and they continue to mature as they travel and as they wait for you in the store. Look out for skin punctures and oozing syrup. Worms have been at work and such a peach is not a good buy at any price.

In buying frozen peaches there is no need to do any testing or judging of your own. You have the Department of Agriculture's guarantee that you are getting just what you pay for and in full measure. The Government has established three grades based on quality, color, odor, size, symmetry, and tenderness and has even specified the best uses for each grade. Grade A (Fancy) is recommended for salads and as a dessert fruit. Grade B (Choice) is also suitable for salads, dessert fruit, or breakfast fruit as well as for use in pies, cobblers, and shortcakes. Grade C (Standard) is a good purchase for use in cooking recipes as well as making flavoring sauces.

In grandma's day the enjoyment of peaches was pretty much limited to the fresh peach season, which isn't long in any part of the country. But the deep freeze cabinet of modern home refrigerators has changed all that. Now, whether you use dried, canned or frozen peaches, the peach season can be extended throughout the twelve months of the year. About one-half the crop has been used fresh in recent years; the other half has been processed.

Dried peaches should be stored in a tightly sealed container and kept in a cool place—the coolest room in the cellar will do although the refrigerator is better. Before using, it is not necessary to soften them up by soaking if they are of good quality. They can simply be immersed in water to just cover, brought to a boil, then reduced to a simmer until the fruit is tender, as you watch the amount of water, now turning into syrup. A little sugar may be needed to give added sweetness. When preparing dried peaches in bulk for household storage and later use, have tight containers ready and plan a space in the refrigerator to accommodate them. They will not ferment if they are kept cool until you serve them or use them in pie or shortcake.

As for frozen peaches, they should be stored at zero

Fahrenheit or below in order to maintain maximum flavor and vitamin values. If stored in the ice-cube compartment of the home refrigerator, which does not maintain a temperature as low as zero, they should be kept no longer than two weeks.

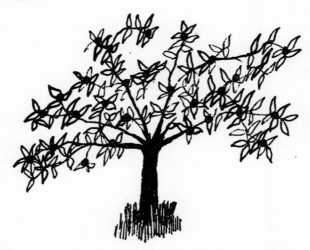

Frozen peaches in the package can be thawed at room temperature or in a pan of cool water. For even thawing the package should be turned several times in the process. A one-pound package of peaches packed in syrup requires six hours to thaw on the refrigerator shelf, several at room temperature. Leftover thawed peaches should be cooked and stored in the refrigerator; not refrozen.

Here are some peach recipes that are creative rather than routine:

Peach Butter

In the state of Georgia where peaches are abundant some forgotten kitchen genius asked herself one day, "If apple butter is good wouldn't peach butter be even better?" She started a trend that has become a state-wide enthusiasm. You may use either clingstone or freestone. Whichever, the fruit should be ripe and perfect—no spots or blemishes.

4 pounds of peaches	⅜ cup sugar for each cup of
2 cups of water	pulp
2 teaspoons cinnamon	1 teaspoon cloves, if desired

Peel peaches and remove pits. Cook peaches in water until reduced to a pulp. Add sugar, cinnamon, and cloves, if desired. Cooking time is approximately three hours on low heat. Pour into hot, sterilized glasses, and cover with paraffin, in the regular method of home-cook canning.

The yield is one and a half quarts.

Peach Pickles

Have you ever felt that joy of accomplishment when you line up a half-dozen or a dozen Mason jars of preserves on the kitchen table before setting them on a high shelf or, like treasure, stowing them in the preserve cabinet in the cool basement? Here's a recipe for pickled peaches which will make you positively glow with well deserved pride.

6 pounds of peeled peaches	3 pounds granulated sugar
1 pint of vinegar	1 pint of water
1 tablespoon of ginger	2 tablespoons crushed cloves
4 sticks of cinnamon	salt

Peel peaches, first giving them a quick dip into hot water then a plunge into cold water. This makes them easy to peel. Cut peaches in halves, remove pits, slice or quarter them. To prevent fruit darkening during preparation drop fruit into water containing two tablespoons each of salt and vinegar for each gallon of water. Wash and drain in cold water just before taking the next step.

Put one pint of vinegar into the preserving kettle, add hot water, bring to a boil and skim. Add the spices tied in a cloth bag. Put the peaches into the boiling mixture and cook them about one minute or until they can be pierced with a broom straw. Lift peaches from the liquor and pack in jars. Fill up jars with boiling spiced vinegar. Seal the jars and place them in a simmering hot water bath. Set them aside to cool slowly.

That's it. When you open one of those jars in the weeks or months to come as a relish to go on the plate with any meat or fowl dinner you will be well rewarded for your time and satisfying work in putting up this great and delicious fruit in pickle form.

Peach Jam and Peach Jelly

If peach pickles make the dinner more zestful, peach jams and jellies do the same for breakfast. They contribute an epicure's delight when spread on muffins, toast, flapjacks, or, if you wish, put a spoonful or two over a bowl of oatmeal and cream in place of sugar. Watch the family go for that combination.

Here's how to lead up to that great moment. Make sure you are buying yellow-fleshed peaches for your jam. By name they may be Halehaven, Cardinal, or the Dixie type of Alberta. Avoid the white-fleshed peaches because they are inclined to brown.

First, peach jam.

For each pound of peeled and sliced peaches use three-quarters of a pound of granulated sugar, the amount depending upon the native sweetness of the peaches. Crush the peaches and combine in a container, a large bowl perhaps, making layers of alternate crushed peaches and sugar. Let this mixture stand until some of the peach juices are extracted from the flesh, a matter of three or four hours or until the sugar is thoroughly dissolved. Transfer to a cooking kettle, place on a low fire and bring to a slow simmer, stirring constantly until the mixture is somewhat thick and syrupy to the spoon.

In the meantime, you have sterilized jars or jelly glasses in piping hot water and have let them stand in the water to keep these glass containers warm so that they will not crack upon receiving the hot jam. Fifteen minutes should do it. Pour the hot jam into the containers and set them aside to cool slowly, uncovered. When cool, seal the glasses with paraffin tops (or you may have used jars with screwcaps) and tuck them away in a coolish place until, one by one, they are used to give that wondrous, gala flavor touch to a good breakfast.

Now, peach jelly.

Peach lovers in those areas where peaches are plentiful often do not favor the use of peaches for jelly-making, preferring to use this tender fruit for jam, marmalade, conserve, or pickles. However, it is possible to make a delicious peach jelly, translucent and firm to the spoon. It might be well for the beginner to try it on a small scale at first, with a pound of peaches to a pint of water. Peel and cut up the peaches, put them into the heated water. Taste for sweetness and add granulated sugar to offset the tartness of the peaches you are using. The sweet, fully ripe freestones need less sugar; more will be required for the less ripe clingstones. Boil rapidly, constantly stirring, until all the peach parts have disintegrated. Pour the hot brew into a jelly bag and hang bag above a bowl to drip. Do not squeeze the bag. Let the sweetened juice drip slowly. Skim the cooling jelly from time to time to prevent ending up with a somewhat tough jelly. While it is still warm dip the coagulating jelly into glass containers and let cool slowly. Cap with melted paraffin and set them in your special treat cabinet.

Peach Fritters

If you like to hear protracted applause here's the way to win it from the folks you cook for. First, stir up a good fritter batter and set it aside while you peel and halve maybe a half-dozen yellow-fleshed peaches. Sprinkle the halves with sugar, or a little kirsch, rum, or cognac if you care for the taste of these flavors. Let the treated peaches stand for about thirty minutes to give them time to form a flavored peach juice in the bowl, when they will have thoroughly absorbed the flavors you have added. Pour the peach syrup into the fritter batter, stirring it in. Dry the fruit and dip, a piece at a time, into the fritter batter. When all have got their batter-jacket fry the fritters, a few at a time, in deep fat at about 370 degrees until the fritters are golden brown. Drain on absorbent paper, arrange fritters on a platter, or individual plates, and sprinkle with a little sugar.

If you are a real fan of peach dishes, and if the fresh peach season is with you, there are some delicacies that you won't want to miss. Some of them demand a hot oven but, even so, they will reward you well though a mid-summer temperature holds sway.

Peach Shortbread Tart

3½ tablespoons quick-cooking tapioca
¾ cup sugar
¼ teaspoon salt
¼ teaspoon nutmeg
1¼ cups water

4 cups sliced fresh peaches
1½ tablespoons lemon juice
1 baked 8-inch shortbread crust, cooled (see next page)

Combine tapioca, sugar, salt, nutmeg, water, and 1½ cups of the peaches in a saucepan. Cook and stir over medium heat until mixture comes to a boil. Remove from heat. Let stand 15 minutes. Then stir in lemon juice and remaining peaches. Cool. Before serving, fill crust with peach mixture. Yield: one 8-inch tart.

Shortbread Crust

½ cup soft butter or   ¼ cup sugar
   margarine   1¼ cups sifted flour

Mix butter and sugar with pastry blender or fork. Add flour and mix until crumbs are formed. Then mix thoroughly with hands until soft dough is formed. Press evenly into bottom and sides of an 8-inch round cake pan, 1½ inches deep. Prick bottom with fork. Bake at 325° F. 35 to 40 minutes or until lightly browned. Cool shell in pan. Remove carefully. If shell sticks, heat gently a few seconds over low heat. Fill shell just before serving.

Deep-Dish Fresh Peach Pie

6 cups (about 3 pounds)   2 tablespoons butter or
   sliced fresh peaches   margarine
1 cup sugar   pastry, using 1 cup flour
1½ tablespoons quick-cook-   salt
   ing tapioca

Combine peaches, sugar, salt, and tapioca. Turn into a 1-quart casserole. Dot with butter or margarine. Cover with pastry rolled to ⅛-inch thickness. Trim, turn under, and flute edges. Cut a small gash in center of crust to allow for the escape of steam. Bake at 425° F. 30 to 40 minutes or until crust is brown. Serve warm or cold. Yield: 6 servings.

Peaches in Rose Wine

3 cups sugar
6 cups water
few drops of red fruit coloring

8 whole ripe unpeeled
  peaches
1½ cups Rose wine

Boil sugar and water together in a deep kettle; add coloring to make delicate pink. Drop peaches into boiling syrup. Cover and cook gently for 10 to 15 minutes. Peaches should be tender, but not soft. When they may be pierced easily with toothpick, add wine. Turn off heat and let stand, covered, in kettle for 10 minutes. Ladle peaches into glass bowl or serving dish and pour syrup over them. Serve warm or chilled. Yield: 8 to 10 servings.

All-in-One Peach Cake

5 canned cling peach halves
⅓ cup shortening
½ cup sugar
½ teaspoon vanilla
2 eggs
1 cup sifted cake flour
1¼ teaspoons baking powder

¼ teaspoon salt
1 tablespoon canned cling
  peach syrup
¼ cup sugar
½ teaspoon cinnamon
¼ cup chopped roasted
  almonds

Drain canned cling peaches and slice thin (sliced peaches should be sliced in half). Cream together shortening and the ½ cup sugar and vanilla. Add eggs and beat until light. Sift together flour, baking powder, and salt. Add by thirds to first mixture, beating after each addition. Add canned cling peach syrup. Spread half of batter in oiled, floured 8-inch layer pan. Cover with peach slices. Spread remaining half of batter over peaches. The batter will barely cover at this point. Cover with mixture made from the ¼ cup sugar, cinnamon, and almonds. Bake in moderate oven (350° F.) for 45 minutes. Serves 6.

Golden Pie

1 cup sliced canned cling
  peaches
4 tablespoons cornstarch
6 tablespoons granulated
  sugar
¼ cup orange juice

1 tablespoon grated orange
  rind
1½ cups syrup from peaches
½ teaspoon salt
pastry for double 9-inch
  crust

Combine cornstarch and sugar. Add orange juice, orange rind, peach syrup, salt, and peaches. Mix well. Cook until thick, stirring continuously. Pour into pastry-lined pie pan and cover with top crust. Bake in a very hot oven (450° F.) 25 to 30 minutes. Serves 6 to 8.

Peach Refrigerator Cake

½ pound marshmallows
½ cup orange juice
1 cup heavy cream (to be
  whipped)
½ cup ginger ale
sponge cake or ladyfingers

8 sliced peaches (fresh
  peaches, peeled, cored
  and sliced)
½ cup chopped crystallized
  ginger

Cut marshmallows in quarters, add to orange juice and stir over hot water until almost melted. Cool slightly; add ginger ale. When slightly thickened, fold in ¾ cup cream, whipped. Line a spring-form pan with waxed paper; arrange layer of cake or ladyfingers, whichever you want to use, on the bottom, next a layer of peaches, then a layer of marshmallows until there are three layers of cake and two of fillings. Chill in refrigerator overnight, unmold, garnish with remaining peaches, cream, and ginger. Use *fresh* peaches wherever possible.

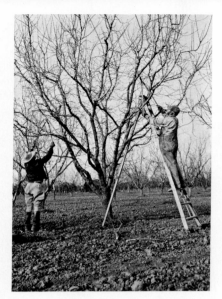

The California cling peach story. Tree pruning is done during dormancy.

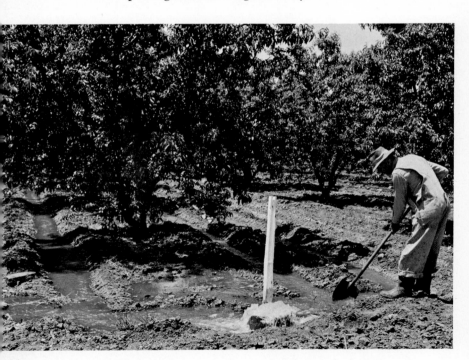

Peach trees require constant irrigation prior to and during the bearing season.

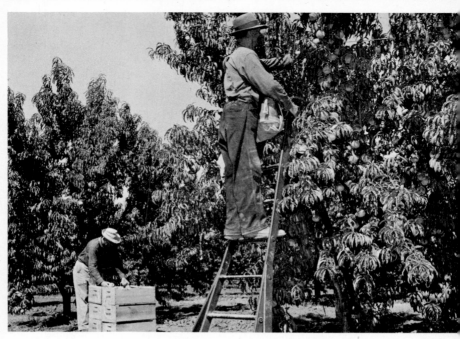

Harvesting takes place from July to September. Most of it is done by hand.

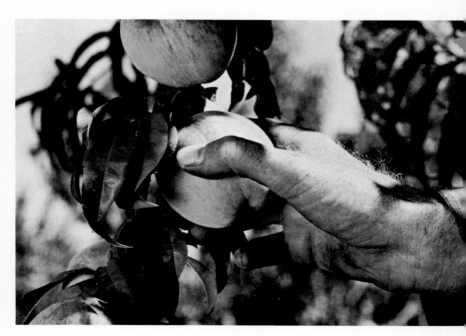

The minimum diameter of a cling peach is 2⅜ inches, but sizes often run to more than 3 inches.

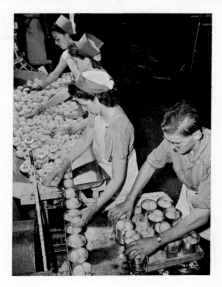

On the cannery lines, cling peaches pass hundreds of eyes in one continuous inspection during processing.

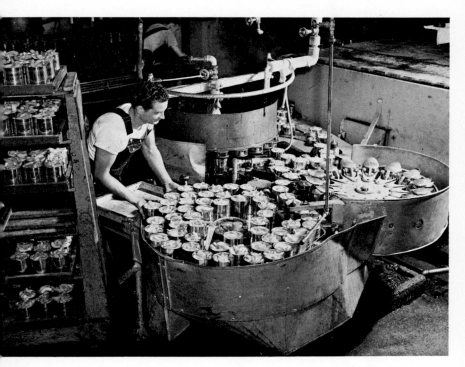

After being filled to the rims with slices or halves, syrup is added to each can.

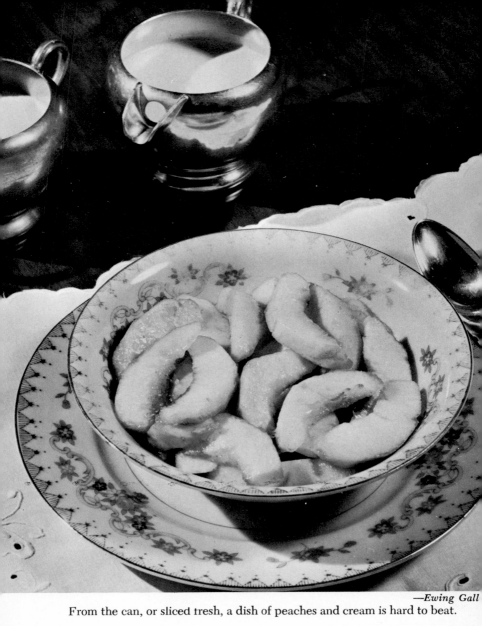

—*Ewing Gall*

From the can, or sliced fresh, a dish of peaches and cream is hard to beat.

Peach Chutney

It's good with chicken or with pork dinners. This will make about 7 pints of chutney, which is put up in sealed sterilized jars.

5 pounds of firm, ripe
  peaches
1 pound seeded raisins
½ pound chopped dates
2 cups tarragon vinegar
¼ cup lime juice
1 lemon

2 to 3 cups of sugar, depending upon ripeness of
  peaches
½ cup candied ginger,
  coarsely chopped
½ cup chopped nuts—any
  type, to suit your taste

Pare and cut peaches into small pieces. Add raisins, dates, vinegar, and lime juice. Quarter lemon, remove seeds, slice thin; add to mixture. Cook until peaches are soft, stir to prevent thickening. Add the sugar. When mixture is thick add ginger and nuts. If you want a more gingery taste, add a teaspoon of powdered ginger as well.

You might call that a homemade relish, although the name of the recipe is Peach Chutney; but, after all, chutney is a kind of relish.

Peach Dumpling

¾ cup granulated sugar
1 teaspoon cornstarch
½ teaspoon cinnamon
1 cup of water
1 tablespoon fresh lemon
  juice

1 package of refrigerated-
  type biscuits
2 diced, peeled ripe peaches
2 tablespoons butter
light cream

Start oven (400° F.). Combine the sugar, cornstarch, cinnamon, and water; cook for 5 minutes or until clear. Remove from heat. Add lemon juice. Cut each individual biscuit into four pieces, roll each piece into a 4-inch circle. Add a dot of butter to each circle, and put a little of the diced peaches in the center of each. Gather up dough over the peaches and seal, and place in a baking dish. Pour syrup over these, and bake for 25 minutes. Serve with light cream, while warm. You should have about 5 perfect dumplings.

Some French recipes, Americanized, from *Je Sais Cuisiner* by Ginette Mathiot:

Peaches in Wine

Preparation time, 10 minutes—2 hours before serving.

6 peaches	or champagne
½ pint sparkling white wine	¼ cup powdered sugar

Peel the peaches. Cut in quarters. Put in bowl. Pour the wine over them and sprinkle with the powdered sugar. Let it marinate one or two hours. Serve cold.

Peach Mousse

Preparation time, 10 minutes.

3 peaches	⅓ cup sugar
½ pint whipped cream	sponge cake

Put through a fine sieve 3 perfect peaches, peeled and stoned. Add the sugar and the whipped cream carefully. Place in a compote dish and surround with the sponge cake cut in pieces. This dessert can be prepared in advance, but if so, one must add to the peach purée a tablespoon of gelatin softened in a little water.

Peaches Bonne Femme

Preparation time, 15 minutes—Cooking time, 40 minutes.

6 good peaches
¼ cup butter

6 slices bread (may be stale bread)
¼ cup sugar

Butter a casserole. Butter the slices of bread. Peel the peaches and cut them in halves. Take out the stones. Arrange peaches in casserole with the bread, sugar and dot with remaining butter. Sprinkle with a little water and bake in a slow oven for 40 minutes. This may be made with canned peaches, using syrup instead of water to moisten the dish.

Peaches Melba Style

Preparation time, 30 minutes—Cooking time, 25 minutes.

6 peaches
1 pint milk
5 egg yolks
1 pint water

currant jelly
¼ cup almonds
½ cup sugar

Peel peaches and poach them in a syrup made with water and half the sugar. Put them in a bowl, cover them with a layer of currant jelly, and cover with the almonds which have been blanched, chopped and toasted.

Make a soft custard with the milk, the remaining sugar and the yolks of the eggs. Let it chill slightly. Pour the custard around the peaches and chill several hours.

Peaches Columbine

Preparation time, 20 minutes—Cooking time, 30 minutes.

6 peaches   Some preserved fruits—cher-
⅔ cup rice cooked in milk   ries, angelique, etc.
⅛ cup sugar   ½ pint madeira sauce

Prepare the rice, making it rather firm. Poach the whole peaches in boiling sugared water, drain, peel and cut in half and remove stones. Stuff each half peach with a little rice, and put halves together again. With a spoon put the remaining rice in the center of a round plate, pressing into egg shapes. Arrange the peaches in a crown around the eggs made of rice, decorate with preserved cherries, angelique, etc. Cover with madeira sauce.

Commercial Canning

Although Americans take for granted that they can fill their pantry shelves with first quality canned goods, such an ability represents a way of life not to be found anywhere else in the world. It is due in part to the abundance of food in this country, and in great measure to the skill and determination on the part of the canners to provide the finest products available, under constantly advancing modern methods.

Peaches and pears were canned commercially as far back as 1863. However, it wasn't until the marketing developments of the early part of the twentieth century that canned fruits became available in both quantity and variety. Today the canning of fruits is a giant industry. Over 115 million cases of fruits are packed annually.

Peaches respond most acceptably to the processes of modern canning. The soil and climatic conditions of California, Oregon, and Washington are ideally suited to the cultivation of fine fruits. Over 90 per cent of all canned fruits are grown and packed on the Pacific Coast, and over 90 per cent of all peaches canned are grown in California. This does not mean that other states do not produce a remarkable quality of peach—take, for example, Georgia, whose beauties are unparalleled in the markets.

As soon as the fruits are delivered to the cannery, they undergo the most rigorous tests for quality. And as they go through the various canning operations, they are inspected again and again.

It would be a great benefit to all housewives who use canned fruits to pay a visit to one of the canneries which are operated by the dominant companies in the field. In this industry all run model canneries and welcome the opportunity to demonstrate their efficiency to interested consumers. Many things become clear when canning is demonstrated, including the value of labeling. Good labeling, which means good *descriptive* labeling, is important as a guide to good buying, since information about the product is clearly stated and is pertinent.

The history of canning is a fascinating chapter in the growth of modern industry the world over. Modern canning begins with Napoleon's time, when, in an effort to provide his soldiers with proper food, he offered a prize for someone to come up with a way to preserve it. A French chef, Nicholas Appert, as a result of this offer, won not only that prize but a far greater reward—he goes down in the annals of cookery as The Father of Canning. His experiments, founded on trial and error, had to include war on heat, moisture and air, which prompted him to put food into wide-mouthed bottles, filling them to the top to exclude air, corking them tightly, boiling them in a kettle and then cooling them. He was the first (although at this distance of 150 years it hardly seems possible) to recognize the need for sealing the bottles tightly before boiling them. He also worked out different cooking times for different products.

Luckily, in connection with his prize, M. Appert had to write a book explaining his methods. This has become the Bible of the canning industry: *The Book of All Households, on the Art of Preserving Animal and Vegetable Substances.*

Through the years as the methods of canning have improved until they have reached a state of near-perfection, anyone who eats food, serves food, or is concerned about the health of humanity will find an interest in a study of this industry.

Peaches, as a fruit, have taken so kindly to canning that they might almost be regarded as at the head of the class. Anyone who has opened a can of first-quality freestone peaches, with their brilliant red hearts and firm-fleshed yellow halves, knows a certain thrill which accompanies recognition of a superior product well dealt with.

There are those who, living near peach-growing areas, have opportunities to buy early varieties of tree-ripened peaches directly from growers, but they *still* go to the markets and buy their favorite brand in cans. After all, they can't do the grading, selecting, and guaranteeing that are behind this canned product which is close to the ultimate in peach selection. It must be admitted for purposes of absolute verity that tree-ripened peaches may have a little edge on flavor. The difference must be made by the cook who serves the eventual dish.

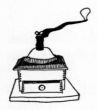

8

The Bean that Conquered the World

by K. Cyrus Melikian
and Lloyd K. Rudd

Coffee is like a glamorous woman, whose ways are endlessly provoking curiosity and interest. Everyone who loves coffee, in a sense, woos it—wants to know more about it and fit it into his daily life for stimulation or restful release, as he chooses.

Recorded history indicates that the story of coffee began in Kenya and Abyssinia (Ethiopia). The coffee trees grew wild in the jungles or forests. Coffee berries fell to the ground and germinated, seedlings emerged, and coffee trees began to spread.

The Arabian mocha coffees still come from Ethiopia and are grown with little attention of a professional agricultural sort; as a result these coffee trees are fairly wild. From year to year and from crop to crop they change somewhat in flavor, naturally. Users of coffee blends must be careful in the use of Arabian mocha, as to quantities and proportions, that is. Our blend has a goodly amount of Arabian mocha, since we regard it as the "wine" of the Levant—the countries washed by the eastern Mediterranean.

Legends about this coffee are legion. Some say it goes back to the time when the Abyssinians moved northward toward Arabia and carried with them the sprigs or seeds of those wild coffee trees. When the Abyssinians were driven out of Persia, they left in their hurried departure many of these coffee seedlings and coffee berries.

Coffee has a pedigree of some 1,400 years. It has been adopted and appreciated by most civilized peoples; it is a daily mainstay in the menus of most countries. As individual and characteristic as the brews are, they have one important element in common: they serve as a mild but delightful stimulant.

The Persians, in common with the Arabians, tasted of the ripening fruit and found it good. When we talk of Persia, we must speak of Yemen, still one of the chief ports for coffee export in the world. Even today, good mocha-type coffees are shipped from Yemen, despite hot or cold wars, and rumors of wars. One wonders if any army can exist without coffee. Modern armies, with their tremendous numbers of stimulant-demanding men certainly have a right to object to much of the brew served under the guise of coffee.

Someone, these hundreds of years ago, had a spirit of adventure and experimented—chewed the leaves, tasted the red berries or cherries, or perhaps the coffee-bean itself, which is the nut inside the cherry. Legend hath it that it was an Arabian shepherd who combined the berries or nuts with water and boiled them. Whoever he was (Kaldi is the name handed down) he is lost in the mazes of antiquity and his identity is gone forever. He might not have been a shepherd but a goatherd and possibly his interest was first aroused by the goats who went about nibbling at the cherries on the wild cherry trees. At any rate, we are indebted to him, because coffee, as we now so gratefully know it, might forever have been lost to us.

The Arabic word for coffee is *khawwah,* though there is no comparable diphthong in English for the "kh" sound. It comes to us as *quawah,* and is usually spelled *kahwa* in our newsprints. There was a time when khawwah also meant wine. But the Mohammedans objected to wine; objected so strongly it was forbidden to the faithful.

The brew from the coffee bean became popular and was served as one does a wine. To this day, throughout the Arab-speaking countries, coffee-drinking plays an important role in society, to say nothing of economy.

We could profit by adopting their coffee-making technique, though perhaps it is too elaborate for our busy, ulcer-inducing existence. Involved preparations go into a proper making of Arabian-style coffee. Coffee is prepared in a little copper container, tin-lined and diamond-shaped, a "jazzvah"—we venture the spelling. The coffee is ground to a fine powdered consistency, to which sugar and water, or even milk with water, are added and is brewed in the jazzvah.

In Clementine Paddleford's column in the *New York Herald Tribune* of March 21, 1959, there was a description of coffee-making, near-Eastern style, at a restaurant in New York featuring these exotic coffees.

Nirvana champagne heads the coffee listing. This is a blending of Javanese, Medellon and Senegalese, these coffees stone ground to brew and sell for 50 cents a cup. Kafe Kuwaiti is an Arabian coffee of finest quality, strong and pungent, for the drinker a solace, a stimulant. Kahwa Turkish coffee is made as it is in Turkish, Armenian and Syrian restaurants. The brew boiled up in a special pot called a racquie, made of copper, nickel-lined, urn shaped with a long handle at the side. The coffee used is the dark grind, pulverized. First the pot is filled with cold water within two inches of the top; measured in is powdered sugar, two teaspoons for a cup. The sweetened water is placed over a chafing dish flame and brought to a boil. The coffee is measured in, one teaspoon for each cup, add a cardamon seed. Let the brew come to a froth, tap the pot, once, twice to settle, return to the flame. Again the brew is let bubble, now tap and repeat the above procedure and once again.

The 'skim' is dipped from the pot and divided into little cups—each must have its portion of the seductive brown froth. Into the pot shake a drop or two of orange water to compel the unruly grounds to settle, then pour.

But to return to the jazzvah: after the mixture is brought to a boil, then allowed to cool, more water is added to fill the jazzvah and brought to a boil. Since specific gravity causes the coffee to settle in different layers, the weak brew at the top of the vessel is poured off. Then the rich coffees at the bottom are poured into small Turkish (or Armenian or Near Eastern) coffee cups.

To serve, you pour the brew in small amounts; a little bit into each cup at a time. You never, never fill the cup fully at first pouring. Probably you will fill one third of the cup, at next pouring bring it to one half; next, two thirds, and finally the cup is full. You'll find it is frothy on the top, a little thicker as you go to the bottom. After you have savored the flavor and finished the brew, with your left hand (so tradition indicates) pick up the cup and, turning it away from you, place it upside down in the saucer.

Part of Near Eastern hospitality is for the host—provided he is genial and responsive—to read your fortune. Whether Lebanese, Syrians, Persians, or Turks, this is a long-standing custom; all guests are flattered and delighted with this attention. Naturally you hear only the most pleasant predictions. If your host is inventive he will include others present in your fortune, and if you are good at dissembling, you can contribute to your own story to capture the attention of the audience. This group breathlessly awaits its turn, and, if your host has been successful in his crystal-gazing, there will be several who ask for second cups of coffee so that more and more fortunes may be read. Customs such as these surround coffee, and its past is as glowing as its future.

Over the centuries enough has been learned of coffees of all lands to build up to an impressive history. Kave, or coffee, was used as an herb by medicine men in antiquity; it served as a cathartic, and for a basic in an herb cellar or closet. So valued was it as a curative, it enjoyed a special aura of its own—was it not the gift of a Divine Being? Of course, because it was healthful and stimulating and never intoxicating. It made brackish water seem pleasant and refreshing. The coffee plant seemed to prosper without much encouragement, proof that Allah wanted his devoted ones to drink coffee or he would not have made it so readily available. Look at Yemen, a place of sandy soil, and still the coffee plant flourished.

So the use of coffee spread. It was not the clear, brown brew later to win favor with most of mankind; it was made by boiling the freshly picked leaves and cherries, with water. It was a bitter but stimulating drink. Later the fruit was sun-dried and husked, and the seeds roasted.

Kaldi, the Arabian herdsman, probably had no difficulty in convincing the abbot of a nearby monastery that those frisking goats of his got that way from nibbling at the cherries. The abbot, it is somewhat unreliably reported, tried them himself and finding them surprisingly exhilarating had stumbled on the great secret—how to keep his monks awake during their long religious ceremonies. We can only regard this old monk's tale as apocryphal, but it does serve to bolster up the theory that coffee can and does stimulate, does titillate, and in a modern world is a device adopted by employers to increase the productivity of their employees.

In the real beginnings of coffee preparation, grinding the seeds began approximately in the year 1400. Someone in Persia liked the idea of coffee, and with a somewhat greater knowledge of chemistry the Islamic peoples became really devoted to brewing coffee. When visiting temples and mosques, they drank it while making their prayers. The monks, it is said, after they had had their daily quota, went around offering it to the people at their devotions. Coffee was indeed a favorite of the holy men, and coffee-drinking in public was accepted and approved.

So we come to the origin of the coffee-house. A gathering-place for students, a haunt of professional people, artists and lawyers, a focal point for discussion, relaxation, and naturally gossip. Here were the true devotees: they drank the coffee, they read their fortunes, they found coffee to be fun. So, indubitably, the first coffee-break dates back to 1475, when there is recorded evidence of the first coffee-house, known as Kiva Han.

In Turkish, coffee house is *Quavah Kanes* (or *Khanes*) —in modern Turkey *kaveh* probably is considered correct. The Turks were wise in their preparation of coffee and substantially improved it—indeed started its modern development by the method in which they dried and roasted coffee. Then it was ground with a mortar and pestle, boiled in water and strained through silk. Its flavor was preserved by decanting it into earthen pots. This, we definitely believe, was the origin of the concentrate as we know it now. Portions were reheated and served, flavored with cinnamon sticks or cloves and served in china-type cups. Sound good? It sounds delicious.

Since the Islamic peoples were forbidden the release that comes from alcoholic beverages, it is natural that coffee-drinking became a firm part of their living habits and is retained to this day. The coffee-house became the center of social life. Entertainers, musicians and dancers, were hired to amuse the customers; and the more serious-minded gathered to discuss politics and religion. The music was probably made by a douvil, a drum and a zournah, a reeded, fluted shepherd's horn, supplemented by a violin or an oud, a mandolin-type instrument. Customers could take their choice of being entertained by professionals or stimulated by esoteric conversation. Not very different from what goes on today in such gathering-places.

It is a reasonable conjecture that Europeans who traveled to the Near East or the Middle East found coffee-drinking most pleasurable. If they visited Syria, especially Aleppo, the second largest community of the country, they were impressed by the black, inky beverage. Constantinople, a great trading center, served it in quantities, and a visiting botanist, Leonhard Rauwolf, in about the year 1575, took it back to Germany. Coffee-appreciation spread to the Dutch through their maritime interests, which also stimulated its acceptance by the Spanish and the Italians. The Italians, specifically the Venetians, loved coffee and wanted to trade for it with the East Indians, as the trade routes were developed more and more.

In Europe coffee was valued chiefly for its medicinal properties and was prescribed for many different afflictions, even for reducing swelling in the body and certain stomach disorders. It had virtues in the eyes of the physicians of calming the violent and stimulating the passive or exciting men to deeds of passion and daring.

The Italians were the first Europeans to regard it favorably as a social beverage; they removed it from the medicine chest, and by 1675 dozens of coffee shops sprang up in Venice, patronized and supported by the upper-class citizenry. The Italian word *caffe* was attached to many of these public houses, and the most famous, the Caffe Florian, was opened by a prominent Venetian, a highly regarded citizen and diplomat. He was also a politician, which probably accounted for the success of his venture since it was frequented by his following.

While the upper classes loved their coffee, the clergy were denied it. At one time by Papal decree, not only the clergy but all Catholics were forbidden to drink it. It was regarded by the Pope as an invention of the devil, because for Mohammedans, forbidden to drink wine, coffee had become the brew, the "wine" of Islam, therefore, Satan's own black potion.

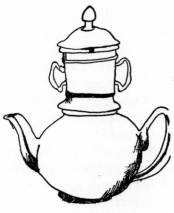

While this theological dictum was in force, coffee was making inroads into France, via Marseilles. Merchants, for purposes of self-interest, and soldiers, travelers and sailors, for reasons of sheer sensual pleasure in the concoction, were as avid as a modern promoter to "push" coffee further and further along its historical way.

Louis XIV, who reigned from 1643 until 1715, was presented with coffee by a Turkish ambassador. The palace nobles took it up with a vengeance, and it became a mark of social distinction to drink and serve coffee. With the example of the French court, it was only natural that Hungary, Servia and Bulgaria, near neighbors of Turkey, followed suit. One of the great coffee centers then came into existence and has remained ever since—Vienna, Austria.

Northward the tide of coffee swept on. It held its own in the Near East, but the north was claiming its share of coffee-lovers. The king of Denmark began to drink it daily, and while it was sold, following the usual European pattern, in apothecary shops and prescribed by doctors, midwives and chemists, it eventually made its way into general use as a beverage of distinctive flavor, highly valued as a stimulant.

Coffee reached England in the seventeenth century. It was first sold in London about the year 1650, and until the early 1800's and the emergence of the London clubs, the coffee-house was the hub of English social life; masculine social life, that is. The response of the women to this rash of coffee-houses which kept their husbands away from home was to take action. A petition was circulated against coffee on health grounds: it was a lethal beverage, dealing poor health and untold illness to its users. Actually this was a feminine revolt against the stag life that coffee-drinking engendered.

However, the coffee-house had a firm hold on the habits of the male population by this time, and around 1725 there were almost two thousand coffee houses or taverns in the London area. The acceptance of coffee was not confined to the aristocracy by any means. Every class of society was drawn into its orbit, and every guild had favorite gathering places where coffee was the chief brew. Since London was then a small community, coffee-houses literally dotted its landscape. At one period, London consumed more coffee than any other city in the world.

Vogues have a way of running their course, disappearing from the scene with as little reason as they appear on the scene in the first place. It is a phenomenon of civilization advancing, if that's the word. And even though coffee-drinking had in this period penetrated to the nethermost ends of the social structure—one evidence is that coffee-house prices were one or two pence a cup—the drinking habits of the populace underwent, in England, a gradual change.

But not before the coffee-house had placed its indelible stamp on literature. Dr. Samuel Johnson literally swilled his coffee at the Turk's Head, and who can say that many of his social observations, as in "Rasselas," say, were not coffee-inspired? He had distinguished company in Boswell, Burke, and Garrick, who were all great coffee drinkers, and their activities indicate that they derived more than usual stimulation from the brew.

The decline of public interest in coffee-drinking is a whole saga in itself. Not only in England, but all over Europe its influence had made itself felt. Johann Sebastian Bach produced a Coffee Cantata, which musically embodied the emotions felt by women protesting the coffee-consumption of their men. For some reason women retained the original opinion of coffee as a medicine longer than men, eventually crediting it with dark, dank properties. Actually theirs was simply a social revolt: they just didn't want to be ignored in favor of the coffee-house frequenters.

In Germany, coffee ran neck and neck with beer in beverage consumption. The beer industry was a dominant factor in German economy, and in 1775 Frederick the Great issued a manifesto to slow down the flow of money to foreign merchants supplying green coffee to his country. It was believed that it was ruining the beer industry, and certainly it was a potent rival.

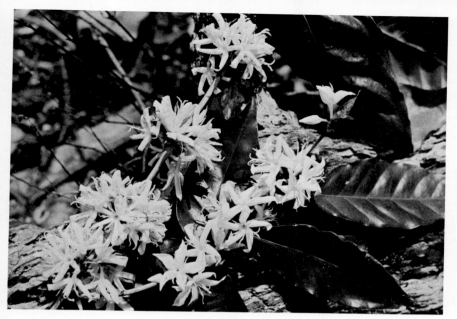

Blossoms of the coffee tree resemble those of orange trees in both color and fragrance. After flowering, the fruit—the coffee cherry—begins to form.

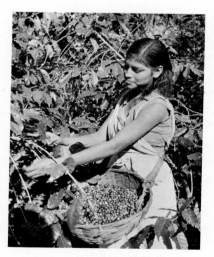

Workers must hand-pick nearly two thousand coffee cherries to provide enough beans for one pound of roasted coffee. Each cherry contains two beans.

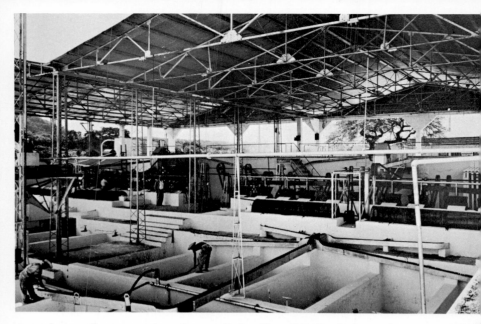

A modern coffee processing plant, called a "beneficio," which employs wet method processing. Here the outer and inner skins of the coffee cherry are removed, leaving o the two beans enclosed in a tough parchment.

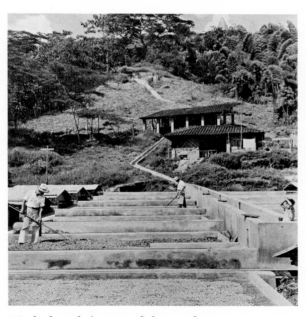

Washed and fermented beans drying in an open patio. During the day, to assure uniform drying, beans must be constantly turned.

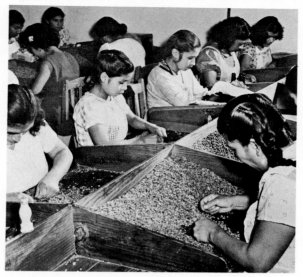

Parchment and final skin are removed from beans by machines at milling plant. Hand sorting removes discolored or defective beans. Perfect beans are then transported to warehouse where they are graded, tested for quality and placed in bags.

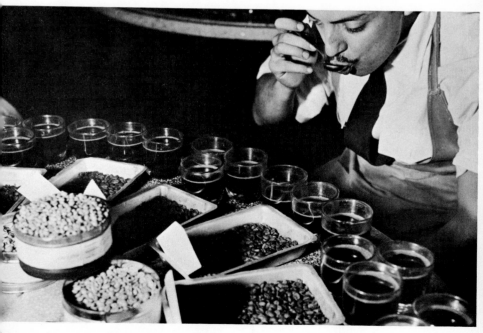

ere a taster tests the grade of coffee. The round cans contain green coffee from a ocessing plant. In trays are roasted beans from same plant, while glasses hold coffee brewed from roasted beans.

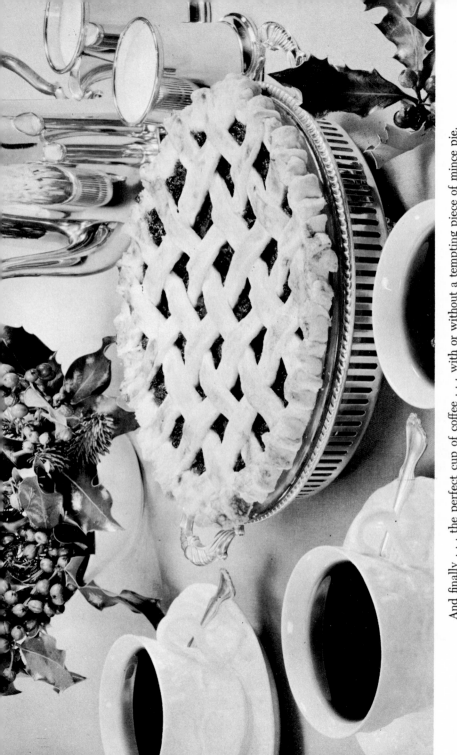

And finally . . . the perfect cup of coffee . . . with or without a tempting piece of mince pie.

It was in Germany that the Kaffeeklatsch was born, and thrived, eventually becoming as important to Deutschland as tea-time is to Britain as a daily routine or ritual. Although it was formally observed at a different time of day, the Kaffeeklatsch corresponds to the coffee-break in the United States. It was the essence of *gemütlichkeit*, and this time the ladies took over. They made of it a moment of high social importance, and in rich, elegant homes as well as in lowlier domiciles, this rite was observed each day. Some of the greatest *kuchen* in the world emerged from the observance of this set-aside moment of the day; cooks outdid themselves both in Germany and Austria to make the Kaffeeklatsch a great occasion.

In America the coffee-house became a popular meeting place about the time of William Penn, around 1680. In those days it is recorded that a pound of coffee cost five dollars. It was green coffee and when roasted shrank about 12 per cent, which, in effect, added some sixty cents to the cost—an expensive item. The Colonists, prior to the American Revolution, were tea drinkers, and it took the oppressive and excessive tea taxes to alter the beverage-drinking habit of the new nation. So the ultimate tea-boycott against England and the Crown's retaliation which led to the Boston Tea Party was the kick-off to general coffee-drinking in America. Colorful records of the time reveal that the Union Street Coffee-House in Boston became the patriotic gathering place for discussing strategy and, since tea was a nasty word, coffee became king. Such men as John Adams, James Otis, and Paul Revere were doubtless in the vanguard when this change-over from tea to coffee took place.

As time marched on, we became the largest consumers of coffee in the world, today absorbing about 70 per cent of Latin America's annual crop, for example.

With the advent of prohibition, coffee sales soared. It

was amazing what prohibition did for coffee consumption. If any industry profited by these arid years, it was the coffee business. When the Eighteenth Amendment was repealed, more coffee was being consumed than ever before. The coffee habit became firmly established during the years 1919 to 1933, and succeeding generations have followed suit.

Men in the armed services have grown to regard coffee-drinking as an essential part of their daily routine, not that the coffee served them is reminiscent of home and mother. The United States Navy has a high per capita consumption ratio, possibly the highest in the world. Sailors like coffee on tap round the clock, an appetite which arises from the fact that the men work on eight-hour watches. Watches are four hours on, four off, and what sailor can do without his frequent tot of coffee?

The coffee-break in America has become such an important part of the business day that employers, at first bewildered by its universal acceptance, realized suddenly that no office or firm could really get going on the morning's business until time out for coffee and "Danish" had been permitted. They gradually came to believe that a happy employee was a more productive employee, and if coffee would keep 'em happy, well, keep 'em happy. Besides which, the employers like the coffee-break for themselves. Now many an office, particularly in the big cities, has two coffee-breaks in an eight-hour day—mid-morning and midafternoon. Sometimes the coffee is made in the mailroom and available all day. Sometimes instant coffee is served. (These powdered coffees account for some of the substantial increase in coffee sales, both wholesale and retail.)

In world coffee production, Latin America leads, producing 85 per cent of the total. The remaining 15 per cent is divided among countries like Java, where the output is small; Hawaii, practically nothing, though perhaps as a new state the coffee production may be stepped up; Ethiopia, which raises even now a substantial amount; Kenya, a substantial percentage. Indeed, the African coffees from the Ivory Coast, Gold Coast, and West Coast are fast showing signs of becoming important factors in coffee economy and the world scene.

Brazil, as the largest coffee producer in the world, providing over 50 per cent of the world's supply, has many economic problems as a result of growing coffee. Many coffee drinkers don't realize that it takes five years to get a coffee tree to bear. The coffee cherries, inside of which is the nut or bean, do not mature under five years. The bean must be roasted and ground, and that means there are many steps from the harvesting of the cherries to your cup of coffee. It is obvious that this takes a prodigious amount of work. This means hand-handling, treated in a different manner in each of the haciendas, faciendas and ranches on which coffee is grown. Labor commands little reward.

The average yield of coffee from each tree is at most two pounds of roasted coffee. You can see that you must have forests of coffee trees in Brazil to supply those millions of pounds of coffee to the North American market alone. Literally, millions of bags of coffee come from these Latin American countries under conditions of handling and packing which seem unnecessarily laborious as compared to our agricultural ways.

It has been about 140 years since Brazil first began producing coffee. In 1818 the country's first substantial export was around 75,000 pounds. Java and small areas of India produced about 15,000 pounds—even then Java was quite a factor in export sales.

The coffee industry may be held responsible for the radical ups and downs in Brazil's economy. There are many tragic elements in the economic history of Brazil; many evils may be laid at the doors of the coffee growers and distributors. Now, however, there are many government price supports. The complexities are as great as in our own Department of Agriculture. Many assists to the growers have been worked out, and despite the elaborate systems in monetary exchange, the present situation is better than it has ever been, although permanently stable prices are still almost impossible to conceive of in Brazil and Colombia.

Colombia produces about 30 per cent of the world's supply of coffee, although it is a fairly small country. Her coffees are relatively different from the Brazilian varieties.

The Dutch control Java, and their method of introducing coffee production into that country forms one of the most diverting chapters in coffee history. They virtually sneaked or smuggled coffee beans in for cultivation, and since they were so scarce, laws were passed to prevent taking them out—they were contraband. Java became a great coffee-producing area for the Dutch chiefly because the climate was ideal for its development. Coffee may flourish in temperate climates, contrary to popular belief. It is not necessary to grow coffee in the steamy heat of the tropics, though this is thought by many people to be a requisite for its production. The importance of tropical cultivation of coffee berries is that the grower is able to get two crops—one big and one small yield a year. The smaller is called the catch crop; the larger is the regular yield and is the profitable one when the year's crops are in.

There is little comprehension of the part played by the blender in the process of bringing the coffee from the plantation or hacienda to the consumer. The blender (roaster or mixer may be the name you are familiar with) is a company rather than an individual. Blending is a fine art, but there is a great deal of hocus-pocus about this phase of coffee processing. Naturally, the purchaser wants the best blending of coffee types to produce the finest brew—the balance and composition to insure the most acceptable flavor. The blender company employs a high-priced professional, an expert. You might think of him as a front man for the coffee industry, and since the blender is in a constant guessing game to determine what the customer wants, this kind of expert advice has been cloaked in mystery.

Since Brazilian coffee represents 50 per cent of the entire world production, it is not remarkable that Brazilian coffees appear in almost every blend. There are several kinds of these coffees:

First, there is Santos, then Paranas, then Minas, Bahias, Rios, Victorias, and Pernambucos. The experienced buyer will decide what proportion of each is necessary for his needs.

The "milds" are a distinct group of coffees. Seemingly best grown in Latin America, there are varieties which come from Africa, Java, and even Hawaii. Most milds come from Colombia, Mexico, Guatemala, and Venezuela.

The coffee blender is concerned with the "chop," a means of sampling which is identified on each bag of coffee. This "chop" number tells the purchaser just what he needs to know. The coffees in each bag are going to be the same, since they have been through a cupping test. The blender has analyzed strength, acidity, body, color—in a word, what is present in every coffee blend.

This sampling technique is very important, particularly in quality control. Much publicity has been given the ritual of coffee-tasting. The tasters sit round tables flanked by brass cuspidors. They take mouthfuls of coffee, savor each, then use the cuspidors, sometimes frowning and solemnly shaking their heads. This method of tasting is romantic, but instrumentation is taking over and soon the physical means of testing could be a thing of the past.

In buying coffee there are certain essentials the blender looks for. The purchaser may search for an "acidy" coffee. Acidy coffee is slightly sour-tasting, somewhat sharp and quite distinct in flavor. This is a characteristic of certain mild coffees. What the blender is striving for in taste may be obtained only by combining five or six acidy coffees to produce just the wanted flavor. Long periods of storage increase coffee's acidity.

Roasting lowers coffee's caffeine content somewhat, although a popular misconception is that the darker you roast coffee the more stimulating the brew. Actually, this is not quite true. Whether the roaster gets a light cinnamon, a dark Italian or a French roast, the caffeine content is constant and so is the stimulating strength.

What *is* a good cup of coffee? It may be 50, 60, or even 70 per cent Santas with 30 per cent Colombian. By Colombian, we mean the mild coffees—Manizales, Armenia, or the Medellins. The super-patriotic Colombian thinks there is only one kind of coffee in the world. The Colombianos take great pride in their mountain-grown coffees, but perhaps they are best when blended with other types. At Rudd-Melikian we use a particularly large amount of Colombian in our coffee and coffee concentrate, expensive as they are, with the conviction that they make a splendid contribution to the blend.

Armenian coffees come from Colombia. Armenians settled there at one time, though they certainly are not there any more.

Manizales is a famous type of Colombian mild, and this represents a large percentage of the coffee Colombia markets in the United States. Generally these coffees are not sold unblended; this is because, while they are smooth, they lack the acidity and pungency supplied by other coffees of different sorts and other climates.

Coffee turns rancid fairly quickly after it is roasted and ground, and in order to keep intact its volatile esters, it is best to keep it in the refrigerator or a container with an airtight lid.

Now we'd like to show you the great versatility of coffee; the many ways it can be used in beverages and as a flavoring in recipes.

Coffee has been party to many marriages. Some of them have been most felicitous indeed; many have been romantic and exciting; and all of them have had their devoted adherents.

The subject of coffee can hardly be done justice to without a review of the part Cafe Espresso has played in the coffee-making of the world. Until a few years ago it was relatively unknown in America, but its fame was spread by the GIs who went to Italy and discovered its virtues, even though coffee itself was in short supply. Italian Espresso machines are made in Milan, and tourists traveling in Italy, Spain, and Switzerland became familiar with them and grew enthusiastic about the somewhat exotic brew which flowed from their taps.

Chrome-plated, the machine bristles with intricate taps, handles, valves, and spouts and was not to be found in America until after the war. Now, from Mulberry Street to North Beach, from Atlantic City to San Francisco, numbers of fine coffee-houses and restaurants have them, and make a feature of Cafe Espresso. The vogue has spread to the point of manufacturing small Espresso machines for home use, electrically operated, such as are featured by Abercrombie & Fitch in New York. The Espresso machine has become to a degree a present-day substitute for the old Anglo-Saxon coffee-house, and in London and New York it is looked upon as a heady and fashionable way to prepare coffee. In our opinion, it is a temporary enthusiasm and no one can venture to prophesy how long the vogue will last. At the moment, though, Espresso is important, since it inspires good conversation and serves as a focal point for coffee-lovers who regard the Espresso urn as a symbol of escape, a logical successor to the coffee-house. It is a sophisticated drink at the moment, largely because of the limited production—essentially it is a one-cup-at-a-time service. The coffee used in an Espresso machine is fine drip-type, and about a teaspoon or a little more, about four ounces, is measured for one cup of coffee.

Any Espresso coffee-house worthy of its name will offer its patrons an impressive number of coffee drinks, not all of them Italian. Whether Espresso is served in large cups, demitasses, or small glasses, starting with freshly brewed Espresso, or cafe, you may create variations which are not too difficult to achieve. Here are some typical

Espresso Recipes

Cafe Anisette: Espresso with a little anisette or anise added, in a quantity to suit the guest. This is really a cold-weather drink, since it is warming, as is *Cafe Anisette Royale,* which is the same drink with a topping of whipped cream for that extra touch of richness.

Cafe Borgia: Of the legends that surround the famous Borgias, one of the most pleasant (and least lethal) drinks served in their famous palaces was devised by one of their chefs. It combines equal parts of hot chocolate, made with milk, and coffee, finished with a little cream and a flourish of grated orange. In a second version, bittersweet chocolate is grated over whipped cream, along with some orange and almond slivers. If the invited guests were courageous enough to drink anything in company with the Borgias, these drinks may have been delightful enough to blind them to any substance dropped surreptitiously from a signet ring into their cups. Those were surely the days of glamorous—if dangerous—hospitality.

Cafe Espresso with Liqueur: Served with brandy or almost any liqueur of your choice—creme de menthe, kümmel, Cointreau, curaçao—it is an ideal climax to a formal dinner. Just choose the liqueur which best suits your character or the mood of the moment, always taking the season of the year into consideration.

Cafe Espresso with Rum: This is a variant on the age-old rum-and-coffee drink which has been a favorite of gourmets for generations, to which, for a spicy taste, a touch of cinnamon has been introduced.

Cafe Strega: In the cup or out, Strega and Espresso blend companionably. It's effective to serve Strega in its own liqueur glass, with a demitasse of Espresso—sip one and then the other, the flavor of both is enhanced.

Cafe Tonico: After a rich and generous repast, the tang of bitters seems absolutely right. Put a dash of Fernet Branca Bitters in to make the coffee with a tonic freshness.

Cafe Zabaglione: In the top of a double boiler, over boiling water, combine some egg yolks with sugar and Espresso, stir the mixture together until it is foamy and thick and serve in a warm glass.

Cappucino: This drink combines equal parts of Espresso with hot boiling milk (*leche*—the Italian-Spanish word for milk) and you have a warm-colored drink the shade of the light-brown tunic worn by Capuchin monks, hence its name. With a little cinnamon and nutmeg, and served in a six-ounce cup, it is frothy, light, and easy to drink.

Ciocco Laccino: Equal part of Cappucino and hot chocolate to each cup are topped with some whipped cream to which a scattering of bitter chocolate adds a decorative touch.

Espresso Romano: For the drink of the Eternal City, drop a twist of lemon peel into a glass of steaming Espresso. Be sure you have a sterling silver spoon in the glass, so it won't crack.

Other coffee recipes for party drinks:

Cafe Caccala: To each cup of freshly brewed coffee, add one jigger of creme de cacao and top off with whipping cream.

Cafe Cointreau: To each cup of coffee, add one measuring teaspoonful of grated lemon peel, then gently stir in one jigger of Cointreau.

Cafe Nectar: In a blend combine approximately three to three and a half teaspoons of coffee concentrate and water, a little coffee ice cream and Angostura bitters, beat well. This will serve three or four people.

Cafe Royale: A fine after-dinner coffee drink—it's just a piece of sugar in a demitasse filled with strong coffee to which a little brandy is slowly added. If done properly, the brandy will rise to the surface, and then it may be ignited to burn for a few seconds. It should be well stirred before sipping.

Cafe Tropicala (iced): Fill an electric blender with some finely chopped ice, add one and a half teaspoons of coffee concentrate and one rounded measuring teaspoon of fine granulated sugar (4X). Blend until thick, serve at once for a fine, cool drink.

Coffee Ice Cream Soda: If made with a concentrate, add a little sugar, some cream, coffee ice cream, and fill a tall glass with this mixture and sparkling water.

Frosted Coffee Hawaiian: For a flavorful drink, com-

bine three or three and a half teaspoons of coffee concentrate with a little water; stir in some soft coffee ice cream
and pineapple juice. Proportions should be to taste and
number of people to be served.

Iced Coffees: There are infinite ways to prepare iced
coffees, but a coffee concentrate is mixed with cold water,
poured over ice, and served with a little honey and
whipped cream, and dusted with cinnamon and nutmeg.
This is, obviously, Honey Iced Coffee.

Irish Coffee: Put a jigger of Irish whiskey in a glass.
Fill with strong hot coffee to within a half inch of the
top and add whipped cream.

Mocha Shake: Ideal for the picnic kit. Mix one and one-
third cups instant nonfat dry milk crystals with three
cups ice water; stir lightly. Add four teaspoons sugar,
four teaspoons instant coffee powder and three tablespoons chocolate syrup; blend. Add two cups crushed
ice; pour into a thermos bottle. Shake before pouring.
This yields eight servings.

Trader Vic's Coffee Grog: One of this famous restau-
rateur's specialities, has acquired a wide following. It
requires half a cup of strong coffee, which can be made
from approximately two teaspoons of coffee concentrate,
and about four ounces of water. Now comes the magic:
half an ounce of light rum and half an ounce of either
imported or domestic brandy, and a dash of heavy dark
Jamaica rum, a small piece of lemon or orange peel, six
cloves, and a sprinkling of cinnamon. The ingredients
are combined in a saucepan and heated quickly. It is
served in a special heavy mug, which looks a little like
the old-time shaving mug, previously rubbed with a little
butter. Cream and sugar are added to taste.

Viennese Coffee Frost: The greatest of coffee-lovers,
the Viennese, are responsible for a delightful coffee frost,
which is made with cold water and concentrate. For ac-

cent, powder some cinnamon sticks and cloves, some all-spice berries, with crushed ice, some lime and sugar syrup to flavor. Serve in tall glasses, with a topping of whipped cream.

Mexico has used coffee with imagination to make a delightful cordial. South of Mexico City and in Guatemala, mild coffees are grown. These have been blended to produce a coffee liqueur or cordial called Kahlua, presently popular. The back label on the Kahlua bottle makes several interesting suggestions as to serving.

Many people are surprised to learn that coffee is a prime ingredient in the preparation of meat sauces. Here is a fine steak barbecue sauce:

⅔ cup strong coffee, made in concentrate

⅓ cup butter or oleomargarine

2 teaspoons Worcestershire sauce

1½ teaspoons dry mustard

1 tablespoon lemon juice

1 teaspoon sugar

dash of tabasco

Combine all the ingredients together in a saucepan, heat, stir until the butter melts, then brush over your steak, as it broils, or use it over pork ribs. This is a wonderfully flavorful barbecue sauce.

Italian Meat Sauce

1 pound of ground beef

1 medium onion (chopped)

3 ounces chopped broiled mushrooms

1 clove garlic (minced or chopped)

2 tablespoons Italian olive oil

2 cans tomato paste

½ teaspoon sugar

½ teaspoon oregano

¾ cup coffee, medium strong

To the olive oil, add the onion and garlic and brown; add the meat and stir with a fork or mixing spoon until brown; add the tomato paste and some tomato soup; add the coffee and sugar and simmer for half an hour; add the mushrooms and oregano, simmer for another five minutes. Serve on a thin spaghettini or spaghetti with grated Parmesan cheese. This makes an excellent Italian meat sauce, simple to prepare and delightful to savor.

Coffee goes well with gravies. Take, for instance, a pot roast of beef brown gravy. To a quarter-pound of suet, sautéed in a Dutch oven, or a large kettle until it is dried out, add about a 4-pound pot roast, rolled in flour, season it with salt and pepper, and brown on all sides to retain the fat. While the meat is browning, add some onion slices and a cup of strong coffee, cover it with about 3 cups of water, simmer over a low heat for 3 to 4 hours, depending on the cut of meat. The time usually allowed is an hour a pound. If necessary, the meat is turned several times in the course of the cooking, and also, if necessary, the gravy is thickened.

Coffee flavoring is ideal for puddings. Coffee Bavarian is a great favorite with the children; so is coffee ice cream, either bought commercially or made at home. A jellied coffee soufflé is delicious, as is a Mocha surprise pudding. Frozen concentrate gives a good tangy flavor in eclairs and cream fillings and is labor-saving.

Mocha Eclair

Here is a party eclair, finger-sized, which takes a little time but is rewarding. The pastry bag comes into use— make with a flat tube, about a half-inch wide. The eclairs are baked on a buttered baking sheet, and filled with a

mocha cream filling; the top is iced with a mocha confectionary icing. Here's how you do the mocha cream filling:

1½ cups milk	½ cup sugar
⅓ cup coffee, strong	¼ cup sifted flour
4 egg yolks	

Prepare the egg-and-sugar mixture, beat until light,
then fold in the flour; to this add the milk and coffee, stir
until it turns into a creamy consistency in a saucepan. Do
not allow it to boil. Cool the mixture, stirring as you cool
it, then put it into a filling or pastry bag and fill the mocha
eclairs. The mocha confectionary icing is made with 2
cups of sifted confectionary sugar; add 2 tablespoons rum
and 2 or 3 tablespoons of strong coffee (concentrate),
1 ounce unsweetened chocolate, and 3 or 4 tablespoons of
black coffee. Melt the chocolate in the black coffee and
continue to beat the icing until it is smooth and shiny.
Put a teaspoon of icing on each eclair, smooth it on with
the backside of a teaspoon or the blade of a silver knife,
occasionally dipped in hot water.

Footnotes on Coffee

Americans are becoming connoisseurs of coffees, going
even to the great lengths of home roasting and blending.
It isn't too easy to buy unblended green coffee, but with
some effort it can be obtained even if you have to go to
a select group of importers in New York City. In Italy,
the story is a different one: most coffees are bought in
the green state and home-roasted in a frying pan with a
cover. It takes a bit of doing, since the roaster has to be
expert to avoid burning the coffee bean. Americans find
Italian coffee heavy for the most part; this is because the

coffee actually is burnt during the roasting process. Coffee is described as a heavy Italian roast when the coffee oil sweats to a fine shinyness and the bean is burnt. Sometimes this Italian or French coffee is known as a "sweet roast."

Coffee doesn't behave too well and in fact reacts rather badly to temperatures over 500° Fahrenheit. Under average roasting conditions the coffee bean will expand two and a half times its green bean volume. If you are an amateur, but at the same time would like to roast your own coffee, you should try for a color which might be described as medium brown. Whatever roasting device you use may be of your own choosing, but the important thing is to keep your eye on the beans rather than the clock. Grinding should occur only at the time the coffee is to be brewed. Therefore, roasted coffee should be kept in a good, tight jar in the refrigerator since ground coffee flavor is highly volatile and perishable. Green coffee has almost unlimited keeping qualities, but when baked or roasted it becomes perishable and must be used quickly and handled carefully. The volatile aromatic esters and the coffee oils and acids blend together to form that superb taste so distinctive of coffee. Brewing coffee indicates only that water has been passed through ground coffee beans to extract the volatile flavoring materials and oils and the soluble solids. The result is actually a concentrate incorporating the extracted flavors of the roasted beans.

When you think in terms of a coffee concentrate, you are ordinarily considering controlled production conditions where coffee is brewed or percolated automatically, and the flavoring substance extracted from the bean. The resultant coffee concentrate is rushed into a freezer and shock frozen. With all its flavor "locked up," frozen in cans and kept at low temperature storage, you will have all the factors which make sense in terms of frozen coffee.

Coffee, of course, to the gourmet, as well as to the house-wife, can mean many different things. If you are an old-fashioned coffee drinker, a perfect brew, according to the Coffee Brewing Institute, can be made by using two tablespoons of ground coffee for each cup to be brewed. (A cup of brewed coffee is considered to be six fluid ounces.) If you decide to make five or six cups in a coffee pot, then you can add one more tablespoon, the proverbial "one for the pot." The sensual pleasure derived from the marvelous aroma of brewing coffee prepares the palate for its ultimate enjoyment, but don't forget that this delicious fragrance means that good coffee flavor and taste are going up in steam. In addition, it actually does "burn-out." Coffee burn-out is a technical expression for the flavor deterioration which takes place when coffee brew boils, or is even kept hot for twenty minutes or longer. Therefore, the secret of good coffee is to brew each cup fresh every single time.

We in America are able to enjoy the world's finest coffees in our daily cup. One of the chief reasons for this is that our country does not put an import duty on coffees. Let all the countries in the free world produce coffee, and ship it to us without tariff or duty, say we!

Since in America we try to promote trade, instead of just giving aid, we buy these agricultural products from our Latin American and Central American coffee-producing neighbors, as well as from West Africa and North Africa, East Africa, the West Indies and the East Indies —thus we get the best of coffees. As a large producer of concentrated coffee, we of Rudd-Melikian are naturally interested in other kinds of coffee, but because of our interest in trade, we do get the best coffees.

In Europe, coffee has often been in short supply, and many substitutes have been introduced to the market.

Chicory is a familiar one; in England even turnip tops were brought into play. The shortage of coffee during the war was quite serious and the pitiful substitutions were, for the most part, vile. Coffee was stretched with all sorts of devices, but every time the real bean was available it found adherents in every class of society. Germany, until recently, had a tremendously heavy duty on coffee, which is sold by the gram. Actually, it was almost a contraband item, known only to the black market. At this time, in Free Europe, coffee consumption is increasing at a tremendous rate; more people are drinking coffee in greater and greater quantities.

Coffee drinking has become a ritual. Not only is it an after-dinner beverage, it is drunk during meals. The day starts with a strong breakfast brew, and midmorning has its own moment when coffee is king—the coffee-break!

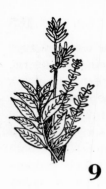

9

"Better A Meal of Herbs..."

by K. Cyrus Melikian

A phrase from the Bible sticks in my mind, perhaps not quite accurately: "Better a meal of herbs where love is than a stalled ox and hatred." So always I associate herbs with love, although I regret to say that it occurs to me that a stalled ox might well furnish the basis for a fine oxtail casserole. As I got to know more about herbs and discovered for myself what amazing and versatile fragrances they could produce when combined with basic meats, poultry and fish, and grew to recognize the lift they give to cooking, I remained in awe of their potency—and that goes for spices, too.

The Bible is replete with references to the subtlety and effectiveness of spices and records such impressive moments as when the Three Wise Men brought to the infant Jesus gifts of frankincense and myrrh. I have always been impressed by the resin gums which are so much a part of antiquity and these are two costly ones. They occur over and over again in records of commerce and part of their pervasion has to do with the value placed upon them from almost the beginning of recorded history. They have their place in religious ritual. In mythology they have important reference: Adonis, for example, was said to have been the offspring of a myrrh tree.

No doubt about it, herbs were famed in song and story from the earliest times; mythology and legend have surrounded them; great writers have extolled their properties and virtues. In Elizabeth I's age, herbs were given significance and character. Shakespeare rendered them forever important: in *Hamlet,* the distracted Ophelia strewed her flowers and herbs, and said the immortal lines: "There's rosemary, that's for remembrance . . . there's fennel (flattery) for you, and columbines. There's rue for you, and some for me. We may call it herb of grace o'Sundays. (Rue represented both sorrow and repentance and therefore became the herb of divine grace.) Oh, you must wear your rue with a difference!" Also in *Hamlet,* reference is made to "sallets"—salads—which Shakespearean authorities say were always "highly seasoned" in the state of Denmark.

So seasoning of foods to add piquancy has had a noble, romantic, pleasurable connotation reaching back into deepest antiquity.

Herbs and spices are always bracketed together, though in cooking they have separate functions. What they have in common is to provide a fillip to the prepared dish. For the most part herbs belong to the meats, or dishes of substance, which may include fowl or fish and tossed salads, while spices can step up cooked fruits, breadstuffs, and desserts to new exalted highs. And as for preserves: what can be added to a well-flavored peach, for example, when gently cooked and preserved to give it celestial, ambrosial flavor, but cloves, studding the sides of those symmetrical halves to furnish the perfect accompaniment

to familiar dishes and add strangely exotic accent to unusual combinations?

I realize that in America it has taken a matter of generations of blending cultures to inject interesting food flavorings into menus. But now, with our consistent experimentation in the test kitchens of great food companies,
painstaking research on the part of the big-circulation
women's magazines, early training in home economics in
our schools and colleges, we have made progress. Now in
many a kitchen there are herbs, peppers, spices, seeds,
and seasonings which even the young and inexperienced
cook wants to use, but sometimes doesn't know quite
how or in what proportions. Her hand floats above the
jars and she thinks to herself, "Should this go in that
stew?" and rushes to her cookbook. Often enough she
reads that her dish needs a pinch of this, a dash of that.
But what's a dash? What's a portion to be added? She is
more apt to overdo it than not; and finds out, too late,
that her brand-new husband just *hates* paprika, curry,
or nutmeg. I can only hope she doesn't stop seasoning
things, because discovering and exploring individual tastes
is what has made great cooks.

Examine the ancient spices which have persisted as the
greats in seasoning foods. First, pepper. There's hardly a
meat or main course dish which doesn't respond to the
addition of pepper, in some form or other. When the
Orient first let its mark on trade, pepper was a staple
article, establishing a link with Europe. It came from a
small East Indian climbing shrub with bright red, flavorful berries. It inspired many things, that expensive item,
pepper, even the opening of sea routes to the distant East.
Royal gifts were made of the precious substance—they
were regarded as favorably as jewels as a token of esteem.
In today's kitchen, whether that of a great hotel, restaur-

ant, or an individual home, to be without pepper would be to paralyze a gastronomic operation.

Next, ginger and saffron. Ginger is best known to urban Americans in Chinese cooking, but it has an amazing number of other uses. Back in the days of Marco Polo, its fleshy, buff-colored rootstock, grown in the warm regions of Asia, was a source of wonder and delight. This pungent and aromatic root is found now at its best in Jamaica, British West Indies. When ground it makes mouth-watering cookies, gingerbread and buns, and whole it can really make the difference between good and indifferent chutney, pickles, conserves, and even apple sauce. Turmeric is botanical brother to ginger. Combined with prepared mustard, its bright yellow color is what good cooks have learned is a dramatic ingredient in mustard pickle.

Crocus flowers—their stigmas, that is—are the source of saffron, native of Egypt and the Mediterranean. To make an ounce of saffron the pistils of four thousand flowers are used. Caution in adding it to foods is important, since it has a most distinctive flavor and might easily produce a dish *not* fit for a gourmet. It is one of of the most flavor-contributing of the spices, a chef's joy if added in proper quantity. It is a basic ingredient in some Creole and Near East dishes.

No kitchen today should be without curry powder which can turn dull leftovers of meat and poultry, among other things, into brilliant chef's dishes. The ritual of curry, served East Indian fashion, is one valued by cooks and hostesses with real ambition who love to assemble seemingly endless accompaniments in small bowls, group them around the main curry dish or platter and serve for gala events. East Indian curry may make a most dramatic buffet supper, and unless the guests suffer from peptic ulcers, is usually a resounding success. Called the "salt of the Orient" curry is a blend of turmeric, coriander, caraway, several kinds of pepper, ginger, and many another sharp and distinctive ground powder from roots or flowers.

Before I go further with suggestions for uses of specific herbs and spices in daily cooking, I'd like to give a few simple words of advice on buying and keeping them. Important to the wise cook is that she buy small quantities at a time, since they lose their flavor if they are permitted to get too old. Also the type of container they are kept in is vital to their preservation; they should be housed in an airtight small metal or glass container, and stored in a good, average temperature. They should never be exposed to a drying heat, moisture, or air. Whenever possible, they should be fresh-ground. Hungarian paprika, for example, provides almost double the piquancy if ground just before using. This special attention which may seem to many like an unimportant detail may make or break fine meat or chicken dishes—goulash, for instance, one of the most rewarding of the flavored beef dishes. It may be difficult to find shops which deal in freshly ground spices, but they are always available in the big cities, or through the mails.

Careful measuring, no slapdash treatment, should be the rule in cooking with spices. Their virtue is to enhance, rather than smother flavor, and nothing is so disappointing as to be served a dish where either the herbs or the spices have taken over to destroy or render ineffective the natural flavors of the foods. The process should be a delicate one. With foods that require long cooking, spices are generally added near the end of the cooking cycle rather than when the dish is first put on. One reason is that spices turn bitter if cooked too long. Quite the reverse is true of spices for uncooked foods. They should be added well in advance of serving; if they are chilled, they should be allowed to penetrate to the last morsel. These are the cardinal rules, and so easy to remember there should be no failures in taste-provoking, seasoned dishes.

Good, serious, gourmet-minded cooks mentally separate herbs into categories—fine herbs such as basil and rosemary and thyme; robust herbs such as mint, dill or sage. Rosemary leaf came originally from southern Europe, but is now grown in the United States. It is not unlike sage or thyme but is delicate in flavor and finds a welcome home in meats, soups, fish dishes, and salads. Powdered rosemary is effective with vegetables, eggs, stews, sauces (particularly fish sauces), even contributes a mellowness to the positive and distinctive flavor of kidney stew.

One of the pluses in herb-cooking is that you may, even in the city, have your own herb garden. The use of fresh summer herbs add zest to a midyear menu as nothing else can; when your tired summer appetite needs a real stimulus you can find excitement and taste thrills in your own garden. Not that dried or packaged herbs are not as good as fresh—they are, just about. Perhaps a notable exception is mint, which does not dry as well as some other herbs. They must be used, of course, in the off-growing seasons such as a Northern winter.

Mint, at its fresh summer best, marries a julep and makes it sheer heaven; chives are right before they bloom —then they have full flavor. When they are cut, dried, stored and screened before they are hung in bunches, often the flavor is lost. Nothing is so inviting on a hot summer day as a meal preceded by a cooling julep with fresh mint and begun at the table with an iced or chilled soup—perhaps Vichyssoise?—garnished with chives.

I'd like to insert at this point a priceless recipe for mint juleps. Certain bars and hotels have built great reputations on the juleps they serve, and they never divulge their secrets of preparation. There is always a mystery which accompanies the ritual of julep-making, and it is poured carefully, equal care being taken to prevent the guest from finding out what it is. Possibly the julep was handed down from the Virginia cavaliers who moved on to Kentucky because they discovered Kentucky blue grass was the best fare for their fine horses. The julep, associated with mint as well as with bourbon whiskey, came to its finest flowering in that state.

To get on with the perfect mint julep recipe: First of all, you have to house it in the right glass, and that must be chilled. The right glass is a silver julep mug. This is a sterling goblet, about an eight-ounce size. Preferably it should be chilled in a freezer, but if that isn't possible, it can be filled with crushed ice. You know how well sterling silver responds to cooling; it will frost up on the outside. Take three or four fresh mint sprigs, add one teaspoon of sugar and a teaspoon of water, bruise the mint leaves gently with a wooden muddler, stir the mixture until it is dissolved. Pour it in the glass with finely crushed ice, stir it and pour in just one ounce of bourbon. Stir briskly until the frost starts to appear on the outside of the glass—I hope it's a sterling silver julep mug —and then fill it with bourbon to the brim, cut a stem or sprig of mint, set the sprig on the ice, and then put a little powdered sugar over the top. Now if you want to add a strictly French touch, you may add a small part of cognac. The added cognac, however, constitutes the only variation from the straight bourbon julep as described— a combination of two recipes, and great.

More About Mint

Mint is one of the most stimulating aromatic herbs. As I have said it has a wonderful affinity for bourbon whiskey in the julep, a great American institution.

One of the delights in using mint in flavoring numbers of recipes is that you can plant it in your own garden, even in the city, and watch it grow.

Mint was a favorite herb of the Greeks, and there are innumerable legends about it in mythology. One has to do with Pluto, god of the underworld, who turned a lovely young girl into an herb, which was mint. Not a bad fate at all, it would seem.

Its uses apply to many things which are aromatic, fragrant, cooling and refreshing. There is no end to its uses in the culinary arts, which is why I think it deserves a special set of recipes of its own, some of which are given here.

Mint Sauce for Meats

Cook together a mixture of syrup (one-half cup water and one-half cup vinegar with two cups of sugar) and one cup firmly packed mint leaves, run through the finest blade of the food chopper. Blend this sauce well, and store in hot sterilized bottles. After opening, it need not be used all at once, but may be kept for some time.

Mint Vinegar

Shred two cups finely packed mint leaves, mix them well with one cup of sugar, let them stand for five minutes. Bring one quart cider to a boil, add the mint and the sugar mixture and stir constantly—crush the leaves against the side of the pan, and simmer for three minutes. Strain the vinegar through a funnel cloth, pour it into bottles and allow it to ripen for several weeks before serving.

Mint Wine Basting-sauce

Simmer gently for fifteen minutes two-thirds of a cup of claret mixed with one-third of a cup of consomme, with a quarter cup of chopped mint. This is excellent for basting lamb and veal.

Mint Chutney

Heat two cups each of sugar and vinegar and two teaspoons each of salt and mustard. Add one and a half cups each of firmly packed mint leaves and raisins, six small onions and one pound of peeled tart apples, a half-pound peeled tomatoes, all finely chopped and boil the chutney for twenty minutes, stirring occasionally; pour the chutney into sterilized jars and seal.

Candied Mint Leaves

Wash and dry large and perfect mint leaves, and carefully brush each leaf with egg white using a small camel's hair brush. Dredge the leaves with a fine granulated sugar and let them dry on wax paper in a cool place. Serve the leaves as a confection or use them to garnish for iced dishes—sherbets, puddings, and cakes.

Mint Jelly

Slice thickly enough green apples, without removing the peel or core, to make two quarts; cover the apples with one quart water, bring the liquid to a boil and cook the apples. Cover until they are soft, strain them through a jelly bag until all the juice is extracted; discard the pulp. Pour one cup boiling water over one cup firmly packed mint leaves and let the leaves steep for one hour. Press the juice from the mint and discard the leaves. To each cup apple juice, add two tablespoons mint extract and bring the juice to a boil. Add three-fourths cup sugar for each cup juice and boil rapidly until the mixture reaches the jelly stage, or 220° F. on a candy thermometer. Add a few drops of green food coloring and pour the jelly into hot sterilized jars.

Minted Baked Apples

Wash and core six apples, preferably Rome Beauties. Peel the upper quarter of each, place a few mint leaves in the bottom of the baking dish, and arrange the apples on the mint leaves. Fill each apple with two tablespoons honey, one tablespoon water, half a tablespoon butter and one mint leaf. Cover the pan and bake the apples in a hot oven, 375° F., until they are almost tender. Remove the cover and continue baking until the apples are done; baste frequently with the syrup in the pan.

Mint Parfait

Here's a good recipe. As you know, a parfait, which is like a mousse, requires no stirring as it freezes. Always begin with the sugar syrup. Dissolve one cup of sugar into one cup of water, bring to a boil and boil rapidly for five minutes. Pour the hot syrup over one cup of hot mint leaves and let it stand for one hour. Strain the syrup through the sieve—lined with two layers of cheesecloth —and bring it again to the boiling point. Pour the syrup in a fine stream on to three fluffy beaten egg whites, beating constantly, and continue to beat until thick and cool. Add a pinch of salt, and a few drops of green food coloring, fold in two cups heavy cream, whipped, and freeze without stirring.

Iced Mint Tea

This is also an interesting beverage, showing the versatility of the mint. First, brew very strong tea, using one and a half teaspoons of a tea leaf like an orange pekoe, or some quick frozen tea, about a teaspoon and a half for every cup. This is tea that is already steeped and it doesn't require too much attention. If you are to use an orange pekoe tea, you should bring it to a boil and let it steep for ten minutes. Using quick tea which is an orange pekoe, a Darjeeling tea, you can just mix it with plain water. Then with this you may brew your mint leaves in some hot water, pour the extract of the mint tea with the tea that's been prepared and as you are ready to serve it, put some ice cubes into it, a slice of lemon and some sugar. Put a few mint leaves into the iced tea and dust the mint leaves with some powdered sugar. That gives it an interesting taste and certainly is most refreshing, whenever the weather is warm or whenever you feel warm. It's aromatic, and it's a delightful, cool, tall drink.

People who love garnishes for salads, particularly relishes, will find mint a versatile herb for this purpose. There is a marvelous mint-and-onion relish, which can be used as a salad garnish, or garnish with ground meat, etc.: Chop finely one bunch of mint leaves, discarding the stems; mix an equal amount of chopped onions and finely chopped green peppers. Season to taste with salt and Cayenne, and toss in one third cup of French dressing made with lemon juice. Chill the relish and serve cold. This can be eaten with little crackers, hamburgers, or small sausages.

With present techniques in packaging the flavor-life of delicate fine herbs as well as robust-flavored herbs has been prolonged. But it is important for the cook to develop her olfactory sense so that when she uses dry products she knows they will add the necessary flavor.

My experience has led me to appreciate and welcome the addition of these particular herbs:

Savory: a Spanish herb of the mint family, as a leaf a wonderful addition to certain soups, bread stuffing, beans, cabbage, stewed meats, poultry and, if you like it, boiled mutton. Powdered, combined with mayonnaise, it's a major ingredient of Russian dressing, and certain soups and cold sauces. Some cooks would die before they'd omit savory from a bread stuffing for fowl, and that goes for fish too.

Basil, so appropriately known as "sweet basil," is a leaf which gives an unforgettable flavor when used in salads, and it adds particularly to tomatoes, either served cold or in sauces.

Marjoram is a mint-like herb of great versatility; aromatic, and with oregano (powdered) an essential ingredient in chili powder. If you like sweetbreads, and know how to cook them, use marjoram or oregano, or both. They are particularly good for hot sauces, too, especially in Mexican dishes.

Sage is adored by Americans whose ancestors stuffed wild turkey and know what a masterful taking-over it can achieve in all poultry stuffing. Sage can permeate the cooking (that is, the roasting) bird as no other herb, and it's only the uninitiated who regard it as too unsubtle and distort bread stuffing with anemic, uninteresting flavors. Perhaps many of the reactions of people who really love and appreciate food, however, can be traced to early experiences with improperly blended ingredients, so never judge a guest's reactions until you learn about his preceding gustatory experience.

I'd like right now to tell you that my own personal vocabulary involves the following definitions of those who mainly concern themselves with food—one, complimentary; two, somewhat less so. In my book, the ones who are concerned with food are far more sensitive, no matter in what degree, than those who just live to stoke themselves for the next unhappy problem in life.

I refer, of course, to the terms most generally attached to those who love to eat. Probably the most flattering one for those who take pleasure in eating is "epicure." This implies a fastidiousness in the selection of foods, someone who is a connoisseur of the finer wines, for example, who knows the important vineyards and the "correct" years, and who drinks wine appreciatively, always relishing its bouquet. He is not, actually, a voluptuary. This is a charge with which the famous philosopher, Epicurus, from whose name the noun derives, was unjustly accused.

Next, and almost on a par in many definitions, is "gourmet." This term has come to mean great discrimination in food and great appreciation of it. But it is often attached to those who know the "right" places to eat, rather than to those who have great knowledge of food.

The "gourmand" is usually a lusty eater, who may indeed appreciate some of the finer foods, but who eats more of them than is necessary or even polite and attractive. (Gourmand comes from Old French and means, of all things, "servant." Now how did that get to be a term of food-appreciation? Can it be that the servant in Old France was a food taster, and grew discriminating in protecting his master?)

The lowest of all terms in conjunction with food consumption is "glutton." Immediately comes to mind the greedy overabundant court food service of Henry VIII, who devoured, rather than savored, his foods. No appreciation of food flavors there, what with tossing the bones from which meat had been gnawed over the shoulders of the nobles who ate like the trenchermen they were.

In addition to these four, there is the gayest of all food lovers—the "bon vivant." He is, as of the present day, the airy, cheery frequenter of charming eating places. He is a judge of fine wines, he can name years when the best vintages have been produced, he can order a superb meal with grace and authority, so that captains or waiters, who may set their sights for major tips, are themselves impressed. He *knows*. He is the show-off of food lovers.

I bring up the subject of food appreciation in this chapter because, with the possible exception of the glutton, herbs and spices are sometimes a true test for the sophisticated diner. Show me a man who douses his steak with sauces and so drowns the flavor of prime beef, or one who does not recognize the subtlety of an Idaho baked potato, mashed with chopped chives and crowned with a dollop of butter or who cannot detect the slight lift that rosemary or thyme gives to fish and casserole dishes, and who yet eats with gustatory enthusiasm, and I'd say you are wasting your time in setting your delicacies before him.

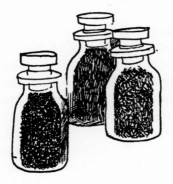

He just doesn't care. But when your dinner companion orders an omelette with *fines herbs* in a noteworthy restaurant, and anxiously consults with the captain as to what might go on in the kitchen and you want to try a new dish (or one new to you), take his advice and let him order for you.

It should be pointed out that in olden times spices were the source of perfumes. Nowadays they belong primarily to food. Think back to Lady Macbeth's tragic admission of guilt: "All the perfumes of Araby cannot sweeten this little hand. . . ."

Spices have long been used for other than culinary purposes. Cinnamon, the inner bark of a small laurel tree originally found in Ceylon, had many uses in the rituals of love and worship. It was, and still is, an ingredient in incense, and Solomon grew it in his gardens. Oriental women of the highest caste perfumed their beds with it. It was the "holy oil" with which the trappings of worship were anointed by priests of many religions. A distillation which was a thick, fragrant oil went into the making of candles for religious occasions. Spikenard was made from a costly, fragrant root used by Orientals to create their perfumed ointments. Certain roots have been found in Great Britain, such as elecampane, a coarse herb of the aster family, often ticketed as "ploughman's spikenard," and turned to practical medical use as a cough medicine. In America, long ago the Chippewa Indians discovered a medicinal property in an American spikenard, of the ginseng family, which they brewed to their own satisfaction for a cough remedy.

I close this chapter with listings of herbs and spices.

Angelica (also angelique): Any one of a large number of herbs of the carrot family, used as oil for flavoring for liqueurs (roots and fruit); and as a perfume. Leafstalks may be candied.

Anise: An herb of the carrot family, originally from southern Europe, having carminative and aromatic seeds; also aniseed. Ground, they lend delicious flavor to salads, and sea food dishes, notably shrimp and crab. Whole they belong on sweet rolls, cakes, cookies, and coffee cake in baking.

Balm (lemon balm): A balsamic resin, specifically certain plants of the mint family, cultivated as a garden herb; an aromatic oil for anointing, as well.

Basil: Sweet, also known as Leaf, originally from India and Persia, now grown in the U. S. Widely used in French and Italian dishes. Delicious flavoring in soups, stews, fowl, meat loaves, and meat balls.

Bay Leaves: Now grown in the U. S., formerly from the Mediterranean regions, have a pungent aroma, which is sweet, and are important seasonings for beef stews, fowl, soups, tomato dishes, and as stuffings for fish and fowl. Almost indispensable for American roast turkey bread stuffing.

Borage: European herb, used medicinally and as a salad.

Burnet: Any of the genus of herbs of the rose family.

Camomile: Often referred to as German Camomile, any of a genus of the aster family, contains a bitter medicinal principle used as an antispasmodic or diaphoretic (ability to induce perspiration.)

Caraway: Originally from Holland and North Africa, the seeds add pungency to soup stocks, and are greatly used in rye bread, sauerkraut, new cabbage, and meats such as pork, kidney stews, and liver. Of the carrot family.

Cardamon: East Indian herb, with seeds which are sweet and aromatic used to flavor breads, cookies, and pastries. Of the ginger family, the seeds are also used in medicine.

Celery Seed: Ground, they are good with salads, fish, tomatoes, whole or in juice, and salad dressing. Whole, they are a delightful accent for soup, stews, and potato salad. One more relative of the carrot family; much of the ground celery seed comes from a variety grown in the south of France.

Chervil: A delicately pungent herb, which lends importance to fish sauces, egg dishes, salads, and soups. Aromatic.

Chives: Often mentioned in this book because of their effectiveness in supplying a sharply distinctive flavor to any number of dishes, both hot and cold. Allied to the onion family, but much more delicate.

Coriander: The ground seeds of this Old World herb are used in gingerbread, spice cookies, Danish pastries, meat sauces, roast pork, and beef broth. From the carrot family, it was native to the Meditteranean, but is now grown in Africa, Asia, Holland, and the United States.

Costmary: A pansy-scented herb of the aster family, a distinguished potherb. Often referred to as Bible Leaf.

Cresses: These are any of those prolific members of the mustard family which make such superb-looking and -tasting garnishes and seasonings. Water cress, which is as pure as the clear running water it grows in, marsh cress, bitter cresses, rock cresses, and winter cresses.

Cumin: Grown all around the Mediterranean including Egypt, it has a caraway-like odor, but a warm, aromatic taste. Many root vegetables are improved by its addition, but chiefly it is used in stews and roast meats. A dwarf plant, it is cultivated for its seeds, and it also is of the carrot family.

Dandelion: Abundant as a weed, this nevertheless has a wonderful essence, since it is of the chicory family. Often prepared like spinach, since chicory is cultivated as a salad plant. A European perennial.

Dill: Here another of the carrot family, a European herb (the anise of Scripture) now grown in the United States. It is most important in pickling (dill pickles are standard in all delicatessens), also for fish, meat soups, salads, eggs, and German-fried potatoes.

Fennel: A most delightful, fragrant East Indian plant of the parsley family, which, of course, means of the carrot family, that ubiquitous source of herbs. Scandinavia has made it peculiarly its own for hot breads, cakes, and cookies. But many Spanish and Italian dishes would be flavorless without it in baked fish and potatoes. It can also be brewed as an aromatic tea.

Flagroot: It is often referred to as "sweet flag" and comes originally from India. While a condiment, it is also a medicine. In New England, candied roots, cut in rings, are used in custards; also, macerated, are important in wine bitters.

Garlic: Though you'd hardly ever think of it in association, garlic is a European bulbous herb of the lily family. It has been widely used in Europe for generations of cooks, and accepted in America because of the fine cooking instincts of many transplanted French and Italian cooks. Many a dish requires garlic browned-in-oil as a base. Here are some garlic variants: *Garlic Flakes:* Dehydrated, these flakes have many times the strength of fresh garlic, and should be used sparingly; if added to a dry mixture they should be soaked for fifteen minutes in cold water. *Garlic powder:* for a touch of garlic, added to meat dishes, or fowl and fish; also to salad dressings, potato salad, and Italian sauces. *Garlic Seasoning Salt* and *Ginger Garlic Seasoning Salt:* produces another flavor good on hamburgers, ground sirloin, lamb, and most roast meats.

Geranium: Usually thought of as a garden plant, it is also an herb of significant flavor. Identified as Herb Robert, or cranesbill, it retains its pungent odor when used as a means of stepping up stews and certain exotic fowl dishes.

Good King Henry: An English herb whose shoots are used as a substitute for asparagus, it is an arrow-leaved potherb, common enough to be regarded as a kitchen herb.

Horse-radish: It's only the root that's important, but this is *very* important for a sharp, tangy sauce that is highly approved as a flavor-making addition to serving with sea food, including oysters, clams, shrimps (served cold). Horse-radish sauce made with sour cream and served with boiled beef is a wonderful delicacy. This is an herb of the mustard family and grows tall and coarse.

Leek: The floral emblem of Wales, this is a cultivated biennial of the lily family, closely related to the onion, and with similar culinary uses. Its leaves, however, are flat, larger than "green" onions, and the bulbs are smaller. Very succulent.

Lemon Verbena: The versatile verbenas produce this small South American shrub with lemon-flavored leaves, useful in many exotic dishes.

Lovage: Once more the carrot family takes a bow, since lovage, a European herb, is mixed with other herbs to add zest to stews, meat dishes, and cold dishes.

Marigold: There are many kinds of marigolds, all of the aster family; if you are familiar with them only as garden flowers you'll need to ask your herb-and-spice merchant how to use this plant in cooking. Adds a fine flavor, though.

Marjoram, Sweet: A perennial herb of the mint family of France. Used in stuffing for fowl and fish, chopped meat, meat balls, sauces, and salads. Powdered, it adds much to stews and soups. Also known as Leaf Marjoram.

Mustard: Here's a big family of plants, which include cabbage and cresses. A yellow powder of mustard seed mixed with liquid may be either a condiment or, of all things a rubefacient (causing redness). At one time it was thought to be a counterirritant to congestion. However, in cooking, it should be thought of as a widely used spice, when ground, with meats, sauces, fish;

highly important in sauces widely used with meats, fish, mayonnaise, French dressings, and cream salad dressings. Whole, the seed is a complement to meats, fish, and as a garnish for salads. Never underestimate the power of mustard.

Onions: Of all the flavors agreed upon by chefs of the first order, onions are at the top. Their origin is in Asia, but every country may produce onions. Of the lily family, it has an edible bulb. Two important types, "Bermuda" and "white," provide the usual domestic fare. They may be prepared in myriad ways, and are a favored addition to stews, roasts, salads—hot and cold —soups; hardly a dish does not benefit by an onion flavor. They are available as: *Onion Chips:* These are dehydrated and are many times the strength of fresh onions. They should be used sparingly. Wonderful for potato salad, fried potatoes, meat loaf, and may also be added to beef stock for a good onion soup. *Onion Flakes:* To supply the flavor of roast onion to gravies for roast meats with potatoes. *Onions, Minced Green:* Tender young shoots may be chopped for garnish and flavor in salads, potatoes, tomato dishes, Vichyssoise. Almost a must for potato salad, cole slaw, cream cheese spread, and certain types of canapes. *Onions, Minced White:* Since white onions are sharp in their pungency, when finely chopped they supply a real flavor to stews, gravies, roast meats, hamburger, and meat loaf. *Onion Powder (plain and roasted)* and *Onion Seasoning Salt:* Used as directed, these add the necessary "touch of onion" to any of the dishes mentioned above: meats, stews, fish, salads and salad dressings, Italian sauces, fowl, and eggs.

Oregano: A pungent Mexican leaf, which grows in Italy and Spain. Important in Italian and Mexican dishes,

SPICE CHART

	ALLSPICE	CINNAMON	CHILI	CLOVES	CURRIE	GINGER	MACE	MUSTARD	NUTMEG
APPETIZERS and SOUPS	Add 3 whole spice to pea soup or stock while cooking	3-4 sticks in punch or sweet pickles	Add a dash to vegetable or meat soups just before serving	Add ¼ teaspoon to Borscht, Mulligatawny, split pea or potato soup	¼ teaspoon blended with cream cheese for a canape spread		Add a dash to oyster stew	Add ¼ teaspoon dry mustard to cream celery, mushroom, bean or lentil soup	Add a dash to cream vegetable or chicken soup
MEATS and POULTRY	8-10 whole spice added to pot roast as it cooks	Sprinkle a little on lamb or pork chops before cooking	1-2 teaspoons in Chili con Carne or barbecue sauce	Stud with whole cloves before baking ham, pork shoulder or corned beef	2-3 teaspoons to beef, pork, lamb, veal or poultry makes good curries	½ teaspoon mixed with salt and pepper to season		1 teaspoon blended into meat for meat loaf, hash or hamburgers	Add ⅛ teaspoon to beef dishes
EGGS and CHEESE	½ teaspoon whole spice in vinegar to pickle eggs	Add ½ teaspoon to mixture for French toast	A dash on scrambled eggs before serving		A dash added to creamed or scalloped eggs	½ teaspoon blended with croquette mixture	Add a dash to creamed eggs or Welsh rarebit	½ teaspoon added to cheese and egg dishes for zest	Sprinkle generously on eggnogs or custards
FISH	Add 3 whole spice to fish while boiling		½-1 teaspoon seasons sauce for seafood or oyster cocktail	Sprinkle very lightly on fish before baking or add 3 whole cloves to boiled fish	2-3 teaspoons in a shrimp or tuna currie		Add ¼ teaspoon to fish sauces or scalloped fish	A necessary ingredient in deviled crab or crab cakes	Add ¼ teaspoon to fish cakes or other fish casseroles
SALADS	Sprinkle fruits used in fruit salad lightly with ground spice	Flavor cottage or cream cheese with cinnamon and nutmeg. Use as garnish		Add whole cloves to pickled beets used for salads	Add ½ teaspoon to basic French Dressing, serve with chicken salad	Sprinkle on pear halves used in fruit salad	Sprinkle on whipped cream dressing for fruit salad	Add ½ teaspoon whole seeds to cole slaw, mixed vegetable or potato salad	Dust fruit lightly when served with mayonnaise
VEGETABLES	½ teaspoon added to squash or sweet potatoes	Sprinkle on squash before baking	A dash seasons tomato sauce or casserole dish	Sprinkle beets beans, squash or sweet potatoes to season	Try a vegetarian currie	½ teaspoon added to sugar when glazing carrots or sweet potatoes	Add ¼ teaspoon to cream sauce for vegetables	Serve a mustard sauce with onions or green beans	A generous dash in carrots, squash, spinach or green beans
DESSERTS	Use in cakes cookies mincemeat	Use in apple, banana, peach, pear or prune desserts, and spice pie crust		Add ¼ teaspoon to chocolate dishes for improved flavor		1¼ teaspoons added to pastry mix for a pie shell variation	Sprinkle on whipped cream to garnish desserts		Sprinkle on custard and rice pudding

Amounts of spice suggested are for 4 servings.

HERB CHART

	BASIL	CARAWAY	DILL	MARJORAM	OREGANO	ROSEMARY	SAFFRON	SAVORY	THYME
APPETIZERS and SOUPS	¼ teaspoon to each cup tomato juice cocktail or bouillon	Combine with cheese for canape spread or stuffed celery	Add 1 teaspoon to mayonnaise served with raw vegetables	Add a pinch to soup stock during the last hour of cooking	A pinch in vegetable or tomato juice cocktail	¼ teaspoon in chicken, pea or spinach soup	A pinch in chicken soup adds color and delicate flavor	¼ teaspoon added to bean or pea soup, fish chowder or consomme	¼ teaspoon in clam or fish chowder
MEATS and POULTRY	½ teaspoon in beef stew for a subtle flavor	Sprinkle ½ teaspoon over pork roast	Sprinkle on lamb chops before broiling	Sprinkle on roast beef, lamb or veal before cooking	Add 1 teaspoon to Spaghetti sauce	Use to season poultry stuffing in place of sage	1 teaspoon to Arroz Con Pollo (chicken-rice)	½ teaspoon added to beef loaf, beef stew or hamburgers	1-2 teaspoons in stuffing ½ teaspoon in lamb or veal stew
EGGS and CHEESE	A pinch in tomato or Spanish omelet	½-1 teaspoon mixed with ¼ lb. cottage cheese makes a good sandwich spread	Add 1 teaspoon to cottage or cream cheese for a sandwich spread	Add ¼ teaspoon to 4 eggs when making souffles, scrambled eggs or omelets		Add a pinch to scrambled eggs or omelet		¼ teaspoon blended with scrambled or deviled eggs	Sprinkle on shirred eggs—add to cheese for canapes or sandwiches
FISH	¼ teaspoon in water used for cooking shell fish		Add a few seeds to water in which fish is boiled	Sprinkle baked or broiled fish lightly—add a pinch to creamed fish	¼ teaspoon combined with butter to serve with shell fish	Sprinkle fish fillets lightly before broiling or baking	½ teaspoon in Bouillabaisse (a fish and shellfish soup)	Sprinkle a little on baked or broiled fish	Sprinkle fish lightly before cooking
SALADS	¼ teaspoon in tomato French Dressing A pinch flavors tomato aspic	Sprinkle seeds on cole slaw or beet salad	Add 1 teaspoon to cole slaw or potato salad	Add a dash to French Dressing served with a green salad	¼ teaspoon seasons potato or seafood salad			Add a pinch to tossed salads of greens and tomatoes	¼ teaspoon in tomato aspic
VEGETABLES	¼ teaspoon to green beans, stewed tomatoes or scalloped egg plant	Add a few to cabbage, turnips or sauerkraut while cooking	Add 1 teaspoon to green beans, cauliflower or cabbage while cooking	Add ¼ teaspoon to water used in cooking peas, carrots or spinach	Add ¼ teaspoon to cream or tomato sauce	Add ¼ teaspoon to water used in cooking peas, potatoes or turnips	A pinch in the water in which rice is cooked for a golden color	Add ½ teaspoon to beans, peas, cabbage or sauerkraut while cooking	½ teaspoon combined with butter. Pour over beans, peas, spinach, or zucchini
BREADS		Use in rye or pumpernickel bread	Sprinkle on top of rolls or rye bread		Sprinkle pizza with Oregano before baking	Add ½ teaspoon to cornbread or muffin mixture before baking	½ teaspoon added to liquid used in sweet bread gives a golden color	½ teaspoon in biscuit or dumplings	½ teaspoon in biscuits or dumplings

Amounts of herbs suggested are for 4 servings.

particularly effective with pork and tomato sauces, and "hot" bean dishes. Powdered it is a chief ingredient in chili powder, good for sweet breads, hot sauces, and Mexican bean dishes.

Parsley: Another member of the carrot family, this was a native of the Mediterranean region, but now is grown widely in the United States. Perhaps the most favored garnish for platters, salads, its taste is delicate, its aroma distinctive and delightful. Because of its crisp, curly appearance, it lends importance to the less colorful dishes, and adds greatly to soups, sauces, baked fish, all root vegetables, potatoes (especially creamed), and salads.

Rampion: A European bellflower, with an edible tuberous root used with the leaves as a salad.

Rosemary: This is one of those borderline herb-spices; it's a fragrant shrub of the mint family long recognized as of value in cookery and perfumery. If you are interested in checking the origin of the name, it has come from the Latin *rosemarimus,* from *ros* (dew) and *marinus* (marine); however, it is now altered to suggest the rose of Mary. Whatever the origin of the name, it is regarded as the emblem of fidelity and constancy. In the United States, although it came from southern Europe, it is grown extensively. A pleasant, delicate flavor which resembles sage and thyme, but adds much to meats, soups, fish and salads. Powdered, it is in wide use with vegetables, eggs, stews, meats, sauces, kidney stew, and fish sauces; since it is delicate, sometimes it has to be combined with other herbs and spices for greater flavoring strength.

Rue: A strong-scented perennial woody herb, whose bitter leaves are used in medicine. Citrus fruits come from the rue family and the herbs are, when combined with other herbs, most effective in casserole cooking.

Sweet Alyssum and *Sweet Flag* or *Calamus:* The first is a European herb, a perennial; the second a marsh herb with a pungent rootstock.

Saffron: Saffron is described at some length earlier in this chapter; powdered, it is *the* important accent in making bouillabaisse. Gourmets love it; guests appreciate it when it is used to flavor fish, shellfish, soups, boiled rice, curries, and fish sauces. The secret in cooking with it is to use it sparingly .

Sage: Sage has such an agreeable pungency that it seems to belong to many soups and meats, but most of all to bread stuffings whether for pork, fish, or fowl (first of all). Possessed of a fine, spicy aroma, it takes over in kitchen odors, promising the best of things to come. In two guises: leaf and powdered. When powdered, it combines with parsley beautifully for cooking vegetables such as Brussels sprouts, cabbage, turnips. But also it belongs in stews and with any boiled fish dish.

Savory (leaf and powder): Here is another representative of the mint family, this time from Spain, but it is conceded that the best savory is grown in Dalmatia. It is widely used in soup, bread stuffing, beans, cabbage, stewed meats, poultry, wild game, and boiled mutton. Powdered, it is excellent for mayonnaise and Russian dressing, egg dishes, soups, cold sauces, bread stuffings for fowl and fish. Also known as Summer Savory.

Sesame: Ali Baba and the Forty Thieves have made the Sesame of fiction familiar to the cooks of the world. It is an East Indian herb which produces a flat, small, honey-colored seed, delicious in flavor and so ideal for toppings on rolls, breads, cookies, cakes, and candies. It also yields an oil used as food.

Shallot: An onion-like plant, with small clustered bulbs, used like onion for flavoring.

Sorrel: Any number of plants bearing this name have a

sour juice; and the acid-tasting leaves, properly treated make for a good herb flavor in cooking.

Tarragon: Here is a delicate pungent herb with a slightly acid flavor, a favorite of gourmets. In America it is best known in a vinegar; and now is famous for flavoring turtle soup, eggs, meat sauces, salad greens, and vegetables. For sauce Bearnaise, it is a true requirement. With veal, fowl, and sweetbreads, most chefs think it is definitely indicated.

Thyme: A shrub native to southern Europe, now grown in the United States. Most cooks regard it as in the forefront for fowl, veal, gumbos, bread stuffings, fish sauces, shellfish dishes, meats. For root vegetables, it is unparalleled. Thyme belongs to the mint family, has a special pungency of its own.

Woodruff: Notably important for flavoring wine, this small, sweet-scented herb, European in origin, has other uses in cooking special dishes; used also in perfumes.

Wormwood: Now we come to the fabled genus Artemisia with its twin associate, gall. Absinthe contains oil of wormwood.

So close in taste sensations are herbs and spices that they are often blended by expert chefs and cooks. If a generality about them is acceptable, it might be that herbs are sharper in flavor, while spices are sweeter. But even this distinction may be broken down in practical cooking. Take, for example, whole pickling spice—this is a blend of herbs and spices, used for pickling and relishes. Poultry seasoning is a blend of herbs and spices, and is perhaps most frequently found in modern kitchens. It is a time-saver in making bread stuffing; it can step up the prepared stuffing, or if stale bread is used, it can supplement the sage, thyme, marjoram and other herbs the cook-in-a-hurry wants to include: Here are some favored spices:

Allspice: The berry of the tree of the myrtle family, given its name because it might be a blend of cinnamon, nutmeg and cloves. But it isn't. Delightful for cooky-making, spice puddings, relishes, pickles; indispensable for tomato catsup, and wonderful in mince pies. It comes both whole or ground; whole, it should be used sparingly, but even game and meats profit by its presence.

Cinnamon (ground and stick): This comes from the inner bark of the cinnamon tree, with an unforgettable aromatic scent. Originally from Ceylon and the southwest coast of India, Malabar, this is a must for apple pies and sauce, indeed all apple desserts; sweet rolls; cinnamon buns or "snails"; coffee cakes and sauces for game. The stick is used in sweet pickling, preserving and for hot toddies, hot rum drinks and often makes the special flavor for after-dinner coffee.

Cloves (whole and ground): These represent the most "married" of spices, since they are so frequently used together. Whole, they belong on baked ham, and perfectly complement beef consomme, venison, preserves and baked apples. You can add a dash of ground cloves to hamburger, or to meat or veal loaf, and deviled meat, Swiss or planked steak. Whole cloves, of course, as we've said, go with ham, but you can also sprinkle ground cloves on the surface; a touch while basting. Ground cloves are fine with rhubarb and apple butter. Not many amateur cooks think of cloves in conjunction with meats, so this creates an unusual combination of flavors.

Ginger (ground or whole): Now, ginger is listed as an herb, but it is so sweet and spicy that it is usually thought of as the most obvious spice in the kitchen cabinet. It is tropical: Asiatic and Polynesian in origin; its pungent and aromatic rootstalks when ground are widely used in baking. Oriental dishes, most Chinese cooking, in fact, profit by ginger; curries are enhanced by it. And do not forget that American favorite—gingerbread. Now grown in Jamaica, B. W. I., ginger comes uncoated and unbleached. Whole, it is a required ingredient in chutney, pickles, conserves, and it is often used in apple sauce.

Mace (ground): Here is the dried, fibrous, aromatic covering of the nutmeg seed, which comes from the East Indies. Used in pastries, cookies, baked goods, preserves; it lends a fine, definitive flavor to oyster stews and baked fish.

Nutmeg (whole and ground): It comes from the Maluccas, and since the world is shrinking so, it's good to know that one of the headiest of spices originates in the Malay Archipelago. Nutmeg has a slightly bitter taste, but since it is aromatic, it is of great value to custards, puddings, pumpkin, and fruit pies. Try it on cabbage, and a delicate result is obtained. Almost always used as a sprinkled topping for eggnog; wise cooks finish off a dish of cauliflower or spinach with dashes of nutmeg.

Paprika: Peppers are listed as spices; much of the paprika that comes to this country is Spanish, but preferred by most cooks is the Hungarian. This is sweet and mild, and has a decided bouquet—a sharper and more distinct accent than the Spanish. Spanish paprika is decorative in coloring, and has a blander taste. Paprika adds a brilliant, colorful accent to many a dish; also (cooked in) in goulash, meat stews, and highly spiced dishes. Veal Paprika is developed around it. Best of all is its sharp, clear coloring—it makes many a bland dish look appetizing, including canapés. If possible, it should be freshly ground—in big cities this is not difficult to find.

Pepper (Cayenne): The name derives from the region of its growth in South America, and it is one of the sharpest, most distinctive of the pepper flavors. Meats and sauces, egg dishes, salads, fish, shellfish, benefit from the recognizable content.

Pepper (Creole): This is grown in Louisiana, and is similar in effect to Cayenne. Hardly any Southern or Creole cooks omit it from their dishes.

Peppercorns (Malabar black): A fine black pepper, valued by gourmets and rightly so, since it is in somewhat short supply. It comes from a small area on the Malabar Coast of India. Used always whole, ground with a peppermill.

Peppercorns (Lampong black): Sun-cured, these are also choice; grown in the Netherlands East Indies. Ground, these are the most important single spice for seasoning for egg dishes, fish, game, meats, poultry and vegetables. Should be sprinkled discreetly on fish, shellfish, and vegetable salads, vegetable juices, fish, game, meat, and poultry stews. Never should be omitted from Virginia ham. Cracked, they make for a sharper, more pungent pepper flavor. Whole, they are for your outsize peppermill.

Pepper (white): Since pepper comes from a climbing shrub, the dried berries yield black pepper, which when divested of their outer coatings yield white pepper. Many chefs prefer to use white pepper in stews and casserole dishes, since it has a special sharpness all its own.

Peppers, Red Bell: When dehydrated and diced they are important in egg dishes, meat loaf, potted meats, and stews.

Peppers, Green Bell: Diced or ground, they are widely

used in spaghetti sauce, string beans, eggplant, and certain liver dishes.

Herbs, peppers, spices, seeds and seasonings can be grouped because they are the fillip—the final stimulus to *bon appetite*. Wise cooks accept their aid in turning out dishes to be remembered.

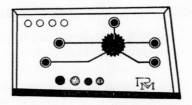

10

Cooking at 186,300 Miles
per Second

by K. Cyrus Melikian
and Lloyd K. Rudd

That's fast! It is the speed of light, the speed
at which the sun's rays cover the 93 million miles from
the sun to the earth; and it is the speed of radioactivity, the
speed of electronic microwaves that do a good measure
of today's cooking in tiny fractions of time.

Here's the way electronic microwave cooking works. At
a touch of the controls the oven is ready to receive the
roasting pan or casserole, pie or cake pan, but the heat
does not come on until the oven door is closed; this door
may be transparent. The degree of microwave activity
is adjusted to the nature of the item to be cooked. Time
signals flash when the cooking is done, indicating that
the microwaves are completely shut off. If the item requires basting or turning, the opening of the oven door
immediately discontinues the microwaves so that there
can be no danger to the cook in reaching into the oven.
Nor does the cook need pot-lifters or any other protection
from a hot utensil. That is because the cooking containers

used, whether plastic, paper, china or glass, do not become hot from the microwaves. It is only when the microwaves reach the item to be cooked that they become heat. The vessels remain cool, unaffected by the waves, and the oven air remains cool. Only the food receives the heat. Perfectly even cooking is insured because the microwaves penetrate the food from all angles.

As for the nutritive value of microwave-cooked foods as compared to those cooked in a gas or electric oven, elaborate tests have been conducted. It is established that foods cooked in a microwave oven retain more nutrients as well as more flavor. For instance, broccoli retains 14 per cent more vitamin C; tomatoes 7 per cent more vitamin C; cabbage 17 per cent more vitamin C; beef 4 per cent more thiamin and 12 per cent more riboflavin.

In the matter of the time required for preparing a dinner, the domestic cook may hang up his or her apron for most of the day. A meal, no matter which meal, is the work of a mere jiffy as contrasted with older methods, and there's no clock watching. For instance, cereals, sixty seconds; two-layer cake, six minutes; bacon, ninety seconds; bowl of soup, sixty seconds; baby's bottle, fifteen seconds; baked potato, four minutes; five-pound roast, thirty minutes; turkey, five minutes per pound. A complete frozen dinner can go from the freezer to table in just four minutes.

Electronic domestic ranges are available on the market today. All the kitchen needs for its installation is dependable electric current. There are several manufacturers who make ranges with electronic microwave ovens for domestic installation. These firms produce similar equipment for commercial cooking on a large scale.

The innovation of the microwave oven brings with it all sorts of advantages to the chef, whether domestic or commercial. The kitchen, large or small, is never heated up by microwaves as it is when they do their work in a regular oven. No blast of hot air issues from the oven when the door is opened because no hot air has been generated.

Since the utensils in which the oven food is cooked are not affected in any way by the storm of microwaves, they can be lifted from oven to table and the food served directly from them. A roast may be cooked on a platter, vegetables in a glass casserole, other foods on plates or saucers, or even on paper plates. Hence there is no tiresome and heavy wash-up job on pots and pans after the meal is over. That's like giving real holidays to Mrs. Housewife.

In regard to the economy of microwave cooking, the speed at which things get done cuts down the amount of electric current or gas volume required to accomplish the same cooking job otherwise. If the serving of a dinner is unavoidably delayed—things are done and getting cool —the cooking dishes can be placed back in the oven briefly and, without losing any flavor or food value, be heated and served as deliciously as if freshly done. In the case of leftovers they can be reheated in the microwave oven to a state of deliciousness exactly the same as when originally served. A Sunday roast warmed over on Tuesday evening will be just as juicy and enjoyable as when it was first put on the table.

If one is thinking of microwave cooking in the field of the domestic kitchen the electronic microwave oven is a marvel of cleanliness. In cooking foods that spatter the item can be covered by a paper plate or a towel. The oven will stay clean indefinitely. If spattering or spilling over does occur the oven can easily be wiped clean, since the spattering does not become charred and fixed on the cool oven walls—a real advantage to the housewife.

Microwave energy as a means of quick food preparation is used in another way when it comes to serving hundreds of people simultaneously. In large industrial plants, particularly, where scores of hungry workers need well-prepared hot food at breakfast, lunch or dinner times, methods and vending machines have been designed and perfected to give workers hot platters comprising full, well-flavored, nutritious meals in almost no time at all. The same service is available to schools, offices, institutions, meeting halls—wherever large numbers of people gather. In this use of microwave energy the food platters offering a wide choice of well-balanced meats and vegetables, appropriately flavored and garnished, are first cooked to perfection in commissary kitchens, then deep frozen pending distribution to the vending mechanisms which have been installed in the specially equipped dining hall. The frozen platters are rushed by refrigerator truck to the food vending machines where they are kept at a refrigerated temperature.

When the proper coins are deposited in the machine, the food is dispensed and microwave energy is automatically available. The platters of food are unfrozen in moments and, at a signal from the machine, the hot platter is ready for the table and, like cooking in the domestic microwave oven, can be lifted out with bare hands, since only the food itself has been heated and the platter remains cool. The food, the gravies and sauces involved, are all as freshly delicious as if they had come straight from a cooking oven, even though the actual cooking was done, perhaps, days and days before.

As examples of what the hungry person would find quickly available: hot platters containing meat, Brussels sprouts, and macaroni and cheese; fish, asparagus, and mashed potatoes with a pat of butter; frankfurters with baked beans; meat balls with spaghetti in tomato sauce; and many others. As for the cost of a substantial meal the hot-platter microwave-equipped vending machine can offer a nourishing meal for as little as thirty-five to sixty cents. That would be hard to match at a cafeteria or restaurant.

Great skill and cooking experience are required in the preparation of the hot meal platters previous to the original cooking. For instance, the very arrangement of the various edibles on the platter has an effect upon the appetizing appearance of the meal at the time that the purchaser takes it from the vending machine after it has been heated to the exact point of serving.

To illustrate, protein items cook more slowly than other foods and must have a greater proportion of cooking heat. They should be arranged so they quickly absorb heat. Instead of using a thick slice of roast beef on a variegated platter the meat should be cut into slices of less than one-quarter inch thick. It will then reach doneness at the same moment as the green vegetable that is cooked with it.

This same element has to be borne in mind in connection with the microwave heating of the fully cooked and deep-frozen platter at the time when it is wanted by the customer. Microwaves, transformed into heat, will penetrate the more quickly absorbent foods on the platter in less time than the foods of more solid composition and, unless correctly planned at the point when the platter is originally arranged, the platter could have, when served, certain portions slightly underdone or slightly overdone.

A further expertness is called for in the use of garnishes such as parsley, paprika, pimento, and others that add to the attractiveness of the meal and give it color. Such condiments, although they have only small food value, must be so used as to make the meal as tempting in appearance as one served fresh from an oven under the supervision of a professional chef.

Thus it is an intricate and painstaking business to produce an assortment of nutritious well-balanced platters involving the arrangement of the various foods on the platter, the cooking of them at exact and unvarying temperatures, the deep-freezing of the cooked platters, and their delivery, still frozen, to the electronically equipped vending machines installed in the far-flung locations where thousands are to be fed, simultaneously, breakfast, lunch or dinner. A group of recipes will be found at the end of this section as examples of the care and meticulousness with which the platters and casseroles must be prepared and refrigerated by the commercial machine vending companies in order to insure the perfection, nutrition, and acceptability of each dish, right up to the time of serving.

The grocery store customer who buys for home consumption such items as commercially prepared dinner platters or any frozen and packaged vegetables, fruits or meats will find that ordinary oven heat, gas or electricity, will thaw and warm them to servable temperature in a matter of minutes. They are, for the most part, not deeply frozen as are the platters that are stocked in the vending machines. But if a home kitchen is equipped with a microwave oven the time required for thawing and heating to serving temperature would be a matter of seconds and the automatic shut-off of the microwave oven would eliminate watching the range and attending to the heating job.

It could be said that the wonder of food as it comes originally from Mother Earth is now, as never before, matched by the wonder of electronics in the form of microwave cooking which brings food to the consumer with all of its values intact—vitamins, proteins, minerals—deliciously, attractively and almost instantly.

Mass Feeding and the High Frequency Cooker

What do Americans like to do better than anything else? Sometimes, it would seem they like to get together in groups, often running into thousands of people, the mutual attraction being food and more food. Certainly it is difficult to summon a crowd or promote a rally without holding out the promise of good food and lots of it. As a point of fact, certain stockholders' meetings where no food was served brought about a revolution among those who attended, who declared they would bypass their dividends and sell their stock if they couldn't get something to eat at the long, sometimes boring sessions. No one denies the relaxing effect of food on a tensed-up audience and many attribute the success of meetings to the fact that those in charge have recognized this primitive fact.

Depending on the size of the crowd, this has often presented problems in the past—now somewhat reduced by modern methods of cooking and serving.

Suppose the "party of your choice" planned a political rally, and you were placed in charge of the details of preparation. How would you go about it? Many professionals are available to assist you but you must be familiar with the means to eliminate the possibility of guessing wrong and winding up with a complete or at least a partial flop. That's no good for the "party."

Among the skilled and wise operators in the food field is a standout in the person of Chef John Brefini. He has had a vast background in feeding the multitude, since he was for years executive chef of the Statler Hotel chain, and thinks of food in terms of tons of produce and hundreds of dishes, rather than individual service. He has developed a number of basic helps to the person confronted with a mass-feeding project, and is able to answer the questions which rise in the mind of a one-time operator, who must produce food in sufficient quantities for the occasion. Suppose, for instance, we take a political gathering, an outdoor affair which about 5,000 persons are expected to attend. This may be the estimate—the hoped-for attendance. Two things may happen. Weather is always a most important factor. What if it should rain? Will just half that number turn out? Or if it is unusually fine, will there be 7,500? Fewer rather than more are likely to turn up, since between the time of announcing an event and the event itself, even the most dedicated may be lured away by distractions which have nothing to do with political convictions.

If you are a novice at ordering for such a mob, perhaps you do not realize that many a commissary may be taken over for a few hours while the kitchens are not in use: for example, in many parts of the country the Howard Johnson chain of restaurants. If your meeting is within range of one of their establishments, you may order your menu, and forget the worries. You don't have to consider waste; if you have food prepared for a certain number of people, it need not be thrown away. The country over, there are commissaries able to take care of your food order. You won't be confronted with the need to keep it hot over a steam table or outdoor oven or fireplace. The food may be prepared in advance by skilled people twenty-four hours before the event is scheduled rather than by temporary help. At a commissary you have proper tooling and mechanization to cut down labor costs in the preparation of food.

Food prepared in advance may be purchased advantageously under proper market conditions, which means good prices for seasonal items and values which will amount to savings for the group or committee for which you are arranging the shindig. You have time enough to shop around for the best values.

On the day of the Great Event the frozen food may be stored in a low temperature truck and merely doled out as needed. Now if the conditions make for a discrepancy in the numbers you have counted on, due to weather or conflicting dates, there is no loss if the food is prepared and handled in this fashion. If there is an overflow in attendance and more food is needed, it is ready and the situation is met. But it should be remembered that those on the committee for arrangements should buy from a contract packer or commissary operator who would take back the food if it is not used—which is possible since it is in a frozen state.

Here is where the high-frequency cooker comes into play. How do you reheat the food quickly? Twenty to twenty-five seconds of time in an ultra high frequency cooker designed to handle such a food load would be adequate to take care of each portion to be served, therefore the key to this mass feeding problem is to have a battery of microwave heating devices. Ten such devices would take care of thirty to forty persons a minute.

If your rally is in the daytime, the hours might be between eleven and two, so in three hours the group could be fed. If it comes later in the day, the same amount of time should be allowed to see that everyone is taken care of with nourishing food and picnic specialties. These specialties might include:

Barbecued sandwiches	Pizza pies
Hamburgers	Roast pork sandwiches
Roast beef sandwiches	Hot dogs
Cheeseburgers	

and variants of these, as well as poultry items, sea food, either entree or sandwiches. There might also be codfish cakes with sauce, fried chicken, small luncheon steaks, or veal cutlets with sauce.

Many of the big commercial packers—Wilson and Seabrook Farms, to name two typical ones—can supply many different items, and therefore purchasing should not be too difficult, even if the numbers are large.

Also, it should be noted, the ultra high frequency cooker can be furnished as self-service, so that the customer can put the food into the oven himself. The cookers work only when the door is closed, and the magic button is pushed. Instructions accompany the cooker.

Chef Brefini has been hailed as one of the cooking greats of all time and is known among his peers as the "modern Escoffier." Escoffier, I venture to say, might be baffled by the means employed now to produce his delectable effects gastronomically, but he would welcome the time-saving and labor-saving that goes into serving many, many hungry people.

Rigid standards and requirements in the preparation of foods for later cooking and deep-freezing have been adopted by all purveyors of automatic meal-vending machines. The greatest exactitude and precision are practiced in selecting ingredients to insure the nutrition and palatability of each combination hot platter as well as its tempting appearance when reheated by microwave energy for serving and to keep the food from any possible taint of bacteria.

Here are some sample recipes now used by large-scale vending-machine operators that illustrate the high degree of exact measurements followed by the commercial chefs in cooking for the mass feeding market. These proportions are printed here to demonstrate the complete uniformity of the meals to be obtained from a vending machine hot platter service, and are for commercial rather than domestic use.

Basic Brown Sauce (Espagnole)
A. Stock

½ pound hard wheat flour
15 pounds bones (half beef, half veal)
¼ pound beef fat
14 quarts water

1¼ pounds mixed vegetables (carrots, onions, celery)
1 No. 15 can tomatoes
¼ ounce thyme
¼ ounce mixed whole spices

Brown bones in a medium oven until light brown. Add flour; add beef fat at this time so that the flour will not burn and to make a light roux. Add vegetables and continue to braise until the whole has been well browned. Remove from oven to a 20-quart stock pot, add water and simmer for 24 hours. Add spices, salt and pepper to taste.

B. Sauce

10 quarts beef stock
¾ pound roux (brown, 1:1 butter fat and flour)
1½ cups beef stock

4½ tablespoons stabilizer W13 (a commercial emulsifier) or 3½ tablespoons arrowroot starch

Mix stock and roux and bring to a boil. Simmer for ¾ hour skimming the top from time to time. Add the stabilizer to the cup and a half of beef stock, then add to the stock mixture 5 to 10 minutes before removing from the heat. Season to taste. The depth of color can be adjusted by adding caramelized sugar or other ready-made ingredients such as Touch of Beef, Flavor Glow Dark, Kitchen Bouquet or Maggi.

Broiled Scrod

Scrod, broiled	5 ounces
Mixed vegetables	3 ounces
Parsley potatoes	2½ ounces (2 pieces)
	10½ ounces

Scrod: Roll in bread crumbs then brown on both sides under a broiler. Cool to 40° F. Cooked temperature of scrod should not exceed 125° F.

Vegetables: Cook separately string beans, peas, carrots and lima beans and cool to 40° F., then mix.

Assembly: Assemble the previously cooked components on a non-compartmented plate. Shield with aluminum foil.

Chicken Croquette Dinner

Cheese potatoes or mashed potatoes	2½ ounces
Peas, cooked	3 ounces
Chicken croquettes (2) deep fat fried	4 ounces
Veloute, supreme, or fricasse sauce	2 ounces
	11½ ounces

Duchesse potatoes: Duchesse potatoes are formed by forcing the mixture through a star-shaped pastry tube into a mass which is about 3 inches long by 1½ inches high. This can be done conveniently on a sheet pan and the pan placed under a broiler to brown. The finished product is then cooled to 40° F. before assembly into dinners.

A standard chicken croquette recipe is used. Shape the croquettes and dust them in a ready-mix breading. Dip in a mixture of two parts of water to one part of ready-mix, and roll in light bread crumbs. Fry in fat at 325° F. until golden brown. The shape of the croquettes is a matter of choice, but they should not exceed ¾ inch in height.

Add the sauce to the plate and arrange the croquettes in it. Add precooked peas and a portion of Duchesse potatoes.

Fried Chicken Dinner

White sauce (basic béchamel)	1 ounce
Tomato brown sauce	1 ounce
Fried chicken (2-3 pieces)	4½ ounces
Lima and corn Mexicaine	3 ounces
Au gratin potatoes	2½ ounces
	12 ounces

Fried chicken: It is preferable to use 2¼ to 2½ pound chicken friers cut into four portions; parboil whole then cut into portions. Season the parts with salt and pepper, dust in a ready-mix breading, dip in a mixture of one part ready-mix bread to two parts water, and roll in light bread crumbs. Fry in fat at 325° F. until fully cooked. Cool to 40° F.

Au gratin potatoes: Use any standard recipe. Garnish with a mixture of grated cheese, bread crumbs and paprika, and brown lightly under a broiler. When assembling the dinner, spoon potatoes with care to preserve the garnish. Cool to 40° F.

Spread the brown tomato sauce on the plate and place the white sauce in the center of the brown sauce. A non-compartmented plate gives the best appearance. Arrange the chicken pieces on the sauce. Add the portions of vegetables and potatoes. Shield the edges of the plate with aluminum foil.

Chicken Pot Pie

Sauce

1¾ gallons chicken stock
1 pound roux
1 tablespoon stabilizer W13

Roux is prepared by blending equal parts by weight of shortening and hard wheat-flour and cooking slowly until a grainy finish has been reached. Add the hot chicken stock and cook about one-half hour. Blend the stabilizer with one cup of cold chicken stock and add to the sauce 5 to 10 minutes before removing from the heat. Do not boil, after the stabilizer has been added.

Filling
¾ ounce carrots, cooked, diced
¾ ounce potato, cooked, diced
½ ounce onions, silver skin
1½ ounces chicken fowl, cooked
5 ounces sauce
½ ounce peas, cooked
1¾ ounces pie crust

Crust
1 pound shortening
2½ pounds flour
2 eggs
½ teaspoon salt
1 teaspoon cream of tartar
1 teaspoon baking soda
1½ teaspoons sugar
1 cup milk

Blend flour and shortening thoroughly with cream of tartar and baking soda. Beat eggs, add milk, sugar, and salt and blend well. Roll to ¼-inch thick and cut to size to fit casserole. Bake at 350° to 375° F.

Place pie ingredients in casseroles and add sauce. Freeze. Pie crust should be frozen separately and the frozen pie capped with the crust. Overwrap and return to the freezer.

Braised Beef à la Mode

Sliced cooked beef	3 ounces
Sauce	2½ ounces
Carrots	2¾ ounces
Noodles polonaise	3 ounces
	11¼ ounces

Beef à la mode: A true beef à la mode must be marinated for 24 hours before cooking. A modification was used in this dinner. A basic pot roast recipe was used. Diluted red wine—about 3½ cups—and a No. 10 can of tomato cauce was added for each 2 gallons of brown sauce.

Carrots: One inch lengths of carrots ½-inch thick.

Noodles polonaise: Cook noodles and add chopped hard boiled eggs, chopped parsley, grated cheese and bread crumbs browned in butter.

Inplant Feeding—The Automatic Cafeteria

In this fabulous electronic age, many new words have been added to the vocabularies of every literate human being in the world. And of them all, perhaps the one most nearly affecting the greatest number of people is "automation." Automation may turn a wage-earner into a statistic; or it may be the source of one of the greatest of benefits.

Retail selling of food has gone through any number of phases. Why there are today some people who remember when there weren't any supermarkets! One of the most dramatic of the developments of the past few years is the growth of the automatic vending machine business. Starting as a humble little operation involving, for the most part penny gum and peanuts, it has become a giant servitor despite a number of setbacks. For example, during World War II production of vending machines was prohibited—a circumstance which for four years halted the development of these machines. But the imagination and creative ability of American inventors and businessmen emerged from this deep freeze to advance far beyond the period when they were so abruptly restrained in their forward march from paper-cup soft-drink vending machines to include such products as cigarettes, candy, ice cream, sandwiches, hot foods, milk, coffee, soup, salads, and desserts.

Automatic selling today is big business. In 1949 it was just less than a billion dollars in volume (from a slow start of thirty million in 1925). And the National Automatic Merchandising Association offered an educated guess than by 1965 it will produce for the industry between four to five billion dollars.

In the trade magazine *Inplant Food Management,* October 1958, William S. Fishman set forth his practical and comprehensive view of automatic merchandising in an article entitled, "The Push-Button World." The material was based on a talk before the Research and Development Associates Food and Container Institute.

Here are some of the points he made:

> Merchandise vending first became popular in public locations; i.e., locations where the general public moved, such as restaurants, transportation centers, gasoline stations, etc. Public location vending is still the predominant market. However, captive locations such as schools, offices, institutions, industrial plants, have become a major area for installation of merchandise vending machines. Currently, the industry is about equally divided between these two types of operations. The newest development in automatic merchandising is the automatic cafeteria.
>
> Less than three years ago, a new machine for dispensing hot canned soups and foods was first introduced. During 1957 over six and one-half million dollars in canned foods sales was realized and most of these sales were new business which never would have been transacted except through the use of these new vending machines. Firms like Armour, Campbell, Heinz and many

others have just begun to realize the potential in vending sales. . . .

Automatic merchandising is a sanitary method of food
dispensing. Our machines are equipped with refrigera-
tion or heating equipment controlled to guarantee correct preservation temperatures at all times. If the
heating or cooling units should become inoperative, or
in the event of power supply failure, the machines are
equipped with automatic devices which prevent further
sales until the trouble is correct and spoiled foods removed. There is not a single case of litigation over food
poisoning by products dispensed through a vending
machine to be found in the records of our higher state
and federal courts. . . .

Automation in our industrial plants is on the increase.
This will result in fewer workers producing a larger
gross national product. Thus, many industrial plants
which heretofore have been able to support manual
cafeterias will no longer be able to justify the expense.
Automatic cafeterias will become more in demand. The
shorter work week will also create financial reasons for
substitution of manual serving cafeterias by automatic
selling. The American "coffee break" is a perfect example of how vending solves problems. Thousands of
office and factory managers can testify to the tremendous amount of time and money saved by the installation of coffee vending machines that serve their
employees right on the premises. Day after day in the
Chicago Loop, for example, office managers are install-
ing coffee vending machines, which often dispense
coffee free, to eliminate the twice daily traffic up and
down building elevators to street level coffee shops. In
short, vending is mobile and versatile. It can be taken to
the people where they work.

The trend toward moving to suburbs creates new
opportunity for vending. Suburban living results in less
concentration of people in a given area. The families

live farther from stores and shops. It becomes more difficult for the housewife to purchase the items which often
need replenishing during evening hours, such as milk,
bread, eggs. Here vending has already started to fill the
need. Many large grocery supermart chains are testing
the installation of vending machines to sell a large
variety of foodstuffs. This development will not only be
of service to the patrons but also will enable the supermarkets to reduce their selling hours and operating
expenses by relying on vending machines to transact
business during hours when volume is low. Machines
will literally enable the supermarts to remain in business
twenty-four hours per day and seven days per week
with very little addition to their overhead and operating
expenses. . . .

As the American people devote more hours to leisure,
travel, and play, and fewer hours to work, vending will
offer them food and refreshment as they move about,
just as it is doing so successfully in the factories and
offices. What is an automatic cafeteria? It is usually an
installation of eight to ten vending machines dispensing
the following products: milk, fruit juices, coffee, hot
chocolate, tea, soups, sandwiches, cold beverages,
salads, ice cream, desserts, pastries, and even plate
lunches. The average automatic cafeteria today requires
a capital investment in equipment of approximately
$10,000. Average monthly sales per automatic cafeteria
must be a minimum of $2,500. Ordinarily 350 potential
patrons or more are required to support such an installation. . . .

Many automatic food vending operators have established their own food preparation commissaries where
daily menus are planned, and food prepared and packaged for dispensing through vending machines. . . .

The automatic cafeteria business is only in its infancy,
but it is a healthy, fast-growing baby which promises
to mature into a brand new American industry. We in
automatic merchandising need and invite the interest

and assistance of our friends in the related fields of food handling, packing, and merchandising. To sum up, automatic merchandising is a two billion dollar industry today. Its growth in the last eight years has been at a phenomenal pace. As of now the industry still derives 88 per cent of its sales income from four products: namely, cigarettes, candies, cold beverages, and hot drinks. But, the new phases of vending are growing rapidly. I have barely touched upon the potential for sale of take-home products through vending machines installed in factories, offices, or gasoline stations. The automatic cafeteria already has proved its value. And, automatic refreshment stands are just a step beyond the industrial automatic cafeteria. Our industry is proud to consider itself a growth industry, ready and willing to pioneer into new fields of distribution of products and services to the American public, at work, at play, in the armed services, at travel centers, and wherever people want quality food and refreshment served promptly and efficiently.

The year 1958 is important because it marks the beginning of the vending of hot platters—an innovation made possible only by the combined elements of improved vending machines, microwave heating, and the gradual enlightenment of management who were fighting a losing battle on the operation of inplant cafeterias of the regulation, conventional sort.

The food in the cafeteries was superior in flavor and appearance, and served at surprisingly low cost. But as Robert A. Arnold, a director of automatic merchandising for one of the vending services, told a seminar of industrial cafeteria managers, as reported in the April 1960 issue of *Inplant Food Management*: "Don't consider vending a direct competitor of manual service. Its use is, instead, an extension of manual service."

The informed and intelligent employer has long since

recognized that the well-fed worker is the efficient worker —capable of new, advanced goals in his work. If the employee is provided the proper food service, he will respond to the requirements of his plant as to his own output, and his boss may congratulate himself on providing good, nutritious food, properly prepared—a protection in many instances from intramural dissatisfaction with conditions and general unrest. Who knows how many strikes might have been averted, how many disputes might have been avoided between labor and management if inplant food had been properly cooked and served?

The "meal away from home" has become an important element in the lives of all these workers—62,000,000 of them—who turn out the products which make American merchandising what it is today. Back home, the women who devote much of their time and energies to shopping, planning, and serving the principal meal of the day worry a lot about how their men are being fed when they are out of their sight. They feel concern as to the kinds of food their menfolk are getting; they strive to make their home-cooked meals the best they can. The present truth is that often, in the light of improved cooking and serving methods, the *best* daily meal their men are getting may well be served in the factory or plant.

Not only workers, but children are getting a better break these days. School feeding-programs are being improved at a startling rate, and the hot meal youngsters get in school may provide the nourishment they much need to aid their growth and development both mentally and physically. Of course, some of these feeding programs need a great deal of attention and improvement, because often they have been in the hands of indifferent or uninformed people. Trained home economists, dietitians and enlightened PTA members, all may contribute to improving the over-all picture. If they are agreed that the menu need not stop at hot dogs and hamburgers, for one thing, a great deal will have been accomplished. The young need an early education in the value of the balanced meal.

When the late John Kelly of Philadelphia was in charge of the physical fitness program during World War II under the Roosevelt and Truman administrations, he discovered a startling and alarming fact. Young America, summoned to the wars, suffered from an amazing number of physical deficiencies. In fact, to get many of them into the army, the standards of physical acceptability had to be lowered. Normally, many of these boys would have been classified 4F.

The probing which went on when this condition was discovered turned up the information that when children, these boys had parents who through poverty or ignorance had fed them improperly. It took a war, a devastating holocaust, to bring about the general change in attitude toward the feeding of school children. A really intelligent program of feeding in the schools was then developed—farm surpluses were brought into play and school programs were subsidized. The next generation of young adults will be healthier and their parents will not be held responsible for undernourished, ill-equipped oncoming groups of citizens.

PICTURE CREDITS

INDEX

Index of Recipes will be found on page 243.

INDEX OF RECIPES